IS THIS NORMAL?

IS THIS NORMAL?

JUDGMENT-FREE STRAIGHT TALK ABOUT YOUR BODY

DR. JOLENE BRIGHTEN

First published in the United States in 2023 by Simon Element,
an imprint of Simon & Schuster Inc.,
First published in Great Britain in 2023 by Orion Spring
an imprint of The Orion Publishing Group Ltd
Carmelite House, 50 Victoria Embankment
London EC4Y 0DZ

An Hachette UK Company

1 3 5 7 9 10 8 6 4 2

A CIP catalogue record for this book is
available from the British Library.

ISBN (Trade Paperback) 978 1 3987 1756 5
ISBN (eBook) 978 1 3987 1757 2
ISBN (Audio) 978 1 3987 1758 9

Printed in Great Britain by Clays Ltd, Elcograf S.p.A.

www.orionbooks.co.uk

To those who have ever felt the need to explore the Internet, bookshelves, or thoughts of their friends in a quest to understand what's normal. May this book provide the answers you're looking for and a plethora of interesting conversation pieces.

CONTENTS

IS THIS NORMAL?

INTRODUCTION

Why are we afraid to say "vagina" in public? And why don't we talk louder than a whisper about sex? Why do myths like "You can get pregnant any day of your cycle" persist through each generation? And why can't most people identify the clitoris? Simple: We're not taught about them. More specifically, we're actually taught not to talk about them. Society teaches us, from a young age, that our bodies are a great source of shame and guilt, so why would we want to talk about that? Even worse, the medical community has further stigmatized normal sexual desires and practices, pathologizing them simply because they deviate from what is socially acceptable to acknowledge: hetero sex with the intention of making a baby.

When I launched DrBrighten.com, a website to help educate women about their hormones and health, I received emails with questions that ran the gamut: Was it normal if their periods hurt so bad, or if their PMS made them all but quit their job when their coworker chewed with their mouth open, or if irregular periods meant they had to use the pill for the rest of their life? In my clinical experience, there isn't a patient who doesn't need to have at least their menstrual cycle explained, or their anatomy clarified, or be assured they aren't the only one who experiences the symptoms they have every week. Menstrual stigma, along with the experience of being dismissed by medical providers, has discouraged women from seeking these answers. This leaves a lot of women suffering. While hormone-related symptoms can affect upward of 90 percent of women, 60 percent of them will never seek help from a provider. What I've experienced in the online landscape is an explosion of women seeking advice on not just understanding their body, but how to care for it and solve their own hormonal woes.

When I first started anonymous "Ask Dr. Brighten" Q and As on social media, I received thousands of questions about sex, far more than any other topic. And it seemed I was getting the questions people really wanted to ask their doctor but hadn't: Is it normal that I have pain with sex; or why do I smell down there; or is it normal that I want to have sex only a couple times a month? I wanted to understand why women were coming to me on social media rather than to their provider, so I created a survey in which over 86,000 people responded. What I discovered was that only 37 percent felt comfortable talking to their medical provider about their sex life. When asked if they felt their provider would judge or shame them for asking sex-related questions, 57 percent reported they did. Only 21 percent felt their provider could address the concerns they had related to sex. We're all curious, confused, and looking for answers, but with very few trusted resources to turn to. It is a serious problem when many people feel they can't ask a medical provider what's normal when it comes to sex. And who can blame them when most of women's medicine feels like an assembly line of speculum insertions and a quick swab of the cervix. The vagina, the vulva—every last bit of it feels so far removed from sex.

But for those who do manage to voice their questions about sex, the answers they receive from the average doctor often don't just fail in offering help, but are laced with the provider's own sexual misunderstandings and internalized shame. It's unsurprising given that inclusive sex education (beyond just STI and pregnancy prevention) is practically void from medical school education, leaving patients to take to the Internet in search of answers. Plus, it's rare to find medical providers competently trained in sexual health. When I look back to my own medical training, which I would classify as sex positive—we attended lectures from medical experts and members of the kink, LGBTQIA+, sex worker industry, and survivors of sex trafficking—but even with that, I was never taught the answers to some of my patients' more in-depth questions. So after medical school, I decided to pursue clinical sexology and sexual counseling training.

It's through this additional education that I've been able to answer the most heartbreakingly common question I receive daily, also the simplest: "Is this normal?" The answer, for the record, is most often "Yes!" Cycles that aren't exactly 28 days? Totally normal. Uneven breasts? Normal and healthy. Finding you can orgasm only on your own? Normal, but also fixable (if you want!). You know what's not normal? Feeling like you're riding an uncontrollable roller coaster of emotions leading up to your period, being dependent on pain meds just to survive those few days of cramps, or fearing pooping yourself or bleeding through your clothes every single month. As important as it is to know what's normal, it's equally important to know the things we've been accepting as "normal" that aren't: the "lady problems" that women have been discouraged from talking about but are in fact *treatable and manageable* symptoms of hormone imbalance. Here's one of the biggest takeaways of this entire book: **Putting up with PMS, mood swings, cramping, pain with sex, disinterest in sex, or other "female" problems is not what you have to do if you happened to be born with ovaries—and any doctor who tries to tell you otherwise is plain wrong.** Write that down!

It's not hard to figure out why so few people understand what the heck is going on with their body, how sexual desire really works, or even basic anatomy. Only eighteen states in the US mandate medically accurate sex education, and thirty-nine require abstinence be taught for pregnancy and STI prevention (twenty-nine of which require the abstinence-only approach be stressed).[1] *If it is not medically accurate then it's not accurate.* And only ten states require that sex ed be inclusive. I know what you're thinking: Surely, these statistics must be outdated? They sound straight out of the 1960s. Sadly, these statistics are from July 2022. If abstinence-only worked, and depriving people of an accurate education about their body made for a healthy population, we wouldn't see the staggering rates of teen pregnancy, sexual assault (only eleven states require education on consent), and people not understanding the basics of their biology, which ultimately leads to unplanned pregnancies, thinking suffering with period pain is normal, and wandering through life with the baggage of shame and insecurities.

In this book, we're going to talk candidly about what your sex ed teacher should have said but didn't. I'm going to do my best to answer all those "woman part" questions you've always wondered about, didn't think to ask, or were too embarrassed to ask. TMI isn't a thing in my world. I have provided you a resource to help you understand your body; navigate your hormones; and release any expectations, embarrassment, guilt, shame, and negative feelings that you have around sex that may prevent you from truly embracing and enjoying it. But this isn't just some anatomy textbook you never had. If you're reading this book, you don't only want to understand what's causing you pain and discomfort, you want to solve it. That's why I've also included a 28-day program to restore a healthy cycle, optimize your hormones, and help you get the pleasure you deserve.

In creating the content for this book, I've listened to the people who have trusted me in asking their most intimate of questions—my patients, my readers, and my followers on social media—to bring you the most-common concerns and provide the most-sought information. Somewhere between the void of information we're provided, and the myths constructed surrounding sex and our bodies, many of us have arrived at answers about what's "normal" that aren't entirely accurate. Anxiety and embarrassment flourish when we aren't given medically accurate information about our bodies, let alone a reliable place to ask questions. You and I are about to change that.

NOTE TO THE READER

We don't discriminate here, but because this is a medical book, we have to give a few caveats. Please note that in almost all the research discussed, we're talking about assigned female at birth (AFAB) individuals. When it comes to the talk on sexual desire, sexual response, and parts we all share, there's a high probability it can apply to everyone who is experiencing it—although research on sexual health is seriously lacking, so I can't say for sure. If you're transitioning female or have already done so, that's totally cool and you can still get plenty out of this book. If you were AFAB and now identify as male or nonbinary, know that there are many things for you to take away from this book and, just like everyone else, individual needs may vary from what is discussed.

Part 1
YOUR SEXUAL SELF

CHAPTER 1
SEX

WHAT'S NORMAL FOR GETTING IT ON?

What do you think about when you think about "sex"? Do you picture getting down and dirty, or passionate lovemaking? Is it kinky and adventurous, or sexy and soulful?

Regardless of our age, education, or lifestyle, how we think about sex is shaped by society, our experiences, and everyone around us. I hate to break it to you, but no matter how open-minded or independent you think you may be, your perception of sex and what's normal is not entirely your own. Think about a lot of popular TV shows with coming-of-age characters, like *The Vampire Diaries*, *Gossip Girl*, *Friday Night Lights*, or *My So-Called Life*. These series share a running theme when it comes to sex: making a big deal about virginity—which we'll discuss the scientific validity of—and purporting that when a woman loses hers, it's momentous. While having sex for the first time is certainly a big deal for many people IRL, these shows typically create a tremendous amount of pressure to have the picture-perfect experience. We also never see much in these shows about real-world things like consent, foreplay, safe sex, the need for lube, or the much-feared STIs. Can someone please explain to me how vampires get wet? The influence of these shows, like much of pop culture, sometimes affects us even more than we realize. It permeates my patients' concerns, social media followers' questions, and friends' inquiries at parties with one running theme—when it comes to sex, what's normal?

Ashley, a thirtysomething epidemiology graduate student and part-time bartender, first came to see me for fatigue, hair loss, and irregular periods. Like so many of my patients, the symptoms creeping in were easy to ignore amid her busy schedule until they weren't.

For all new patients, during intake, I do a thorough review of all aspects of health, lifestyle, and diet. One question I ask is whether patients experience any difficulty with orgasm, since the inability to climax can be a sign of an underlying physical or psychological issue. When we got to this one, Ashley dodged the question a bit, explaining the sex schedule that she created to keep her marriage "normal and happy." Every Sunday, she performed oral sex on her husband, and on Thursdays, she and her husband had sex whether she wanted to or not. She believed this is what normal married couples should do, and that without weekly sex her husband would likely cheat. You may have heard something similar, as plenty of self-proclaimed online "sexperts" recommend couples do it weekly regardless of mood or anything else that's going on, in order to create, maintain, or reestablish their sexual spark. While there are circumstances where this can be beneficial (we'll discuss responsive sexual desire here and in chapter 3), the "should" of this situation was stressful for Ashley because "It's another thing on my to-do list."

Now, I'm all for scheduling sex if it ignites a spark for you or satisfies *you* sexually—but not if it's done just for your partner, or some arbitrary calendar obligation. Ashley's sex schedule was a major point of stress in her life. She told me that she often had sex just because she assumed her husband wanted it, that making sure they had sex was part of her responsibilities as a woman and wife, and that sexual frequency was necessary to keep their marriage strong and committed. She wasn't necessarily enjoying it; rather, "going through the motions." She instead wanted the kind of spontaneous desire she had felt when she and her husband began dating—before school, work, maintaining a home, and the rest of married life set in.

Ashley's sex schedule wasn't the cause of her irregular periods, although the stress of it wasn't helping. Through lab testing we discovered she had hypothyroidism, which commonly shows up with fatigue, hair loss, and what many patients refer to as "period problems." After several appointments together, Ashley's energy was returning, her periods were becoming more predictable, and she was battling to keep the wispy hairs of new growth from popping out of her otherwise well-maintained ponytail. Since her primary concerns were improving, I felt OK suggesting she consider having a direct conversation with her husband about their sex life (as I will say throughout this book, good sex starts with good communication). Ashley took my advice and spoke with her husband outside the bedroom. When she told him about her schedule and its stressors, he surprised her by saying he hadn't even noticed there was a schedule. He even admitted there were instances when he hadn't been in the mood at all—yep, guys don't want it all the time, despite society's presumption of male hypersexuality—and he often went through the motions, just like Ashley did, because he believed doing so would please his wife.

Three months later, Ashley came into my office aglow. Before she even took a seat, she gushed about her sex life. It had gone from scheduled, predictable, and impassive to engaging, sometimes exciting, and most important, satisfying—not every time they did it, but most of the time. And now she had follow-up questions. She and her husband now had sex when they felt like it, which she felt correlated to certain times of her cycle. Because she was tracking her periods with me, she had noticed that there were some weeks when they didn't have sex at all, and others where they were intimate several times. Which is normal. As we'll review in chapter 9 your sexual desire or libido can fluctuate with your hormones throughout your cycle.

You might not be married or partnered, or maybe you think having a sex schedule is weird, or perhaps you would never dream of working part-time through grad school, but I bet there's part of Ashley's story you can relate to. That's because we all have preconceived notions about what we "should" and "shouldn't" do sexually, like how many times a week we *should* have sex, how many overall sexual partners we *should* have, what kind of fantasies we *shouldn't* have, and what even counts as "sex." Sociocultural constructs are pervasive and powerful, infiltrating our brains like an earworm, even if it's something we don't realize.

ASK DR. BRIGHTEN:

What's normal when it comes to sex?

If you have questions about what's actually normal and what isn't, you're right in line with what I receive from people and patients weekly. I'm asked things like, How many partners is it normal to have; is it normal that the first time hurts; how often is it normal to do it; and what really counts as sex? Allow me to provide insight on these important questions and dispel some myths along the way.

What's considered sex? If I go down on someone, does that count as having sex with them? Or if neither of us orgasms, did we really just have sex?

These are some of the great debated questions of all time, right up there with whether ketchup counts as a vegetable, or if you've been to a foreign country if you've just flown through the airport. The reality is that most of us are living by someone else's definition of what sex is and isn't, which is how we can find ourselves asking these types of questions.

But let's ask some experts. According to top authorities of the English language (looking at you, *Merriam-Webster*), sexual intercourse can either be penetrative or not and includes both oral and anal. Penetration when no one or only one person orgasms is still sex.

While dictionary definitions can be useful as a starting point, in reality, sex exists on a spectrum and can't be neatly defined by one group of people. For example, in the United Kingdom, if you cheat on your husband or wife with a member of the opposite sex, it's considered adultery and legal grounds for divorce. But if you cheat on your partner with someone of the same sex, it's neither adultery nor a legal reason to end a marriage.[1] Every culture's definition of sex is only opinion, circumscribed by age-old biases and social constructs.

Mutual masturbation, frottage (the fancy term for what many refer to as "dry humping"), and tribadism (commonly referred to as "scissoring") are considered forms of nonpenetrative sex. Some people choose to participate in these as a means of pregnancy prevention or because they believe it is a form of abstinence, since no penetration takes place. As we'll discuss in chapter 7, while they can be effective in reducing the risk of pregnancy, these acts may still put you at risk of STIs. Others may not consider these acts sex at all.

I know the "sex exists on a spectrum" answer isn't super satisfying. I get it: as humans, we all want to see our world as easily classifiable and neatly ordered. But sex is really anything that makes you feel, or satisfies, sexual desire and/or arousal. That means sex can include anything that happens on your own or with a partner, and doesn't require you to touch or even be in the same room with someone else. But what sex actually is can only be defined by what it means to you.

At the same time, just because everyone has their own definition of sex doesn't mean it wouldn't be helpful for you to take the time to examine and reevaluate yours, especially if you think it might be preventing you from expressing or experiencing sexual pleasure in the way that you want. One of the goals of this book is to help broaden the discussion on sex so that you discover new ways to embrace and enjoy it that are authentic, pleasurable, and "normal" to you.

When should I have lost my virginity? If I was *x* age, is that normal? Or if I haven't lost my virginity by *y* age, is that normal? *(Fill in the x's and y's with whatever age you want, as I've heard it all, from age twelve to twenty-two to fifty-two.)*

Sit down if you're not already because what I'm about to tell you just might make you stumble, spill your coffee, or go "Holy shit." *There is no such thing as being a virgin, losing your virginity, or the concept of virginity in general*—at least not in medicine or science. According to the World Health Organization, "virginity is not a medical or scientific term," and there's no way to assess or diagnose whether someone is a "virgin," even if they have, in fact, had vaginal intercourse.[2] What this means is that those virginity tests that check whether a woman's hymen is still "intact" have no scientific basis and are, as the United Nations puts it, "painful, humiliating, and traumatic."[3] Sorry, T.I., while I can get down with your music, I cannot get down with the fact that you submitted your eighteen-year-old daughter to virginity tests,[4] and I agree with the many international organizations that see this as a violation of basic human rights. No doctor can accurately conduct a virginity test, as the American College of Obstetricians and Gynecologists has made clear, and there are no medical guidelines to assess or determine virginity.[5]

I know what you may be thinking. We've all heard the myth about how the hymen breaks when women first have sex, that her "cherry is popped," which refers to the mild bleeding that can occur when the hymen is stretched for the first time. But the hymen is not a fruit and can't be "broken" or "popped." Instead, the hymen is a thin piece of mucosal tissue that surrounds the vagina (in less than 1 percent of women, the hymen can cover the vagina).[6] Just like everything else in the human body, the shape and size of the hymen varies from person to person, and some women are even born without one. Your hymen also thins with age and can stretch and even partially tear to accommodate objects like tampons, fingers, toys, and penises. Your hymen can also partially tear from several other activities, too, like some forms of exercise and even vaginal exams.[7] But a stretched or torn hymen never indicates that someone has had sexual intercourse. A torn hymen is not a broken hymen, and a woman who has had sex is not "broken," as this language implies. What's important to take away here is that you don't need to prove your sexual history to anyone. Sure, anyone can ask about when you lost your "virginity" or other details around it, but just like having sex with you, they are not entitled to that info.

While virginity doesn't have any medical or scientific basis, the virgin myth runs deep in our society, causing many to worry whether they were (or are) too young or old when they first initiated sex. Perhaps unsurprisingly, there is no "normal," but I can tell you what's common. According to the Centers for Disease Control and Prevention (CDC), the average age to try heterosexual vaginal sex for the first time is seventeen.[8] Homosexual men are closer to age eighteen, although it's not clear how their first experience is defined, whether through anal or oral sex.[9] Data on lesbians is inconclusive, in part because women who have sex with other women qualify their first sexual experience differently, too.[10] And for nonbinary and trans individuals, the numbers are unsurprisingly lacking. At the end of the day, it's all arbitrary. You can look up all the stats in the world, but whatever age you choose to consensually engage in sex is your normal.

What about the forty-year-old virgin, made legendary by the movie with the same name? Statistically, people who don't experience sex until their thirties, forties, or fifties are outliers, but that doesn't mean they're abnormal. I have one patient, Clara, who at age thirty-eight has never had heterosexual vaginal sex because, as she told me, it just never appealed to her. Instead, she prefers engaging in oral sex with both men and women. I've had other patients with severe endometriosis who haven't had vaginal intercourse for years because it's been too painful (see page 110 for tips on how to help resolve painful sex). Some people with a history of sexual assault or abuse also choose never to have sex, while others—around 1.7 percent of the US population, according to research—are asexual.[11] In short, whatever feels good to you and makes you happy is your normal.

Does the first time always hurt?

When I get this question, it's almost always about having vaginal sex the first time. The idea that it should hurt the first time is a myth that has been perpetuated for generations, likely due to misbeliefs about the hymen. Some people do experience pain the first time, while others don't, but pain should not be the standard we should all expect. We'll explore pain with sex in much more detail in chapter 5, and I'll share some tips to help make the first time (and every time) less painful no matter the type of sex you plan to participate in.

What does it mean to give consent? Does someone have to ask for consent before each and every sexual encounter? And does it count as consent if I've had a few drinks?

Let's get serious here. When you give consent, you agree to engage in sexual activity with someone else. Consent should always be asked for every time you're sexually active in any way, no matter what you've done together leading up to that activity or whether you've consented to the same activity in the past. Just because you're partnered or married doesn't mean this ask suddenly goes away. It also doesn't matter how much someone paid for dinner, what they've given or done for you in the past, or what they might do for you in the future. Consent needs to exist in every type of sexual partnership every time a sexual act occurs.

Consent also must be 100 percent voluntary. If you feel pressured in any way to engage in sexual activity, your consent doesn't count. It's kind of like drawing up a legal document, which won't hold up in court if either party was threatened or pressured to sign it. If your partner ever tells you that you would do *x* act if you really loved them, or that by not doing *y* act it means you'll hurt them, that's pressure, and whatever you say is not consent. Similarly, if someone continually asks you over and over again until you feel browbeaten into giving consent, you didn't really give it. You also can't freely agree to or refuse sexual activity with someone who's in a position of power over you, like an employer, landlord, teacher, coach, or doctor. All of these are major red flags for anyone trying to have sex with you: heed them.

To give consent, you also have to be mentally and emotionally capable of giving it. If you're intoxicated, high, asleep, visibly upset, or under the legal age, you're not of right mind to deliberately agree to or refuse sexual activity. I find myself frequently commenting in social media posts that someone who's asleep can't give consent. Seriously, it doesn't matter if your partner has a foot fetish that they're too embarrassed to tell you about: they still cannot suck your toes while you sleep. And consent is also never implied: just because you didn't say no doesn't mean you said yes. Equally important and covered in more detail on page 73, genital arousal, vaginal lubrication, or any like physical signs do not negate the "no" of your mind.

What if you've had a few drinks or taken a few hits off the weed pen, but aren't exactly intoxicated? That's when we wade into the gray area. Everyone has a different level of alcohol and drug tolerance, and what impairs one person might not even make someone else feel buzzed. If you feel tipsy but are still perfectly coherent—for example, you're able to say no to another drink—you're likely able to say no to sex, too. But if you're slurring your words, having difficulty walking or getting yourself home, aren't coherent in any way, or won't remember what happened the next morning, your consent doesn't count. If you're the one asking for consent, it's better to always wait until someone is sober than to be one who might induce trauma.

Sex by deception is not consensual. This occurs when an individual withholds information that one may consider important in deciding whether to engage in sex with them or not—marital status, STI test results, job occupation, age, or religion are a few examples. Is it a clear case of rape if someone deceives you? While it is without a doubt morally wrong, many legal scholars have argued that just as fraud to get money is theft, fraud to get sex is sexual assault.[12] But given the outdated perspective that sexual assault occurs only through violent force while a victim screams no, it unsurprisingly hasn't been deemed a criminal act. Regardless of the law, the decision to have sex with someone based on deceit is not consent.

All these qualifications around consent are a lot to remember, I know. That's why I like the acronym FRIES, created by Planned Parenthood.[13] (Also, who doesn't like thinking about fries?)

F-**Freely given:** You aren't pressured, manipulated, or under the influence.

R-**Reversible:** You can change your mind at any time, even if you consent at first.

I-**Informed:** Consent only counts when you know what you're consenting to.

E-**Enthusiastic:** You consent to what you want to do, not to what you think is expected.

S-**Specific:** Saying yes to one activity doesn't mean you agree to another.

If you say no or are unable to say no freely, it's considered sexual assault, which the federal government defines as any nonconsensual sexual activity.[14] Sexual assault includes all unwanted contact that's sexual in nature—for example, if someone grabs any part of your body, forces you to kiss them, or rubs their genitals up against you in the hallway or on the subway. Sexual assault also includes rape, defined by the US Department of Justice as "the penetration, no matter how slight, of the vagina or anus with any object, or oral penetration by a sex organ of another person, without the consent of the victim."[15] Woah! Did we just dive headfirst into legal-speak? Yeah, we did, because it's very serious business, and people downplay it all too often.

Sexual assault and rape can happen in a number of ways, including at the hand of someone you love or live with. It doesn't always occur how we see it portrayed on TV and by the movies. If you've experienced sexual assault, no matter whether it conforms to your idea (or someone else's) of unwanted sexual activity, it's not your fault, and you're not alone. Tell someone you trust and get help, whether from a doctor, mental health specialist, family member, or friend. You can also call the National Sexual Assault Hotline anytime, twenty-four hours a day, seven days a week, at 1-800-656-HOPE.[16]

BUSTING THE "BLUE BALLS" MYTH

There are some not-so-great guys out there who manipulate women into having sex by telling them that they'll get "blue balls" if they don't. For anyone who hasn't come across this before, "blue balls" is slang for the pain some men experience after prolonged sexual arousal without an orgasm. It's a real thing—in medicine, we call it epididymal hypertension—but no one is going to die, suffer excruciating pain, or incur any harm or reproductive damage if you don't have sex with them.[17] Yeah, blue balls can be uncomfortable, like a lot of things in life, but the pain is mild and often passes quickly (not like the lasting pain many women put up with every month around their period, *hello*). What's more, there's plenty that someone can do to alleviate the pain themselves, like masturbating, taking a cold shower, or working out. You're not their doctor, and it's not your job or responsibility to treat them. It's also not your "fault," and you didn't "give" them the condition by being a "tease." If their testicles are actually blue, swollen, and extremely painful, they may have testicular torsion, and the answer there is always the ER, not sex.

How many sexual partners is it normal to have? Do I have to share my "body count" with someone I'm sleeping with?

If you've been asked "What could you buy with your body count?" what that other person really wants to know is how many sexual partners you've had. People make a big deal of it—some of us wonder about (or even obsess over) how many people our partners, friends, or first dates have slept with. Others obsess over their own number or compare themselves to others to try to gauge their level of "normal."

If you fall into this camp, you're not alone. It's normal to be curious about the most intimate aspects of someone else's life or how your own sexual history compares. But the numbers game isn't played the same when it comes to sexual partners for men and women. Well-established gender norms have created one standard for men and a much different criterion for women. Neither does anyone any favors. Having lots of sexual partners for a guy is considered proof of his masculinity, "alpha male status," and virility—this last word meaning both "masculine" and "capable of procreation," which only emphasizes my point.[18] By comparison, women with a high number of sexual partners are viewed as promiscuous, easy, or a THOT ("that ho over there," for anyone who hasn't been on Urban Dictionary). Don't believe me? Just look up the word "slut" in the thesaurus, where you'll find a number of synonyms traditionally associated with women—hussy, harlot, jezebel, bimbo, minx, tramp—and not one word historically used to label men.[19]

Often, in our society, the more sexual partners a woman has over the course of her lifetime, the more negatively she's perceived. At the same time, a high "body count" for men has no negative bearing on their social reception or valuation, according to research.[20] Actually, guys who haven't slept with a lot of women often receive their share of shame or ridicule. Overall, women tend to underestimate their body count, while guys over-exaggerate or round up,[21] with 40 percent of all men reporting pressure to have "many sexual partners."[22]

These double standards are unfair to everyone, setting rigid expectations and condemning judgments that aren't based on biology or reality. While there may be evolutionary differences between why men and women seek out sexual partners, both genders are programmed equally for promiscuity, according to studies.[23] This just makes the double standards on body count even more damaging, and the sooner we get rid of them, the better it'll be for us all.

No matter how many sexual partners you've had, I want to assure you that it's normal. Your body count or "score card" isn't a reflection of your sexual health or happiness, and how many people you've slept with or want to sleep with is your own business. If you want to wait until marriage to have sex and end up having only one partner for life, that's normal. If you're polyamorous or have a triple-digit body count, that's normal, too—just make sure you're practicing safe consensual sex. Everyone's got their own "ideal number," which is great for them, but has nothing to do with you.

Also, nobody's got a right to ask how many people you've slept with. Body count is irrelevant to sexual health if you frequently get STI tested, and you don't need to share your number with someone just because you're in a committed relationship, married, in love, or living together. While honesty is critical in intimate relationships, this doesn't mean you have to reveal every private detail of what you've ever done, especially when doing so feels invasive. Consenting to sex doesn't mean you consent to sharing your entire life story.

While any number of people you've had sex with is perfectly normal, I do get asked a lot about averages. People are curious; I get it. According to the CDC, women between age twenty-five and forty-nine have a median of 4.3 partners with whom they've had vaginal, anal, or oral sex, while men have 6.3.[24] Newer surveys, however, bump the number up to approximately seven for both genders.[25] Let's keep in mind that these numbers are contingent on people being honest, and as we know, the research shows that there's a propensity to round in favor of society's expectations.

How often is it normal to have sex?

The age-old saying "quality over quantity" definitely applies when it comes to how often you have sex. Guess what? However often you're having sex—if the frequency makes you feel satisfied, happy, and connected with your partner—is totally normal. But I'm sure you're still curious what others are doing because, well, you're human. The average American has sex fifty-four times per year, which works out to approximately once a week. But this number is a gross estimate and therefore a little arbitrary.[26] What that really means is that whenever you survey large populations to come up with a mathematical average, it means many people don't hit that average on the nose but fall somewhere above or below that number. In this instance, some folks are obviously having sex several times a week while others don't do it for months at a time. Are you happy? Are you satisfied? A yes to those questions holds far more value than any number on a scale.

If you're in a relationship and aren't intimate as frequently as you'd like, start by having an open and honest conversation with your partner about your desires without placing any pressure or setting expectations. Sometimes, sexual desire in a relationship can fade due to "death by a thousand cuts," or when things that seem so trivial in the moment add up to big issues over time. Like if someone doesn't take out the trash or never does the dishes or forgets to ask about someone's family or doesn't help with the kids when the other has a lot of work. The ongoing additive effect of these actions (or inactions) can create lasting resentment and eventually lead us to believe that our partner doesn't listen to, help, value, care for, or prioritize us or take us seriously. Resentment, distrust, and other relationship stressors can dissolve sexual connection over time. It's best to address them before they build, and/or work with a therapist who can help you and your partner make sure the other feels cared for and valued.

There are times, though, when sexual infrequency indicates a problem outside of relationship issues. When patients tell me that they haven't had sex in months or years, I ask if that's by choice or unintentional. Some respond that they haven't had sex because they feel insecure about their bodies, depressed, or incapable or unworthy of attracting a partner. As I tell them, lots of people experience these internal struggles, and despite what you might feel, you are worthy and capable of being in an intimate relationship if that's what you truly want. For these patients, I always suggest seeing a therapist who can help resolve possible mood disorders or address feelings of inadequacy about being intimate with others.

Some physical conditions like hormone imbalances, autoimmune disease, fibromyalgia, and cancer, along with certain medications like antidepressants and antihistamines, can diminish sexual desire. This is why speaking with a provider is always step one if you find yourself suddenly apathetic about sex or unable to orgasm on your own.

Is masturbation normal?

Masturbation is a totally normal part of childhood development and adult life, despite the stigma around it. There are so many falsehoods around masturbation—no, it doesn't desensitize your clitoris or ruin you for your partner. It's also physically, mentally, and emotionally healthy for you, despite age-old rumors that it can make you insane or cause you to grow hair on your hands (say what?). I'll dive into these myths and everything you need to know about masturbation, including all the sex toys that can turn your woes into Os, in chapter 6.

Is it normal to masturbate if you're in a relationship?

Masturbation doesn't necessarily stop just because you enter a relationship. In fact, research tells us that solo sessions may fuel sexual satisfaction in a relationship.[27] As I will discuss in chapter 6, some people find that masturbation relieves stress, as it releases oxytocin, which counters the negative effects of stress hormones. That's just one of the many of benefits of orgasms and a big reason why people incorporate masturbation into their self-care routine.

Masturbation isn't always a solo event, as is the case with mutual masturbation. During mutual masturbation two or more people masturbate alongside each other or while being watched. Some people use this as an option to stay sexually engaged with their partner when they can't have penetrative sex due to pain (we'll discuss details in chapter 5), recovering from surgery, pregnancy complications, or genital infections; or they don't like the idea of having period sex (although see page 255 on why period sex can be beneficial); or a variety of other reasons. People in a long-distance relationship can use mutual masturbation over the phone or by video as a way of connecting and cultivating intimacy in their relationship. And since there's no risk of pregnancy or STIs, mutual masturbation is a great alternative when you're ovulating and not trying to conceive, or suddenly discover you've run out of protection. Other times, people engage in mutual masturbation simply because they find it pleasurable.

Here are four tips if you're curious about mutual masturbation but don't know where to start:

1. **Communicate.** You don't have to have a formal sit-down talk with your partner—I realize that saying, "Hey, do you want to try mutual masturbation?" can be a little awkward or a complete buzzkill. Instead, you can simply start touching yourself in the bedroom and ask, "Does this turn you on?" An enthusiastic yes is your sign to keep going.

2. **Engage.** Mutual masturbation doesn't mean you have to isolate. Instead, increase intimacy by looking into each other's eyes, kissing, talking, and entwining your legs and arms; or sit or lie on each other, and try other ways that make you feel connected during this experience.

3. **Consider toys.** If you've been wanting to bring toys into your relationship, this can be an ideal time to introduce them and show your partner what you like. Before you pull out a bag of toys, ask for your partner's consent by showing them the toy and asking whether

they're cool with you using it. If you're curious about your options, jump to page 150 to explore the world of sex toys.

4. **Don't forget the lube.** Lube makes all sex better, including mutual masturbation with a partner.

SEX POSITIONS THROUGH THE AGES

Like most things sex, the cultural and societal influences are what dictate your perspective on normal. If you were raised in Western civilizations from the Middle Ages until now, you probably think that missionary position is the norm, so you may be surprised to learn that cowgirl is the leading searched sex position in Japan.[28]

- Ancient Egypt's Turin Erotic Papyrus documents a dozen different positions (not one is said to depict missionary, BTW).[29]
- What is called doggy style today is said to have its origins in ancient Greece.
- Mayans allegedly had twenty or more different sex positions just for doing it in a hammock.
- In Rome, if a sex worker was asked to be on top, then she could command higher pay, presumably for the extra effort.
- Missionary—what so many of the Western world consider normal sex—reportedly got its name when natives of other countries had a good chuckle observing this was how religious missionaries did it. While that story may not be a whole truth, the position was deemed the only acceptable one by the Catholic Church during the Middle Ages, as other positions may challenge the power dynamic of gender roles.[30]
- When it comes to discussing sex positions, the *Kama Sutra*, the ancient Hindu text filled with erotic positions and relationship and life advice, is king. The *Kama Sutra* is so prevalent in popular culture that even WebMD has an article on it.[31]

Is it normal to be interested in kink?

The next time you tell the hostess "Party of five, please" at your favorite restaurant, know that odds are at least one person in your party has participated in what is referred to as kink.[32] So far, everything we've talked about is considered conventional sex: vaginal sex, masturbation, oral sex, kissing, etc. Kink is all the "other stuff," or what is considered nonconventional. Although with 30 percent of people reporting engaging in spanking, 43 percent having public sex, and at least 50 percent of people interested in learning about it, I'd say kink is a lot more normal than is currently acknowledged.[33]

While there's no medical definition for kink, I get plenty of questions about it, and whenever I discuss kink there is always at least one person who voices their concern about the dangers. Kink practices, like all sex, should be consensual. They should also involve good hygiene (we'll be discussing cleaning sex toys and more in chapter 6), STI testing considerations, and being mindful of safety. Outside of that, having sexual preferences or fetishes (sexual fixation on an object or body part) is a normal part of being a human. Before engaging in any sexual activity, have a conversation with your partner to fully understand what you're both consenting to, what's off-limits, what cues you'll use to stop before things go too far, that consent can always be retracted, and any concerns either of you may have.

There are hundreds of different kinds of kink to explore. Here are a few of the most popular varieties:

Threesomes or Beyond: Americans fantasize more about multipartner sex than anything else, according to a large survey conducted by Kinsey Institute researcher Justin Lehmiller.[34] Statistically speaking, this is one of the most "normal" fantasies. But while it may be a common daydream, only 10 percent of women and 18 percent of men report actually ever having had a threesome, per a separate study.[35] No matter how many lovers are involved, before you begin, be sure to discuss what the group hopes to gain from the experience and any activities that are off-limits.

Role-Playing: One-third of all Americans fantasize about role-playing, which is taking a break from who you are in real life to assume another identity and act out whatever erotic fantasy you want.[36] Popular role-play dyads include boss-secretary, cop-criminal, firefighter-victim, doctor-patient, stripper-client, handyperson-homeowner, and two total strangers. Some people take it a step further and decide to dress up or meet in a public space like a park, library, restaurant, bar, or coffee shop. Role-playing isn't just a turn-on: it can also deepen your connection with your partner by increasing your trust, communication, and shared experiences together.

BDSM: Short for "bondage and discipline, dominance and submission, and sadism and masochism," BDSM can involve one partner being dominant over the other. You may be familiar with BDSM as awareness surrounding it has risen thanks to *Fifty Shades of Grey.*[37] I'm not a big fan of the franchise since it got so many things wrong about kink, including the idea that people who practice BDSM have a history of emotional or sexual trauma, and are cold, unfeeling, or even cruel to others. Because according to research, it's actually quite the opposite. Real-life BDSM practitioners don't have any more trauma than the general population and may have more consideration for others, less anxiety and stress, a stronger sense of connection and trust with their sexual partners, and a greater degree of emotional well-being compared to those who don't practice.[38] What's more, BDSM isn't just whips, gags, and red rooms: The kink can be as simple as spanking, or role-playing in a dominant-submissive dyad. You can also restrain your partner or be restrained using a T-shirt, tie, scarf, or pair of sexy panties, in addition to the more stereotypical handcuffs or rope. Physical or emotional pain can be part of the BDSM experience, but violence, abuse, or any activity that's not 100 percent consensual is a form of sexual assault, not kink. If you want to try BDSM with your partner, plan to have a conversation beforehand so you can both set boundaries, receive consent for everything discussed, and agree on a safe word or gesture to stop the activity.

Nonmonogamy: What used to be known as swinging or wife-swapping has come a long way since the notorious 1970s key parties, when couples would drop their car keys in a big bowl at the beginning of a soiree, then go home at the end of the night with whoever's keys they plucked from the bowl. While you can certainly still swing like it's 1972, nonmonogamy today also includes cuckolding, when one person watches their partner having sex with someone else; and polyamory or ethical nonmonogamy, which means having sexual relationships with more than one person at a time. Whatever form of nonmonogamy appeals to you, it's not cheating when you and your partner *both* agree to terms set before anyone gets busy with someone else.

Voyeurism: You like to watch. Or you like being watched. Or you like both. Whether you want to play voyeur or exhibitionist, voyeurism can be fun for everyone, just like how a good Broadway play is enjoyable for both the audience and actors. But for voyeurism to work, it's got to be consensual, meaning other people know you're watching them, or you've received permission to have sex or undress in front of others. Otherwise, watching someone have sex without their knowledge makes you creepy, and submitting unknowing or unwilling folks to your sexcapades is often grounds for criminal action.

TL;DR: SEX: WHAT'S NORMAL?

- From *Beverly Hills, 90210* to *The Vampire Diaries*, we all have sat through our fair share of implicit norms that shape the way we think about and view sex.
- Sex means a lot of things to different people, and however you define it is *your* definition of having sex.
- Virginity is something society decided exists despite there being no science to support its existence. There is no way to medically assess who is and isn't a "virgin."
- Consent for sex has to be asked for before each and every activity and every time, no matter how long you've been with a person or what you've done together in the past.

- No one has ever died of "blue balls," and he will live to see another day if you say no to his sexual advances.
- Men tend to round up while women round down the number of sexual partners they've had, but whatever the number—it's normal.
- Having sex once a week is not the magic bullet for a happy, healthy relationship.
- Sex doesn't always hurt the first time.
- At least one in five people has engaged in some level of kink, and about half of the population are curious about it.
- Whatever your body count, frequency, or flavor of sex is—that's *your* normal.

CHAPTER 2

IS DOWN THERE NORMAL?

TOO HAIRY, TOO LONG, TOO BIG, TOO SMALL (WE'LL COVER IT ALL)

Apparently since the dawn of time, literally hundreds of different slang words and ridiculous euphemisms for a woman's genitals have plagued us. OK, that's an exaggeration—the English language hasn't been around that long. But the euphemisms for the anatomy that must not be named—because heaven forbid we utter "vagina" or "vulva"—have provided us a safe way to talk about a part of the body that many of us have been taught to feel ashamed of or fear, and have allowed us to verbally evade the otherwise "dirty" words. Except that there is nothing dirty or shameful, and when you're finished with this book, you'll understand when to see a doctor if you are afraid something is not normal.

Maybe the most confusing of all the language is the actual word "vagina," since that's how anything down there gets referred to. It's created a culture of people who don't know the inside from the outside, let alone where the clitoris is. In one study, 45 percent of women and almost 60 percent of men couldn't identify the vagina.[1] A recent poll also found that nearly half of all US women couldn't point out the cervix in an illustration of the female reproductive system.[2] If this is you, too, please understand that it's not your failure to own. Not one bit. I mean, where do we expect you to learn this?

The truth is, we're not taught much about female genitalia in school. For years, most sex ed has covered the vagina only enough for us to know where the penis goes during penile-vaginal sex, and to instill fear of sexually transmitted infections (STIs) and pregnancies. It's so taboo in some places that according to one poll, sex educators admitted that they use the word "penis" in class but are too embarrassed to say "vagina" in front of students.[3] This bias is only corroborated and compounded by the medical field, which has historically dedicated substantial anatomy-page real estate to the study of male genitalia, but given far less attention to the female counterpart.[4] What's more taboo than the vagina? Probably the clitoris. After all, it was named "*membre honteux*," which translates to "shameful member," by a French physician in 1545.[5] Yes, people knew about the clitoris back then, but in what I'd call the greatest conspiracy of all time, medicine set to erase its existence. Although the first published autopsy of the clitoris was in 1844 and the first anatomic representation was in the 1901 edition of *Gray's Anatomy* (the book, not the TV show), it was removed from medical literature, leaving all of us, including doctors, in the dark about the greatest pleasure source of the entire female body (more on this soon).

Even in an age where access to information is easier than ever, one recent survey found that two-thirds of young women (Gen Zers) were too embarrassed to say "vagina" out loud to their doctors.[6] With all the stigma and shame that gets tossed around, people tend to get squirrelly when it comes to female genitalia. Take, for example, *Grey's Anatomy*. The TV show (not the book) used the word "penis" ninety-seven times in one episode, but "vagina" did not appear in the script on any episode in the show's multiseason history.[7] Media sure isn't making it any easier for us to talk about down there.

So what's the big deal if I say "vajajay" instead of "vulva"? Flower, goodies, beaver, box, muff, lady garden, concha, clam, taco, hoo-haw, nether regions, down there, la papaya, carnal mantrap, and the one I grew up hearing, "chocha," may not only feel more comfortable, but you also may just enjoy saying them. How you talk about your body is your choice and, also, the euphemisms are fun sometimes. I'm not here to shame you into using anatomically correct terminology at every opportunity. And I'm going to use euphemisms in this book, too. Not because I don't think it's important to say "vulva" and "vagina," but because I can only imagine you reading this and thinking, *How many freakin' times can someone say "vulva" and "vagina"?*

I am here to give you a tour and provide you an opportunity to learn all the parts so you can better communicate with your doctor and your partner and, most important, better understand your body (so we'll use the right terms when it's important).

What lies behind a society only giving permission for euphemisms is a misogynistic and shameful take on normal body parts that creates a perfect situation for insecurities, unnecessary surgeries and procedures, delayed diagnosis, and medical gaslighting to prevail. Shame, fear, and health illiteracy all prevent millions of women from getting the care they need to prevent or properly treat gynecological cancers, along with other potentially life-threatening conditions.[8] Feeling insecure, questioning if your body is normal, and judging yourself can also keep you perpetually out of the mood and sabotage your pleasure and orgasms, as we'll discuss in chapters 3 and 4. Not knowing more about that smell, discharge, bump, or the color of your labia can definitely push you into freak-out mode. So we're going to talk about it—all of it—but first, let's get you acquainted with, well, you.

ASK DR. BRIGHTEN:

Is my clitoris normal?

The penis is essentially a larger version of the clitoris, except that the clitoris is estimated to house over 10,000 nerve fibers.[9] A tiny, yet mighty, structure. And unlike a penis, whose job is to also pass urine and semen, the clitoris exists solely for pleasure. That's it. That's its primary job and, when motivated properly (that is, how you stimulate it), it is the most giving. But let's back it up to that penis part for a minute. Way back when you were a wee one in the uterus, your genitals were not yet as they appear today. Early in the first trimester, there is a surge of hormones that influences what genitals you'll have, based on your chromosomes (XX or XY). Got XY? The hormones flip the switch on penis time. Got XX? Yeah, that extra X don't care. It sees those hormones and is like, *Cool, but I'm gonna keep on keepin' on.* This is what is called homologous structures—these parts have the same origin, but in the end, they serve a different function (see page 30 for the male and female matches). Kind of makes you wonder: If science knows this, why is it that the penis is the standard? Um, buddy, you're the one who took a detour from my perfection, not the other way around. No, seriously, we all start out phenotypically female; in other words, the tissues appear female in the very beginning even though the sex may be XY.[10] These are some of the biological basics of fetal development that, unfortunately, most people don't learn unless they get a biology degree. And just so we're clear, XX and XY aren't the only combinations, but for our purposes, I kept it simple.

The external part of the clitoris (the glans, sometimes referred to as the head) sits at the top of your vulva and matches up with the glans of the penis. Just like the penis, it really loves to be touched just right. This is only the tip, so if you look under the hood—that is, the clitoral hood, the tissue that covers the body of the clitoris—you'll find there's a whole lot more. You may have heard it referred to as a pea-size structure, but the glans and body combined can be anywhere from 2 to 4 cm, on average, and can potentially get bigger the more you use it (fascinating).[11] Within the body of the clitoris you will find it is made of the same tissues and nerves as a penis—the erectile tissue allows it to become engorged with blood, and the nerves are what give your brain the *Oh, so very good* message. Once considered just a tiny little button, we've come to understand that the clitoris is a vast structure (peep the image below). In addition to the glans and body, there are a pair of legs called the crura, along with two bulbs of the clitoris straddling the vaginal opening, which also expand when aroused. All these structures match the biological male counterparts, too.

Clitoral Anatomy

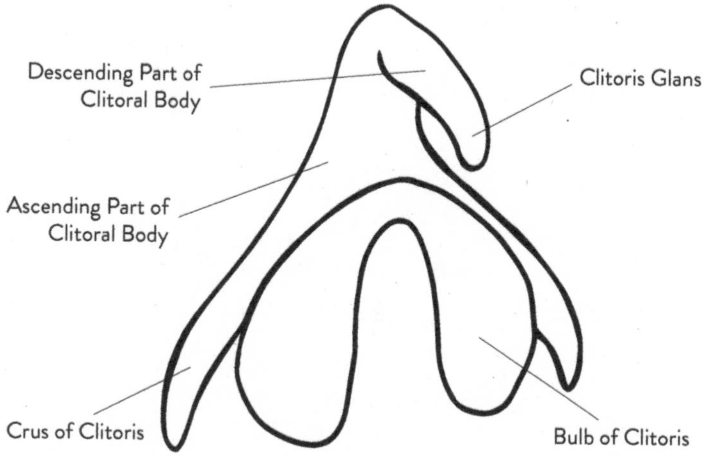

What's the male counterpart for the female genitalia?

These are the matching structures of female and male genitalia. They start off the same but develop different appearances and functions.

XX Biological Female	XY Biological Male
Clitoris	Penis
Crura of clitoris	Crura of penis
Corpora cavernosum	Corpora cavernosum
Clitoral hood	Foreskin
Urethra	Urethra
Labia majora	Scrotum
Labia minora	Urethral surface of penis
Vestibular bulb	Corpus spongiosum
Skene's glands	Prostate

Homologous Structures

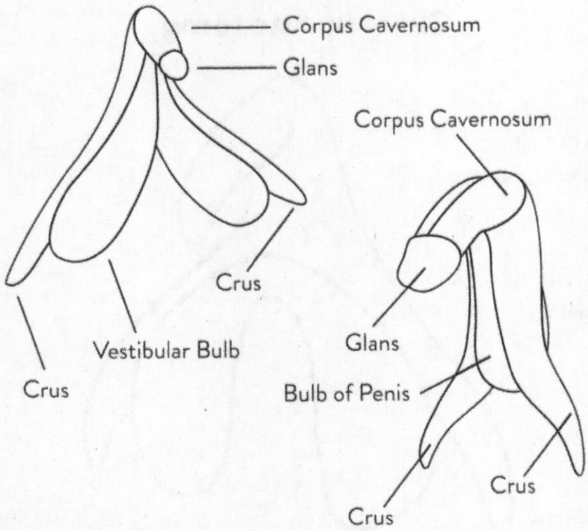

Will the size of my clitoris affect my ability to orgasm?

With an orgasm gap so great (how few women are having orgasms during heterosexual sex we will talk about in chapter 4) that not even the world's best daredevil could jump it, it's no wonder I have patients asking if the size of their clitoris is the issue. When aroused, your clitoris swells and expands in size, which makes a good case for foreplay (hello, pleasure center!) or just stimulating it in general. If you're having issues achieving orgasm, you may need more stimulation or a different kind of stimulation. In other words, it's usually a technique issue, not a "you" issue. I'd suggest exploring differing stimulation methods with your partner, or on your own, which you can skip to chapter 6 for.

While there have been studies stating that clitoral size is associated with orgasm frequency, others have found no relation.[12] It could be that those having more orgasms are seeing their clitoris slightly enlarged, which is normal due to the sexual stimuli. The issue with clit size to be medically concerned about is clitoral atrophy, a condition where it shrinks in size. Head to page 93 for what causes it and what to do about it. If you're wondering if penis size matters, it does, as I explain in chapter 5.

I want to let you in on a little well-kept secret about what will make it incredibly difficult, if not impossible, to orgasm: Worrying about how the bits look. Being self-conscious about any part of your body, but especially your genitals, is like a bucket of water on your sexual fire. In my clinical experience, people who are more confident about what they've got going on down there report a much easier time orgasming. And even when not totally confident, they still find a way to be present in the moment and ride that pleasure for what it's worth. If you, too, would like to wield such confidence, keep reading, because I'm going to give you even more details on what's normal.

Is my clit too big?

Too big, too small, not at all just what you think it should be? Actually, there's a million and one ways to hate on your body, and ain't one of them right. There's a wide variety of clitoral, vulval, breast, and while we're at it, body parts size altogether. And remember: if you're aroused, it is totally normal for it to grow in size. The vast majority of the time when I'm asked this question in my office the answer is, it's normal. In the case of clitoromegaly, which is doctor-speak for a rare condition in which the glans of the clitoris is enlarged (greater than 10 mm), we are far more concerned about what is causing an enlarged clitoris than the fact you have one.[13] This occurs, most commonly, due to exposure to excess androgens (a group of hormones often called "male hormones," but very much a part of normal women's hormone health, as we'll discuss in chapter 8), from applying topical testosterone replacement drugs, exposure to high androgens in utero, or in some cases of polycystic ovary syndrome (PCOS). Should you get surgery to correct it? Hard pass. Considering how it will damage the nerves and blood vessels in this delicate area, it's a no for me. Instead, the underlying cause should be addressed because that is far more serious than the size of your clit.

A CASE OF CLITORAL NEGLECT

Really, though: The Internet was invented in 1982, and the clitoris was "discovered" in 1998. And by discovered, I mean acknowledged. But why did it have to be acknowledged? Well, the clitoris was actually erased from the medical textbook *Gray's Anatomy* by a guy named Dr. Charles Mayo Goss in 1947. Why cut out any knowledge of the clitoris, essentially blinding doctors? Welcome to the deep-rooted misogynistic fear that pleasure without a penis would make men obsolete. Evolution did not make a mistake giving women this pleasure center, as I'll explain in chapter 4, but doctors most certainly have made a large mistake in omitting this information. Today, medical textbooks still remain filled with full-page diagrams of the penis while the clitoris is woefully underrepresented or, in many instances, misrepresented. Fortunately, we are now seeing many doctors, myself included, providing crucial information about the clitoris that is fundamentally your right to know. From being regarded as an inferior "penis" to the signature way to identify a witch[14] (I wish I was making that up), the clitoris has never received the honor it deserves in medicine or society as a whole. We're way behind in not only talking about the clitoris but in understanding it. We've all had a good laugh at the jokes about men who can't find the clitoris. However, this joke shouldn't be as universally relatable as it is. I'd wager that it has never been the intention of a lover to neglect the clit but, rather, the negligence of everyone who should be teaching them that has left them ill equipped, and the butt of a very long-running joke. In chapter 4 I aim to make you more informed than your average doctor about leveraging this pleasure center.

Your Vagina Is the Inside, Your Vulva Is the Outside

I've worked with many women of varying ages who didn't know their labia is different from their vagina, or that their cervix was part of their uterus. It's no secret that female anatomy is much more hidden than our male counterparts', but it sure does seem the specifics have been kept a secret for far too long.

I'd encourage you to get a mirror out and get to know your landscape, especially if you've never done this before. I have a diagram for you on page 34 if you want to compare for location purposes. Use it like a map to locate the landmarks, not a "this is the perfect picture of female anatomy." BTW, I'm going to give you the layperson's terms along with the more technical medical terms; that way, you're well versed in both.

When you first view your vulva, the outside, you'll see there are a total of three holes—the urethra (where pee exits), the vagina, and the anus (from top to bottom, in that order). If this is the first time you're learning you do not pee and bleed from the same spot, you're not the first, nor will you be the last person I come across who didn't know this until I shared. The vulva includes the labia majora and labia minora, or the outer and inner "lips." At the top of your labia minora, just north of your urethra, is the external part of your clitoris that we just talked about. The labia minora forms a border around the vestibule, which extends to surround the opening of the urethra and the opening of the vagina, or introitus. For some, the vestibule can be quite sensitive to touch, even more so if you have vulvodynia, a cause of pain with sex that we'll discuss in chapter 5.[15]

Vulva Anatomy

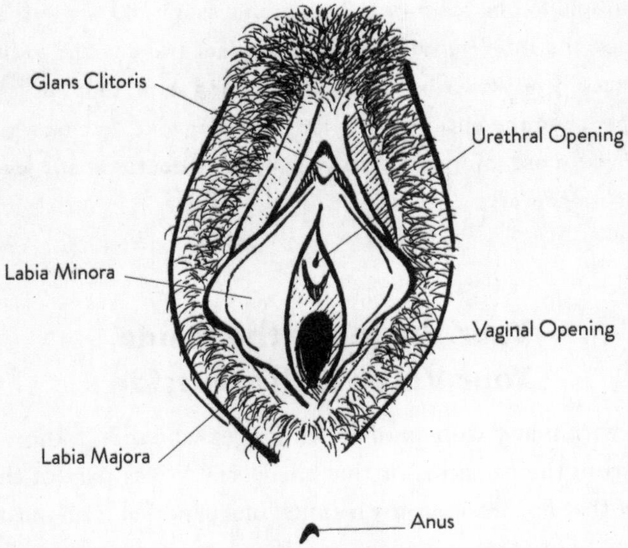

Compared to the vulva, the vagina is a closed fibromuscular canal *inside* the body that no one other than your medical provider will likely ever fully see. The fact that this is an internal structure has led many to mistakenly believe that women's genitals are only an inside job. But as you can plainly see in the mirror, with your vulva and what you just learned about the clitoris, there's a lot going on outside. But the only part of the vagina you see from the outside is the opening to it. There's no such thing as the "outside vagina." The vagina is what bridges both the inside and outside world. It allows for the exit of period blood when your body sheds its uterine lining every month and is how you participate in vaginal sex. It escorts sperm on its way to an egg, and it ushers babies into the world.

At the end of your vaginal canal is your cervix, which acts as a protective door between your vagina and your uterus. The cervix does have nerves and, depending on how you're wired or how it's touched, can be pleasurable or painful. If you've used a menstrual cup or have attempted to get pregnant by monitoring the position of your cervix (among other data), then you know that you can touch it by inserting a finger or two. Your cervix is dynamic, moving during your cycle and with arousal, along with dilating during childbirth.

The uterus, which is about the size of your fist, can stretch to the size of a watermelon by the end of pregnancy. Are you picking up just how amazing your body is? We'll talk about the uterus in much more detail related to your cycle in chapter 9, and how if it is tilted just right, you might end up with a case of "butt lightning" (if you know, then you know, and if you don't, you will soon). Beyond the uterus, you'll find fallopian tubes on each side with finger-like projections (fimbriae) that create rhythmic motions to usher an egg to come inside and cruise on down to the uterus. While a lot of people are under the impression that the ovaries are connected to the fallopian tubes, they're not; they are attached in the pelvis to ligaments. When they release an egg (as we'll discuss in chapter 9), it still must find its way to the uterus.

Female Reproductive Organs

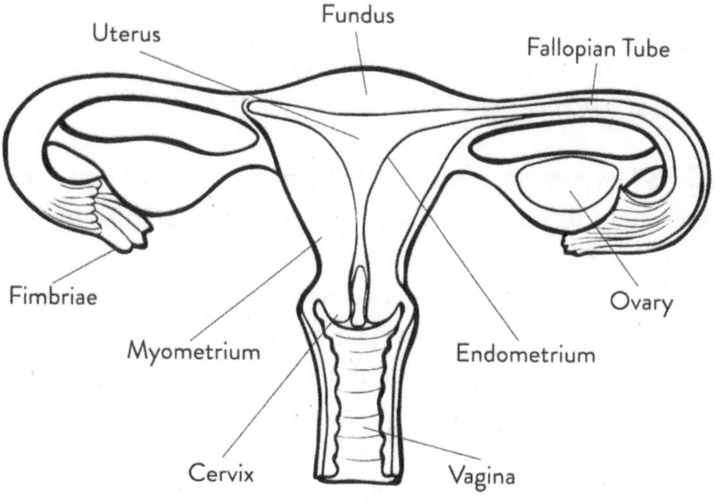

ASK DR. BRIGHTEN

Is the color of my labia normal?

Labia, like everywhere else on your body, aren't uniform in color and that's normal, despite what labia lightening fanatics tell you. Melanin—pigment found in skin—influences the color of the skin everywhere, including tissue down there. Your vulva has more melanocytes—pigment-producing cells—than most other areas of the body, and your labia may be the same color as your thigh or even darker. Your vulvar color can also change over your lifetime. As your hormones change with puberty, so does the color of the vulva, becoming darker for most women. Melanocytes are also particularly sensitive to estrogen, which is why your labia may deepen in hue with pregnancy or lighten as you age. (In case you're curious, estrogen and melanocytes are also why your anus is a darker color.) And just like a mood ring changing colors depending on how you feel, your labia also change color when you're in the mood, thanks to the increased blood flow. Normal labia range in color—pink, purple, brown, mahogany, caramel, eggplant, blush, and burgundy are a few examples—all of which are normal.

While vulval and anal bleaching may be growing in popularity,[16] they're entirely unnecessary and can cause burning, blistering, and scarring, not to mention expose you to some nasty chemicals. There's no medical reason to have this procedure done, and it won't necessarily give you the body confidence you're looking for. What's worse, it could actually rob you of a healthy and pleasurable sex life.

Is the size of my labia normal? If I have an outie, am I normal?

The labia change throughout a woman's life, during puberty, pregnancy, the menstrual cycle, with significant weight loss, and after menopause.[17] No two labia are the same, not between bodies and not even on the same body. An "outie vagina" (you now know it's a vulva, but this is the term people are searching) refers to the inner labia extending past the outer, something over half of women are estimated to have. So it's normal. As we age, it is common for the labia majora to shrink and for the inner lips to become more pronounced. But I get how when you do a Google search to a trusted medical source and come up short on outies, it can feel like they must not be normal. Heck, the majority of medical images are of a white body, depicting symmetry of color and size, and often with no or little hair. We know there's hair (see page 37 for the lowdown on hair). We know different colors of bodies exist. But for some reason, these images get it in our head that symmetry, shorter labia minora, and uniform pink color are the norm. They're not.

What about labial hypertrophy, the medical diagnosis for enlarged labia minora that causes symptoms like discomfort? There are no standard criteria for diagnosing labial hypertrophy—instead it's diagnosed at the discretion of the practitioner. There's a wide range of normal labia sizes, but in some instances, the discrepancy in size can make things downright uncomfortable. Having your labia pulled into the vagina by a thrusting penis, as patients have shared with me, may make sexy time anything but sexy due to discomfort. However, since the labia are full of nerves, responsive to sexual stimulation, and attach to the clitoral hood, there's a case to be made that larger labia minora may make sex more pleasurable. Yes, your body may have devised a way to increase pleasure and generate more orgasms, all while someone else is telling you it's a problem (*rolls eyes*).

If you are experiencing issues like infections, or you feel your labia are causing you pain because they are of significant size, then consulting with a vulvar specialist or a gynecologist is the best place to start. But as I'll share with you on page 41, these surgeries are being performed primarily on normal and healthy vulvas under the guise that it makes them more attractive or enhances sex. Neither claim has evidence to support it. What's even more concerning is that teens, whose bodies aren't even done developing, have been targeted for such surgeries. Performing this procedure on a minor when not medically necessary may be considered female genital mutilation, but when the diagnosis is subjective, there is concern that practitioners are proceeding forward with surgery anyway.[18]

If you're still curious about how much variety there is down there, I recommend taking a scroll through the Labia Library at https://labialibrary.org.au/.

What's normal for hair down there?

Pubic hair is part of the vulva—or rather, it covers your vulva and may extend back toward your anus or down your inner thighs. No matter how much hair you have, pubes are totally normal and, depending on the genetics you were dealt, you may have more than other people. In cases of polycystic ovary syndrome (PCOS) or excess androgens (like testosterone), hair can creep down your thighs or up toward your belly button. If you experience this hair pattern and other symptoms listed in chapter 9, it's a good idea to make sure your doctor is aware.

Pubic hair on the vulva is a heavily debated topic, one where personal preference is often interpreted as either falling prey to patriarchy, sticking it to the man, being heavily influenced by porn, or being a granola kind of gal. Like, when did your vulva pick up a political sign and start a protest? The truth is that to let it grow or chop it down is entirely your decision. Some of my patients report that when wearing pads on their period, with hair removed, their labia is less irritated. Others feel sex is more enjoyable when they are rocking a full bush, while others feel the complete opposite. Make your decision based on what you feel is best for you, and not because someone has told you it's dirty, ugly, or less attractive—it's not. Pubic hair is normal and can help reduce friction during sex and protect against infection.[19] Another benefit: hair may also play a role in pheromones, which may influence sexual attraction (an area still being explored)[20] and stimulating pubic hair during sexual activity activates nerves, providing a pleasurable sensation, so it may be worth the grow-out.

If you do choose to remove some or all your pubic hair, there are a few tricks of the trade (or blade). No one solution is best for everyone, so find the one that works best for you. Here are some things to know about the five most popular methods of pubic hair removal:

Method	Pros	Cons
Shaving	Cheapest; quickest; DIY; instant gratification; can be done anywhere, anytime	Requires daily or weekly upkeep; risk of razor burns and cuts; high risk of ingrown hairs; razor blade should be changed each time to prevent infection; never share razor blades (see chapter 7 for why)
Electrolysis	One-and-done hair removal; no upkeep; no risk of ingrown hairs or infection; permanent	Most expensive; can be painful; requires several sessions; permanent so you can't change your mind; can cause scarring and pigment changes

Method	Pros	Cons
Waxing	Removes hair for six to eight weeks; can cause hair to thin over time resulting in less new growth	More expensive than shaving; requires monthly sessions; exposure to questionable chemicals; risk of burns and skin trauma; high risk of ingrown hairs
Sugaring (a sugar-citric acid mix)	Similar to waxing, but with simple ingredients. Removes hair for six to eight weeks; all-natural; lower risk of ingrown hairs	More expensive than shaving; requires monthly sessions; possible risk of ingrown hairs
Laser	Less painful than other techniques; nonpermanent; effective	Expensive; less effective with darker skin; treatment time is long; requires multiple sessions; can cause pigment changes, scarring, and burns; reduces hair growth

Is the size of my vagina normal?

Vagina size varies from person to person and the length of the canal can vary depending on where you are in your cycle; the uterus is lower during menstruation (the easiest time to feel your cervix), higher while ovulating. The average length of the vagina is between three and six inches, the key word here being "average," because outliers are totally normal.[21] And given its phenomenal shape-shifting properties, this little ol' number is trivial. When you get aroused, your vagina gets longer and wider (a phenomenon referred to as tenting), as your cervix and uterus pull back to make more room for anything incoming, giving you another two to four inches of possible length. Yes, you've been walking around with your very own Mary Poppins bag and you didn't even know it.

But why don't tampons fall out or bugs crawl in? (Serious questions I've had from my patients!) The vagina is a *closed* canal that opens only when things go in (except for the queefing bit, which we'll discuss), yet also can open really wide when welcoming a small human into the world. When you're not in the mood, or nothing like a tampon or other object is actively penetrating your vagina, your vaginal walls are collapsed tight against one another, which is how it remains relatively waterproof when you're swimming (unless you orchestrate just the right move), how tampons stay inside, and why bugs can't ever crawl up there.

Vaginal canals expand thanks to folds of specialized tissue called rugae that line the vagina (rugae are also what allows your stomach to expand). Rugae act like an accordion, allowing your vagina to dilate when necessary. Vaginal rugae, along with the vulva, can atrophy when estrogen levels are too low (commonly seen after menopause), which can cause pain during sex, urinary incontinence, and vaginal dryness. A random cool fact about vaginal tissue: it's the same tissue that lines the inside of your mouth.

Is my vagina loose?

I've heard it said that "a woman's tight is like a guy's soft." Or in other words, skip the necessary stimulation that gets the body aroused and then you'll find a tight (and unwilling to participate) vagina. Vaginas are also tight in the case of vaginismus (involuntary muscle contractions discussed in chapter 5), anxiety, and pelvic-floor dysfunction, and can also be a sign that we're not feeling safe. Tight can also be a response to pain or the cause of pain. I'm not really selling this "tight vaginas are best" mantra that folk chant, am I? Honestly, they've really got it wrong on this one.

Despite this reality, cosmetic surgeries to "tighten" the vagina, otherwise known as vaginoplasty, have shot up in recent years, making it one of the fastest-growing treatments at med spas across America[22] (see more about vaginoplasty and other vaginal rejuvenation procedures on page 41). Then there's the horrific "husband stitch," which occurs when a doctor adds an extra stich while repairing a vaginal tear following vaginal birth, with the intention to make it more pleasurable for a penis. What's worse, these are often done without a woman's knowledge or consent—yes, that's absolutely wrong, if you're wondering—and it doesn't even deliver on its promise. Instead, women who receive the procedure are usually in pain and unable to have sex, and sometimes they believe they are just broken, because their doctor took unnecessary liberties with their body. The worst.

But what about vaginal birth? First, your vagina is resilient AF and, for some, it can return to its pre-birth state anywhere from three to twelve months postpartum. Despite how amazing the vagina and pelvic-floor muscles are, pelvic-floor work can be a tremendous benefit in supporting healing after birth—both vaginal and C-section. But in the early days following those pushing moments, it is totally normal for your vagina to feel "loose." Because, hello, a human head just made its way through, and a lot of accommodations were made for this little one. Just like it took nine months to grow that small human, it can take time to heal from the trauma that occurs to the tissue down there. Perineal tears can take time to heal, too, but no, continual pain with sex after having a baby isn't normal. Some things will be forever changed down there, like there's a lot more tissue folding over in the canal, but that doesn't mean it's a bad thing. I've had many patients report that sex after baby is better than before, which may be due, in part, to how comfortable you are forced to get with the vulva, vagina, and everything else that lies inside. Or it may be an entirely different phenomenon.

Designer Vaginas: Cosmetic Surgery

Let's take a minute to recognize that you are tasked with the ultimate of challenges—loving yourself fully and embracing your body in a society that tells you that you're not only imperfect, you need surgery to fix it. The number of "designer vaginas" has skyrocketed in recent years, as more and more women opt to go under the knife to change the size or shape of their vagina or vulva. The two most popular procedures are vaginoplasty, used to tighten the vagina, and labiaplasty, which shortens the length of the labia minora and reconstructs the appearance of the vulva. While a small number of women undergo these surgeries for reconstructive purposes after suffering cancer, pelvic-floor disorders, vaginal trauma, or a congenital abnormality, a staggering percentage of procedures these days are done strictly for cosmetic reasons, according to market research.[23] Many women who have vaginoplasty do so because they want to be tighter for their partner.[24]

Labiaplasty is even more popular, with a 217 percent increase in the past five years,[25] as women look to turn "outie" labia into an "innie." The most sought-after look is called the Barbie. Yes, the plastic doll void of any vulva features is the standard to which people are holding vulvas. Mattel: destroying women's body image since 1959. While Barbie dolls may make it seem like most women have no obvious genital features, more than 50 percent of all females have visible labia minora (inner lips), according to research.[26] Which means that it's completely normal. What's not completely normal is surgeons taking to social media to influence young women, whose bodies aren't done developing, to undergo an operation for aesthetic purposes, something the American Medical Association has stated is an ethical concern.[27] While these social posts and articles online sing the praises of the surgery, they give little attention to the potential harm, and even go so far as to say side effects are minimal. The American College of Obstetricians and Gynecologists has something very different to say regarding this surgery at any age: "There is no good research to show that female genitalia cosmetic surgeries are safe or work well."[28] On the other hand, the organization notes that procedures like vaginoplasty and labiaplasty can lead to generalized pain, bleeding, infection, scarring, pain during sex, and the need for additional surgeries. And what doctors promoting it don't say is that it can lead to damage of your clitoral nerves and an inability to feel pleasure in this area. When it comes to teens (who were, at one point, the most numerous recipients of this surgery, with 5 precent of all procedures performed on those under age sixteen),[29] let's be clear: operating on a tissue that isn't done developing can have a negative impact that may not even present until much further in the future. Finally, while many people are quick to blame porn for this trend, one study actually found that among the top twenty-five most popular porn videos, only 16 percent had labia consistent with labiaplasty, and 44 percent had labia minora longer than the majora.[30]

ASK DR. BRIGHTEN:

Is it normal if I pee when I sneeze, laugh, or jump?

Nope. Urinary leakage, known as urinary incontinence, needs to be addressed and can be a sign that your pelvic floor needs some TLC. While we're at it, anal leakage isn't normal, either. But both can occur following childbirth, surgery, injury, or from certain habits (like forcing urine out while hovering over the toilet). Two common questions I get around this are why aren't my Kegel exercises working, and isn't that normal after childbirth? See the sidebar for why Kegels are rarely enough. And as far as childbirth goes, it's common in the early days following labor, but if it persists, that's not normal, despite the many mom jokes about how "I just pee my pants now because I've had a baby" blaming it as the trade-off for having a kid. Fortunately, a pelvic-floor specialist can help you get these muscles functioning as they should.

JUST KEGEL IT

Doing Kegel exercises can strengthen your pelvic floor, eliminate urinary incontinence, and improve your orgasms, but they're not the fix-all many make them out to be. Are they an important exercise? Absolutely, for some. But would you go to the gym every day and do only bicep curls to build your arms? No. It's the same thing with your pelvic floor. I suggest to patients who want to strengthen the area, are experiencing pain or incontinence, or have gone through childbirth to see a pelvic-floor physical therapist (PT) who can create a plan tailored to you and your needs, because you may not even need to Kegel. In fact, in some cases, Kegels make things worse by reinforcing or creating imbalances in your pelvic-floor muscles.

Your doctor or pelvic-floor PT may recommend Kegel weights, also called Kegel exercisers or Kegel balls, which are objects inserted inside the vagina to help tone muscles. Be sure to use only Food and Drug Administration–registered versions, and clean them afterward by following manufacturer guidelines.

Is queefing normal? And what can I do about it?

Queef, aka vaginal gas, is the audible sound heard when air exits the vagina. Listen, this is super common and totally normal. In fact, I'm asked this several times a month. As I explained, the vagina is a closed tube. Whether it be from a sex position (or the vigorous nature of the session), your partner pulling at tissues during penetration, or down dogging in yoga just right for air to get in, know that the air must come out, and there is only one exit. A queef isn't a fart, but only you know the exit point, so of course it can be embarrassing.

Is my vagina supposed to smell?

Movies, TV, and commercials may try to sell the idea that you're supposed to smell like vanilla or a freshly peeled clementine, but you're not a fruit. You're a human. Having the scent of a car air freshener is *not* normal—you shouldn't smell like you just got detailed. Yes, vaginas smell, and in chapter 7 we'll cover what's normal and what's not.

Will douching help get rid of odor? What's the best way to clean my vagina?

Your vagina is a self-cleaning machine and is very good at its job. It's kinda like your oven, but with a lot less maintenance because there's no need to clean your vagina, ever (#winning).

Frankly, trying to clean or douche (flushing with liquid) inside can do more harm than good, upsetting the internal ecosystem of symbiotic organisms that live inside your vagina and keep you balanced, healthy, and infection free. You're basically a farmer feeding good little organisms all the time, and cleaning or douching is the equivalent of bulldozing down all the happy creatures that tend to your lady lands. Don't do it!

"But, Doc, I can't live without my coochie cleanser," I once heard a patient say. She was under the belief that she'd be dirty, especially after sex or her period, and would develop an odor. It's quite the opposite, in fact—you may be more prone to developing odor due to infection if you douche. We've been led to believe that our vagina is somehow dysfunctional and needs a specialty cleaner, spray, or other product to be fresh or acceptable. How did we get here? Corporations' need to pivot in the market to keep sales afloat, after years of deceiving women to their deaths. In the early 1900s Lysol was the douche of choice, a throwback to a time before birth control when marketers used "feminine hygiene" as a euphemism for pregnancy prevention.[31] In fact, that's how douching got started way back in the early 1800s, when physicians encouraged women to douche regularly (ironically, they were resistant to washing their own damn hands when it was required of them in the mid-1800s). It was, in part, the old-school Plan B. Warning: It never worked, and when it comes to Lysol, in 1911 there were 193 deaths attributed to using it.[32]

Douching is associated with bacterial vaginosis, yeast infections, sexually transmitted infections (STIs), pelvic inflammatory disease (PID),

Is My Vagina Normal?

Concerned if your vagina is normal?
Take this quick quiz to find out.

- ☐ I have thick, white discharge that looks like cottage cheese.
- ☐ I have discharge with a foul or fishlike odor.
- ☐ I have a change in discharge from what I'm used to.
- ☐ I have itching.
- ☐ I experience pain with sex or any kind of penetration.
- ☐ The area is swollen and uncomfortable.
- ☐ I have pain that is consistent or cyclical.
- ☐ I have persistent and painful vaginal dryness.
- ☐ I experience bleeding when it's not my period.
- ☐ I have problems inserting or removing a tampon or cup.
- ☐ My vulva has bumps, lumps, or has changed color.
- ☐ I feel a bulge or pressure when I use the bathroom or lift anything heavy or constantly feel like I need to use the bathroom.
- ☐ I sometimes leak urine.
- ☐ I have bumps, lumps, sores, or a rash.

If you checked off any of these, then things are not normal, and it's time for a trip to your provider. These are the things that should make you pause, not whether your labia are too big or uneven, or if your vagina smells like a vagina.

inflammation of the uterine lining, and cervical cancer.[33] Some studies have noted a threefold-increased risk of ectopic pregnancy associated with douching.[34] Despite what doctors have said for the past thirty years (yes, I recognize doctors are how all of this got started) and the known risk, one in five women still douches. Among Latinas, it's often our mothers who encourage us to start, making it out to be a mandatory part of womanhood.[35] This is, in part, why douching is highest among Hispanic and Black women,[36] who have been historically targeted in marketing (and society) to believe their vaginas are especially in need of cleaning.[37] It's not true. In fact, your vagina can handle itself and will be healthier and cleaner if you leave it alone to do its job.

What's the best way to wash my vulva? What's all that white stuff I see?

The vulva does need washing and, as we'll talk about in chapter 7, there are sweat glands, like what you find in your armpits, in your groin area. The association with armpits may make you want to take to seriously scrubbing and using some powerful soap, but it's actually not necessary, nor is it advised. The tissue is much more delicate down there, so gently using a washcloth and warm water is best. If you choose to use soap, keep it mild and fragrance free ("fragrance" is code for hormone-disrupting chemicals) to avoid serious irritation. A red, itchy, and tender vulva is nobody's friend.

The "white stuff" you see in the folds of the labia is called smegma, a buildup of natural secretions, oils, and dead skin cells. It can sometimes have a cheese-like texture and, if you don't wash for an extended period, smegma can accumulate and develop an odor. Still, I promise you, it's totally normal and can be easily wiped away using only water and a washcloth. Trouble arises when it's not removed for a long period of time, as it can begin to harden, causing pain around the clitoral hood. Smegma does not mean you are dirty. Healthy oil production, secretions, and the natural exfoliation process, which all of your skin goes through, are totally normal and actually are a sign of health.

RED LIGHT–GREEN LIGHT: THE VAGINA VERSION

Let's play a game of bedroom Red Light–Green Light. Green light is all good for your goods. Red light is, *Betcha gonna land in the doctor's office with this one someday because these things are risky*. OK, listen, I'm all for you having a good time, and supporting whatever you're into, but there are some things that can definitely disrupt your vaginal ecosystem, cause harm (think tearing, scarring, bruising, serious infection, burning, and the unknown), and land you in the ER. I share this list not to shame you, but to enlighten you on the things that patients have shared they wished they'd known before going there.

GREEN LIGHT

- Clean fingers or hands
- Penis
- Nonporous sex toys (see chapter 6 for more)
- Speculum
- Lube (see chapter 5)
- Condoms

RED LIGHT

- Garlic, Pop Rocks, popsicles, corn on the cob, carrots, and any other food item
- Douches, washes, pH-balancing soaps, or anything meant to "clean"
- Undiluted essential oils
- Canola oil or frying oils (opt for olive or almond if you're going DIY instead)
- Chocolate syrup, whipped cream, or anything else sugary
- Vaseline
- Anything that has been in the rectum or had contact with the anus

- Cooking utensils, cell phones, hair dryers, and any other instrument not designed for the vagina
- Alcohol-soaked tampons
- Jewelry or glued rhinestones
- Animals
- Electric toothbrushes or anything else that vibrates that's not designed for the vagina
- Aerosol cans
- Writing utensils
- Glow sticks or anything you'd use for a party

I swear I'm not here to kill the kink, so let's give you some harm reduction best practices. First, when in doubt, please call a doctor, especially if something has not come back out. *Hmm, where did I put my headphones?* (Psst: better toys for this found in chapter 6.) If you suspect something bad has happened, trust your instinct. Second, douching isn't going to undo what has been done and could potentially drive things up farther. Unless your doctor tells you to flush out the vagina, skip this. If you put food in there like whipped cream, chocolate, candy, or other items that dissolve, give your vagina time to do its thing and move it out. If you wind up with funky discharge (like purple, blue, or hot pink), recall what you put in there; for everything else, head to chapter 7. Lastly, be careful with piercings: always check that yours and/or theirs is still intact and accounted for when you're finished.

Is vaginal steaming safe?

Thanks to Gwyneth Paltrow, almost everyone has heard about vaginal steaming, which involves exposing your vulva to a steaming bowl of herb-infused hot water. Proponents say the practice cleans the vagina and can eliminate period pain, infertility, and endometriosis, a painful condition where uterine-like tissue grows outside the uterus (discussed in chapter 5). Um, how good does that sound? Amazing! But ask yourself: If all we had to do is sit over a bowl of steam, why do these issues persist?

Though Paltrow is given all the credit (even by critics), she didn't invent vaginal steaming. It's existed for centuries in cultures across the world. Steaming may help ease period pain by relaxing your pelvic area, but it's not a direct treatment for cramps or bloating. There's no scientific evidence showing that steam helps reverse endometriosis or infertility.

This is to say that I'm against vaginal steaming for the treatment of medical conditions and think it's harmful when people imply you can skip the doctor and necessary treatment and just steam. For some women, vaginal steaming is relaxing and part of their self-care ritual. I've also heard from sexual-abuse survivors that the practice helps them reconnect to and reclaim their genital area. And vaginal steaming is a cultural tradition or spiritual practice for some women, which is a big reason why it's unacceptable for medical providers to shame women who practice it.

Some doctors may advise against vaginal steaming, believing that women will burn themselves. I think it's insulting to insinuate that just because you want to pamper your vulva with a little extra, you're going to get reckless and end up scalding off its skin. Is there the potential to burn yourself? Umm, absolutely, but that's true of any time you come near boiling water or steam. Just like you wouldn't stick your face directly over a boiling pot of pasta, you're probably not going to do the same with your genitals. If things ever feel too hot down there, stop and allow the water to cool. If at any point you do develop issues like red, itchy, or painful tissue, please go to the doctor and discontinue steaming.

DOS AND DON'TS FOR VAGINA CARE

- ***Don't*** **wash inside your vagina.**
- ***Don't*** **douche.**
- ***Don't*** **use soaps with endocrine disruptors (see page 200).**
- ***Do*** **wash your vulva with water and a washcloth,** using only *mild* soap if you want.
- ***Do*** **wear cotton underwear,** which allows your vulva to breathe.
- ***Do*** **sleep naked** or wear loose-fitting shorts or pajama bottoms to give your vulva some friction-free time. If you prefer underwear, keep it cotton and change into a fresh pair before bed.

- ***Don't* wear nonbreathable, tight-fitting clothing** as much as you can avoid doing so, especially if you have an infection, are prone to infections, or have any lumps, bumps, pimples, or pustules that best benefit from this list of dos and don'ts.

Are these lumps, bumps, or acne normal?

As someone who's examined a lot of female genitalia in her lifetime, I can tell you that the vulva isn't smooth, symmetrical, or uniform in color—which is normal. But there are some not normal things you should be aware of like bumps, lumps, pimples, pustules, and warts. While some little blemishes are natural and nothing to worry about, others merit doubling down on how you take care of down there—see the list of dos and don'ts on page 49—or seeing a doctor. Here's a chart to help you decode any changes to your terrain. With all of them, it's important to see your provider. We'll also talk more about herpes and genital warts in chapter 7. (Note: This is not meant to take the place of a proper diagnosis by your doctor.)

How It Shows Up	What It Could Be	What to Do About It
Red bump or whitehead around pubic hair follicle (hair may be visible); can be painful; common after hair removal	**Ingrown hairs** (folliculitis) • See also Herpes, Vulvar acne	Consider gentle exfoliation with exfoliation glove. Discontinue hair removal.
Looks similar to pimples on face; can be painful, painless, or contain pus; usually clears up in a few days	**Vulvar acne** • See also Ingrown hairs, herpes, Molluscum contagiosum (see page 183)	Avoid products with fragrances and spermicides; check laundry detergent. Contact with irritants is a common cause.
Protruding soft skin growths, similar in appearance to skin tags elsewhere	**Skin tags**	Skin tags are harmless but can be medically removed.

How It Shows Up	What It Could Be	What to Do About It
Varicose veins or little blood-filled bumps around vulva; common during pregnancy	**Vulvar varicosities**	A provider can treat these directly and help you address the cause.
White, patchy skin; can be itchy or painful; skin may easily bruise and tear	**Lichen sclerosus**	See a doctor for treatment to prevent skin damage.
Red, inflamed blisters; can be painful or itchy; sores that last weeks; possible fever or flu-like symptoms	**Herpes** • See also Ingrown hairs, Vulvar acne	Meet with your provider. Avoid sex when you have active lesions. Herpes is treated with antiviral drugs (see page 181).
Singular or multiple; soft, smooth, or raised; may look like cauliflower	**Genital warts**	Refrain from sex and see a doctor (see page 183).
Fluid-filled sacs or lumps; often form from blocked glands near vaginal opening	**Vulvar cysts** (Bartholin's cyst)	Apply compress to help drain. See a doctor immediately if you suspect infection.
Lump on vaginal wall; most common following injury	**Vaginal cysts**	See a doctor if painful.
Bulge or pressure; may be accompanied by difficulty peeing or pooping	**Pelvic organ prolapse**	Meet with specialist. Severe cases may require surgery.
Sores that don't heal; changes in skin color or texture; bleeding; lumps or ulcers that don't go away	**Vulvar cancer**	See a doctor as soon as possible.

TL;DR: IS DOWN THERE NORMAL?

- You can refer to your genitals any way you like, but knowing your anatomy and how it all works is incredibly valuable.
- Your clit is much bigger than most people believe, and it exists solely for your pleasure.
- The clitoris is smaller than a penis but is estimated to house over 10,000 nerve fibers.
- The vulva is the outside. The vagina is the inside.
- Vulvas and labia vary in shape, color, and size. They are not symmetrical or uniform in color, and it is totally normal for the labia to be darker (your anus, too).
- The labia minora have nerve endings and connect to the clitoral hood, which is why you feel pleasure when they are stimulated.
- When it comes to hair removal down there, it's not necessary. But if you do choose to remove it, some methods may work better for you than others.
- Queefing is normal. It's just air and, unlike a fart, doesn't have an odor.
- You never need to clean the inside of your vagina. Douching can seriously mess things up and is associated with pelvic inflammatory disease, bacterial vaginosis, and even ectopic pregnancy.
- Washing the outside can be as simple as warm water and a washcloth.
- Glow sticks, cucumbers, candy, and your headphones shouldn't go in your vagina. For the full list of what's safe in and what's out, head to page 47.
- Lumps, bumps, blisters, or sores that are new require a trip to your medical provider.

CHAPTER 3

IS MY LIBIDO NORMAL?

WHY IT'S NORMAL TO BE IN THE MOOD, NOT IN THE MOOD, AND IN THE MOOD FOR CHOCOLATE

As a hormone expert well versed in sexual health, I'm often one of the most popular guests at any party. Here's a recent example. At a baby shower, my friend Jill welcomed me with "I just learned what 'Netflix and chill' means but, apparently, I'm the only mom who isn't able to get in the mood after putting my kids in front of Netflix." *Huh?!?* "Wait, what are we talking about?" Having come late, it seems that I missed the context of the game played. "Netflix and chill means putting your kids in front of Netflix so you and your husband can, *you know*," she explained. I had to step in. "Uh, OK, so Netflix and chill isn't a mom-specific thing, but I love the adaptation to fit mom life. More important, what you just identified is a brake, and knowing your brakes is literally how you get more 'chill' in both senses of the word," I told her.

"Brakes?"

"You know, the things that make your brain go *Shut it down* rather than *Yes, please.* Some of us have more brakes, some of our brakes are more sensitive, and most of our brakes have to be in the off position to make the vehicle go."

Jill nodded in understanding. "I've got a lot of brakes. Like right now my husband is not texting me back about the kids' naps, and that's making me anxious. And once I get anxious there's almost no coming back. Then we get to the end of the day, and he can't understand why I'm not into him, and all I can think of is his not responding to messages, his clothes all over the floor, and how many times I've had to put a coaster under his cup. I know it all sounds stupid when I say it out loud, but these things really get to me. When we first started dating, I felt like we couldn't keep our hands off each other, and all he'd have to do is kiss my neck for me to get in the mood. That's what I want back. Now even all the usual things that used to get me in the mood work only part of the time, and it just makes me feel broken." She ended with a sigh.

"It's not stupid and, in fact, not abnormal or uncommon," I explained. "The usual things that work to get you in the mood are like a gas pedal. While many of us, or our partners, focus on the gas pedal, very few of us recognize we need to release the brakes. I'm curious: Is this anxious feeling worse before your period?"

"That is *the* time that it is the worst, especially as I'm trying to go to bed. Even on days I'm exhausted I find that I'm too anxious to fall asleep," she shared. Jill's experience is a common one, where life and hormones meet to create a pleasure blockade, keeping you from seeing any clear path to sex, let alone getting in the mood. Fortunately, as you'll find in this chapter, there's a lot that can be done to remove the blockade.

What I explained to Jill then is the same thing I explain to the many patients who share a similar story (by the way, friends don't diagnose friends at parties—this was simply knowledge sharing). First, there is a hormone component at play here. Feeling anxious before bed points to adrenal function, while having anxiety that's worse when closer to your period can be a sign of low progesterone. While many experts will claim that hormones have nothing to do with your libido, or that your sexual desire is a hormone-only event, they're only partially right.

The relationship between a woman's libido and hormones is complicated. This intricate balance is, frankly, one of the most fun parts of working in women's medicine for me, but if you're struggling, I get that "complicated" is the last thing you want to hear. Your sexual desire is dependent on a lot of factors in your life, including relationship dynamics and stress. The same factors that can squash your libido can also push those hormones into a stress response (elevating cortisol at the wrong time or for too long), thus compromising progesterone (the chill hormone we talk about in chapter 8)—which can contribute to a decrease in desire and, in Jill's case, an increase in anxiety. To put it simply, your hormones respond to life's stressors and influence your libido, and your life stressors can also pump the brakes on any desire that might be stirring. Why do we talk about so many different factors here? Well, we should address it all if we want to have sex and have sex we enjoy. While that may be overwhelming, know that I'm going to give you tips in this chapter, and guidance in a 28-day plan, to help you get your vehicle where you want it to go.

Trigger warning: This chapter will contain information about sexual assault. While there is an abundance of helpful info in the pages that follow, I don't want you stumbling into this without warning. It may be best to skip to other chapters, or skim this one and leave what you don't need.

ASK DR. BRIGHTEN:

Is my libido normal?

First off, let's get straight on what libido is: your libido is often referred to as your sex drive, which gives the impression that it is a need that is vital to our existence. This is part of what feeds into the insecurities that make us question our normal. To be clear, there is no urgent or vital need when it comes to libido, like there is for hunger or thirst; you won't die if it's not met. For many of my patients, "libido" feels like an intangible term, which makes understanding yours even more difficult. For this reason, I often frame libido for what it is—sexual desire. (FYI: we'll use those words interchangeably in this chapter, since most questions I get are framed in the context of libido.) High sexual desire is categorized as when we think about, fantasize, and experience sexual feelings a lot. It doesn't always manifest as actually having more sex. On the flip side, low sexual desire is what most people think of as a disinterest in sex altogether, but as I'll explain further, that's not always the case. Desire, arousal, and pleasure all tend to get jumbled together whenever we have these sorts of conversations, so let's get on the same page. Your sexual desire happens in your brain or nervous system, and it can be there waiting in the wings, or build in response to pleasure that gets you aroused. Your sexual arousal is your body's response to stimuli that your brain has perceived as erotic in nature. Pleasurable stimuli that you are receptive to, in the right context, need to be interpreted by the brain before any arousal can occur. And that arousal can lead to desire that wasn't previously there. I'll explain more soon, along with a handy graphic to help you understand further.

When I share information about libido with my patients, it definitely leaves them feeling like their sex ed teacher failed them. Most of them have little understanding that your baseline is the metric to measure, that your experiences heavily influence your interest in sex, and that your sexual desire fluctuates. All of which is normal. But knowing if your libido is normal requires knowing what your baseline was to begin with. That's right, tracking your libido over your lifetime is vital to answering, *Is this normal?* Feeling a little unsatisfied? Keep reading, because there's a lot more nuance to this conversation that I'm going to provide in this chapter.

What if I have no libido and never have?

It's entirely possible this is your normal, as is the case in asexual individuals. People who identify as asexual (sometimes referred to as "ace") experience very low or no sexual attraction to other people, or interest in sex, or sexual desire in general.[1] This is different than feeling like you aren't getting turned on or aroused despite wanting to be. A low libido is not the same as identifying as asexual. Although someone may consider themselves asexual, they may still engage in sexual activity or enjoy other acts of affection like cuddling or kissing. Their behavior says nothing about how they identify. Asexuality is a spectrum and, as such, the term can hold different meanings for different people. If your partner identifies as asexual, it is best to ask them what that means for them, rather than assume that you know what it entails. It is important to understand that there is nothing to "fix" in an asexual person—their desire level is normal.

How do I know if my libido is low? Aka your baseline is the metric to measure.

By far, the most common concern about libido I hear is whether it is too low. If your libido has been consistent throughout your lifetime (with the understandable dips that come with stress, illness, etc.), but seems low when compared to others, we're less concerned because it's been your normal. And as I'll explain, there might be a simple misunderstanding of what desire *should* look like. We need to figure out the type of desire that's your normal—spontaneous or responsive. And when you understand this, you'll be able to gauge what your baseline is, to better answer *What's my normal?* However, if your libido downright drops, then we need to investigate. The cause may be a very real medical condition, a new medication, or a change in your life.

Context Matters: Your Experiences Heavily Influence Your Interest in Sex

For most of the patients I see, their desire for sex is influenced by everything that happens outside the bedroom. Dr. Rosemary Basson brought us the Circular Sexual Response model, which helps us understand just how complex the desire to have sex is for women (see graphic below).[2] This model supports the idea that women's sexual desire can be responsive or spontaneous, that context matters, and that factors other than physical stimuli play a significant role in our libido, like the desire for emotional bonding. Remember that Jill's husband's unresponsiveness extinguished her interest in sex?

CIRCULAR SEXUAL RESPONSE

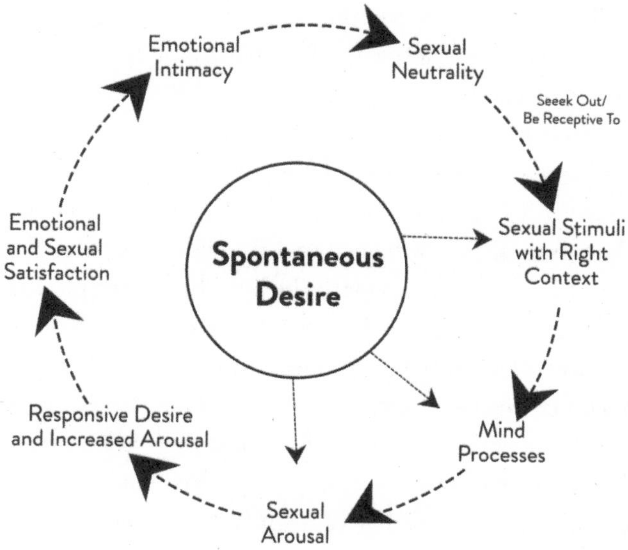

Context matters and needs to be accounted for. Just like your desire changes with your cycle, it also changes with your age, health, stress levels, and relationship status (*muy fuego* in the beginning to more of a slow burn as the relationship matures), as a few examples. While many of us are guilty of jumping to the "baby stole your sex drive" narrative in Jill's story, you may be surprised to learn that I hear about declining libido from women of all ages, in all types of relationships—with or without children. And I tell them what I will tell you: it's normal. In fact, many couples find themselves needing to tend to desire, dampen the brakes, or to ramp up pleasurable stimuli before the brain and body make a shift to what is recognized as the desire to have sex. Louder for the people in the back: pleasurable stimulation (which isn't just physical), when enough brakes are removed, is necessary for sexual desire, and is what leads to physical arousal. These are all things that have likely happened without you ever being aware, and sometimes it's spontaneous and other times it's responsive.

Spontaneous desire is what many (but not all) of us experience at the start of a relationship. I mean, it's part of what is drawing you to this person to begin with. When you see someone and suddenly have an urge to have sex, that's spontaneous desire. It's the most common type of desire we see portrayed in media, which is why we tend to think that's the norm—even though it's not.

Responsive desire isn't the lesser by any means, and occurs in response to pleasure. Pleasure can be mental or physical. Yes, you don't have to be touched to get responsive desire going. In fact, you just need enough brakes disengaged and gas pedals engaged to rev your engine just right. I promise, I'm going to help you identify just that, but before you go skipping to the how-to on me, please keep reading because again, context matters.

Let's take Jill's example and place her in two scenarios. She's already identified her brakes. But what about her gas pedal? She shared with me that watching her husband play with the kids, him bringing her coffee in the morning, seeing him do the dishes, and hearing him praise her hard work all made her feel more at ease and more interested in him. Yes, the events that influence her desire happen primarily outside the bedroom and are either additive or subtractive throughout the day. When I share that this phenomenon is normal with women in a heterosexual relationship, I get an enthusiastic "Yes, exactly what I've been trying to explain to my partner." But with men, it's generally "I had no idea."

SCENARIO 1

Jill's day has been a whirlwind. Her sitter failed to show up, so she had to take one client meeting with a baby strapped to her chest and had to reschedule the rest of her meetings that day. On top of that, her oldest child decided to experiment with making his own popsicles, which instead created a mess of dish soap, orange juice, and crumbled cheese all throughout the freezer and kitchen. On her way to put all his clothes into the wash, she slipped on a pair of her husband's gym shorts, meaning that once again she was left responsible for cleaning up after his workout. Her to-do list had been tripled by the day's events, so when her husband comes home and begins to kiss her neck while she's at the kitchen sink doing dishes, she's unresponsive. He takes that as a sign of her rejecting him, rather than recognizing her brain is in hyperdrive. What happened in Jill's brain is that her husband provided stimuli that under different circumstances would be interpreted as pleasurable and lead to increased sexual desire, but the day's events left her mind chaotic, unable to even recognize pleasurable stimuli.

SCENARIO 2

On a different day, Jill's sitter shows up on time, and all the laundry has been washed, dried, and put away. Her husband managed to land his sweaty workout gear in the hamper. And she had an exceptional day with clients, having met all her deadlines. Her husband picked up takeout on the way home and by some miracle they managed to get all the children down for the night. This time, when he kisses her neck as she's doing dishes, her brain registers the stimuli and says, *Ooh, hello, I like this.* There's no longer so many brakes along the way stopping her from receiving the message that *I like this,* which allows the gas pedal to engage, and the car is ready to go.

These are two extreme scenarios. The days where busy people manage to ramp up desire that brings them to sex they enjoy fall somewhere in the middle. We're not aiming for perfection. The goal is to remove brakes and apply pressure to the gas pedal so that the pleasure you so deserve is achieved. To do that, you need to identify what fuels your brakes and gas.

Sometimes I get responses from men like, "This doesn't take into account what I do all day, and is just another way of making things our fault." It most certainly doesn't diminish what men do in a day. And bro, if all you gotta do is make sure your chonies make the hamper, why wouldn't you just do that?

What's normal, then, spontaneous or responsive desire? Both are normal and neither one is better than the other. That means whatever your desire type, it's totally normal for you.

I want to also acknowledge that if sex hasn't been enjoyable for you, either because it isn't pleasurable, or you can't achieve orgasm with partnered sex, or because you're criticizing yourself, or it's painful, then you may be less inclined to be interested. In addition, if you have a history of trauma or sexual assault, it's not as easy as "just reduce the brakes in the system." Getting support from a trauma-informed counselor, or a therapist who specializes in sexual assault, can make a tremendous difference in not just your sexual health, but your overall health and well-being. One in three women, one in four men, and at least half of transgender individuals are estimated to have been sexually assaulted, so recognize that if this is you, you're not alone.[3] Many of us have work to do in this area, by no fault of our own.

ASK DR. BRIGHTEN:

Why is my sex drive different than that of my partner/best friend/everyone else I know?

You could ask the same of so many other markers of health. Like why is my energy, mood, sleep, period, or appetite different than my bestie's? This sort of variation from person to person, as your hormones fluctuate during your cycle and as "life happens," is all normal.

Let me explain a bit further. When it comes to hormones that influence libido, testosterone claims the crown. If testosterone and libido are both bottoming out, supplementing can improve sexual desire, arousal, orgasms, and responsiveness, while also reducing sexual anxiety.[4] If you're on medications like hormonal birth control, it can result in diminished testosterone and loss of sexual desire. But while testosterone gets the glory, it is not the only libido-influencing hormone: estrogen, cortisol, and progesterone also play a role in both desire and arousal (keep reading, because I've got more to say on hormones). Ask anyone who has been pregnant how shifting hormones impact their libido, and you'll find some folks who are ready to go all the time and others who never want to be touched. For those who cycle, they may notice their desire for sex peaks around ovulation and drops just before menstruation. We'll be tracking these fluctuations as part of the 28-day plan so you can determine *your normal.*

Yes, hormones matter when it comes to desire. In Jill's case, life's stressors were cranking her cortisol, which left her body to prioritize survival over procreation or bonding. The result? Progesterone production declines in favor of cortisol, and anxiety starts to creep in. TL;DR version? Jill's response was normal; relationship issues were definitely weighing on her libido *and* she also had an appropriate hormone response that got in the way of her sexual desire. But giving her a dose of testosterone wasn't going to solve the issue, because at the root of it was stress and relationship factors.

Other factors play into your libido as well. It's influenced by physical health, mental health, past traumas, medication use (see the table below), stress levels, sleep habits, emotional issues, the health of your relationship (if you're in one), body-image issues, alcohol or drug use, your need to bond, how enjoyable you find sex, and even how much or the type of exercise you engage in. This isn't an exhaustive list, either, since nearly everything you do, think, imagine, feel, drink, and eat can influence your sexual desire to some degree. Simply put, your level of sexual desire is different because you're different, as is your lived experience.

MEDICATIONS THAT MESS WITH YOUR MOJO

• Antidepressants	• Beta-blockers and other heart medications	• Hormonal birth control
• Antihistamines	• Cannabis	• Opioids
• Antiseizure drugs	• Cholesterol-lowering medications	• Spironolactone (commonly used for acne)
• Benzodiazepines and other anti-anxiety meds	• Heartburn medication (such as Tagamet)	• SSRIs

What Makes You Want to Hit That Gas Pedal Versus Brakes?

Drumroll, please, because here's the deets on how to apply more pressure to the gas pedal, ease up on those brakes, and get it on. To do that, we need to get our brain and spinal cord—aka our central nervous system—the signals it needs to make the car go.

Your brain is constantly scanning the environment, even when you're unaware of it. What you see, hear, smell, feel, taste, and think are all sending signals that either excite or inhibit your sexual response. Anything your brain registers as sexual in nature will tap that gas pedal. These two opposing systems are what are known as the dual control model of sexual response, as defined by Erick Janssen and John Bancroft.[5] I know that I've been using the terms "gas pedal" and "brakes" a lot, so allow me a moment to give you the DL on what that actually means.

Sexual Excitation (SE) system is the body's "get it on" system, or gas pedal, which we are rarely aware of until we find ourselves in the mood.

Sexual Inhibition (SI) system is the body's "no thank you" system, or brakes, activating when we want to regain our physical and emotional cool, working to decelerate our sexual arousal.

These two systems operate just like the pedals in a car: Providing the right stimuli presses on our gas pedal (SE) and revs our desire, while pushing our brake (SI) slows the roll on the road to sexy town. As it turns out, it's less about the gas and a lot more about the brakes for most women. While you may be thinking *Let's just cut the brakes*, lemme explain why they are a very good thing. Sometimes our brakes stop us from becoming aroused in inappropriate places (um, Thanksgiving dinner table? Awkward) or when your kids walk in (*Damn you, Netflix* *shakes fist*). I think we can agree that an emergency shutdown procedure is warranted when arousal is mismatched with the environment. The brake system is surveying threats, and anything real or perceived will tap those brakes. The threat of pregnancy—as we will talk about in other chapters—is a common one, as is feeling insecure about our body or sexual performance.

But we can change our environment for the signals to the system. This is where the context of the arrival time of that neck kiss Jill's husband placed on her matters, when the inputs of the day have created a situation in which the message of pleasure can be received. In Jill's second scenario, the lower-stress day made her welcome her husband's affection. For you, being available when pleasure rings may mean getting STI testing if you have a new partner (always a good idea), having a solid form of pregnancy prevention so your mind doesn't fixate on the what-if, and spending some time falling in love with your body to enable your mind to be in the moment of pleasure.

Knowing what stimulates our brake and gas pedals is helpful, but it is not as simple as just doing more or less of something. We've got to embrace those things that tap our brakes. And we've got to be OK with how sensitive they are. And on the flip side, we need to be OK with all the things that press on the gas. Plus, to top it all off, we need to be OK about communicating this with our partner. Does this seem a bit overwhelming? That's probably because you'll be doing all this despite having received external messages your entire life that tell you how you *should* function sexually, so it is entirely understandable if you need support from a health provider to do this. (Seriously, this is a topic I could write an entire book on. Fortunately, someone already has, so if you want to go even deeper into how your brain rules your sexual life, I highly recommend *Come as You Are* by Emily Nagoski.)

Back to Jill for a second. "How do I get my husband to understand what my brakes are and what makes me go?" she asked excitedly toward the end of our conversation. I gave her the same exercise I share with my patients: use your smartphone to start a note and jot down the things that are your brakes as they come up in the day—you can even put an emoji next to the ones that are particularly sensitive or hard stops. It's also equally important for you to list all the things that help ease off the brakes and press on your gas pedal. Not sure how to identify those? Neither was Jill. Start by thinking about the times when sex was really good. Seriously, recall the best sex of your life and journal it out. Write down exactly what made it good. Make sure to note what events leading up to it made you so excited. It may take you a few days of just thinking it through before you can really identify your unique accelerators and brakes. Once you've made this list, I recommend that you share with your partner what you've learned. This knowledge can empower you to have not only the sexual desire you want, but the actual sex you want, too. In addition to the exercise I just mentioned, I recommend taking the quiz below to get a sense for how touchy each pedal may be for you. These insights can help you better understand *your normal* and communicate your needs to your partner.

What's ~~Love~~ Hormones Got to Do with It?

If you've ever noticed that midcycle you find yourself thinking about, fantasizing about, or craving more sex, that's all 'bout those hormones. In chapter 8, we're going to get down and dirty with the specifics of testosterone, estrogen, and progesterone. But for now, know that they all fluctuate over the course of your cycle and do influence your sexual desire along the way. If you're thinking you're doomed because your cycles are irregular, know this isn't necessarily the case. My patients with polycystic ovary syndrome (PCOS), a condition in which testosterone is often elevated, sometimes report increased libido despite not having regular cycles. That's because while that excess T is good for the bedroom, it's not so good for the ovaries' ability to function properly. I'll explain more, in chapter 9, about how not ovulating may also influence libido. Testosterone gets an understandable amount of play in this conversation, but it is only one player in this arena. What is too commonly overlooked is the impact of stress, blood sugar issues, thyroid disease, and inflammation.

STRESS HORMONES AND YOUR LIBIDO

Say it with me now: All your hormones are connected. That means if one of them is out of balance, the rest are sure to follow as they try to compensate. Your adrenal glands (along with insulin) are the foundation of your hormone health. Picture a pyramid: at the bottom are your adrenal glands (a set of glands responsible for making stress hormones) and insulin (regulates your blood sugar); just above that is your thyroid hormone; and at the very tippy top are your sex hormones (estrogen, progesterone, and testosterone). While symptoms like decreased libido, acne, irregular periods, and PMS have us wanting to focus on getting those sex hormones to behave as quickly as possible, the answer to resolving symptoms of imbalance for

"How Are Your Pedals?" Quiz

This quiz is an adaptation of the Sexual Excitation/Sexual Inhibition Inventory for Women (SESII-W) and is meant to serve as a guide in helping you understand how sensitive (or not) you may be to certain sexual stimuli.[6] Chances are, if you've read other sexual health books you've come across this tool before because it provides valuable insight. This quiz is by no means diagnostic. Use what you find here to identify how sensitive your brake and gas pedals are.

As you read each statement, write next to it the number that best describes you. Then add up your numbers to get a sense of how sensitive you are to sexual stimuli, versus the things that make some of us want to pump the brakes. This scale has been shown to be useful for women of different sexual orientations and relationship statuses. Before you dive in, I want to be abundantly clear that the results don't mean there is anything wrong with you. They should be used to create more insight and awareness about your sexual desire.

Gas Pedal (Sexual Excitors)

1 = Strongly Disagree   *3 = Agree*
2 = Disagree   *4 = Strongly Agree*

_____ When I think about someone I am attracted to I become sexually aroused easily.
_____ Certain hormone changes definitely increase my sexual arousal.
_____ Seeing a partner doing something that shows their talent can make me very sexually aroused.
_____ Eye contact with someone I find sexually attractive really turns me on.
_____ It turns me on if my partner "talks dirty" to me during sex.
_____ Particular scents are very arousing to me.
_____ *(For this question use the scale 4 = Strongly Disagree, 3 = Disagree, 2 = Agree, 1 = Strongly Agree)* If it is possible someone might see or hear us having sex, it is more difficult for me to get aroused.
_____ *Total (out of 28)*

Brake Pedal (Sexual Inhibitors)

1 = Strongly Disagree *3 = Agree*

2 = Disagree *4 = Strongly Agree*

_____ If I am concerned about being a good lover, I am less likely to become aroused.

_____ Sometimes I feel so shy or self-conscious during sex that I cannot become fully aroused.

_____ If I think about whether I will have an orgasm, it is much harder for me to become aroused.

_____ When I am sexually aroused, the slightest thing can turn me off.

_____ Unless things are "just right" it is difficult for me to become sexually aroused.

_____ If I think that a partner might hurt me emotionally, I put the brakes on sexually.

_____ I really need to trust my partner to become fully aroused.

_____ *Total (out of 28)*

What Your Score Means

Sexual Excitors (Gas Pedal)

Score 1–9: Low Excitation

Sexual stimuli may be something that goes unnoticed, or at least leaves you unaroused. Because you may require more stimulation, introducing mindfulness (a practice of connecting to your body), finding ways to connect more intimately with your partner, and stimulating toys (like a vibrator) may help with your arousal.

Score 10–19: Moderate Excitation

If it is what gets you in the mood and is delivered at just the right time, you'll be aroused and stay there. However, you will need to make efforts to bring in and pay attention to sexual stimuli.

Score 20–28: High Excitation

Lots of things can excite you, even things that don't do it for others, like becoming aroused by food (which is known as sitophilia). While some people may find that stress is a deterrent to sex, you may find sex an enjoyable way to de-stress.

Sexual Inhibitors (Brake Pedal)

Score 1–9: Low Inhibition

Eye on the prize, distractions be damned. You have less sensitive brakes, which means that the usual stuff that might make someone feel inhibited doesn't faze you in the same way.

Score 10–19: Moderate Inhibition

The context in which you receive sexual stimulation will influence your sexual desire. Stress, worry, or the never-ending to-do list can elicit the brakes, as can the first time with a new partner. Look at the areas you marked as high to bring them to your awareness so that you and your partner can address those areas together.

Score 20–28: High Inhibition

Your brakes are sensitive enough that you can have a difficult time getting aroused and staying there. You need to take things slow, set the right scene, and feel relaxed to be aroused. Creating something more closely resembling your "ideal environment," along with cultivating trust and open communication in your relationship can help in easing off these brakes.

As I've described previously, enough brakes must be disengaged for the gas pedal to move the vehicle in the right direction. If you scored higher in the inhibition category, your brakes are more sensitive. Is that a bad thing? No, it's just data about you that will help you understand how to meet your needs and communicate to your partner what you need to become aroused. Many women who find they are in the moderate- or high-inhibition group still have an enjoyable sex life. In these instances, more attention needs to be paid to caring for the brakes than pushing that gas pedal to the metal. It's all normal.

good actually lies in establishing a solid hormonal foundation. I can give you all the tips, tricks, and supplements on the planet to address your sex hormones, but if your foundation is not set right, they're going to take you only so far. The hormonal secret to increasing your desire for sex lies in establishing optimal hormonal health from the bottom up.

Cortisol is the dreaded libido-killin', belly fat–buildin', and pro-aging stress hormone that is easily pushed out of balance. It is necessary for your stress response and to keep inflammation in check. The adrenal glands produce cortisol, along with epinephrine and norepinephrine, in response to real or perceived stress. A lot of different factors can cause these fight-or-flight hormones to go off the rails. You could be sick, you could have lost your job, or you could be playing out what-ifs in your mind. These hormones serve the purpose of helping you survive short-term stress—running away from a predator or fighting said predator, though sometimes instead they cause you to freeze in front of said predator (not very helpful).

Today we don't have to worry about the bear. Instead, many of us are like Jill—working, managing a family, trying to check off an ever growing to-do list, and sometimes cohabitating with partners who aren't doing their share to support such a dynamic. The result is a cycle that causes big trouble for our stress response and can result in hypothalamic pituitary adrenal (HPA) dysregulation. The *H* and the *P* here control both stress hormones and sex hormones. They're found in your brain, so when the brain perceives stress, it (being the incredibly smart organ it is) says, *It's time to make the survival hormones and shut down those sexy-time ones.* I mean, who has time for sex when there's a bear lurking outside? This hormone priority system is also why stress can cause you to miss or delay ovulation, skip a period, or lose your period altogether. Stress hormones can drive anxiety, while progesterone provides a calming effect to the brain. For Jill, the life stress she was experiencing was driving her stress hormone levels up at the expense of her progesterone production. Not only did she lose her desire for the coveted "Netflix and chill," she was also anxious as a result, and unable to fall asleep at night despite feeling tired.

When it comes to stress, your brain and body have their priorities straight with making cortisol and dampening down production of sex hormones. However, you were never biologically designed to be under the unrelenting stress so many of us experience. This is why it's so important we talk about ways to manage stress in order to improve your libido and balance your hormones. If you feel it's entirely unhelpful for a doctor to tell you that all your issues are stress-related and that the solution is to eliminate the stress, I agree. Eliminating stress is easier said than done, especially when we account for past traumas, allostatic load[7] (a term that refers to the cumulative burden of life stress), microaggressions, and the unforeseen. Um, didn't we just experience a global pandemic? Yes, indeed we did. So how you gonna act like we can just wish stress away? I won't even begin to pretend it's that easy. Instead, I've provided you with a list of resources on page 310 to help you manage and process the stress you can't control. In the 28-day program, I'll also be guiding you on the lifestyle changes that love up your adrenals, like blood sugar regulation, improved sleep, and anti-inflammatory foods.

In addition to stress hormones, the adrenal glands produce a glorious anti-aging hormone that goes by the name DHEA (dehydroepiandrosterone if you want to get nerdy about it). DHEA is converted to estrogen and testosterone in the body, which means your adrenals are a vital source of hormones when those ovaries cease hormone production, as is the case in menopause or primary ovarian insufficiency (POI). This is another way in which your adrenals are vital to your entire endocrine (hormone) system. DHEA has also been found to be a key player in our sexual desire and function. Women ages eighteen to forty-four who have low DHEA report experiencing low sexual desire, arousal, and responsiveness.[8] Remember this bit about DHEA because we're going to discuss it a bit later in regard to how it can help your testosterone and libido.

Hormone Hierarchy: How to Heal Your Hormones

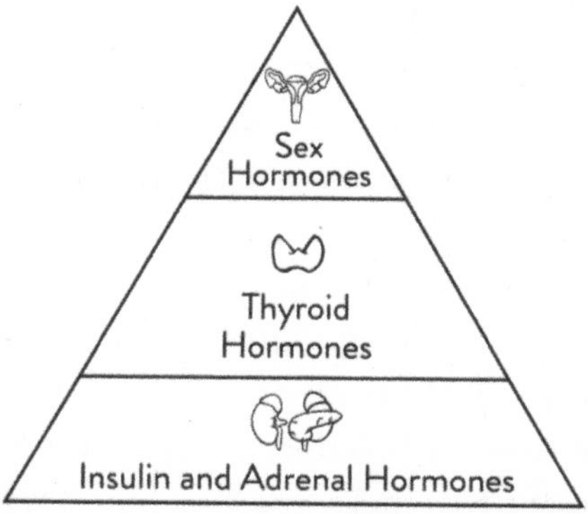

Your adrenal hormones and insulin (blood sugar-regulating hormone) are the foundation of your hormone health. To heal your hormones, you need to ensure you have a solid foundation.

INSULIN AND YOUR LIBIDO

What's on your plate can affect more than one type of appetite. Insulin is the hormone that is responsible for ushering sugar into your cells. You eat, digest, absorb, and then transport sugar molecules through the blood to the cells that need them. Insulin knocks on the cell's door and, if all goes right, that cell invites the sugar in. In cases of insulin resistance, your body will crank out a whole lot of sugar-escorting insulin hormone, but the cells refuse to let in the blood sugar. Over time this leads to chronic elevation of blood sugar, and may eventually lead to diabetes. Screening tests like fasting insulin, fasting glucose, and hemoglobin A1C can help determine if you are insulin resistant or have diabetes. We understand that blood sugar dysregulation and insulin resistance are associated with poor clitoral blood flow and hormone imbalances that can affect your desire for sex.[9]

THYROID AND YOUR LIBIDO

Women are five to eight times more likely to develop thyroid disease compared to men, who have a one in eight chance of developing thyroid disease in their lifetime.[10] The odds are not in our favor, which is why this is information you need to get in on. The thyroid gland, located at the base of your neck, is responsible for creating T4 (inactive thyroid hormone), which is then converted to active (T3) in other areas of the body like your gut and kidneys. Testosterone aids in the conversion of T4 to T3, which plays a significant role in your mood, metabolism, menses, gut motility, energy, and so much more.

Hypothyroidism (too little thyroid hormone) is the most common type of thyroid disorder. Its primary cause is an autoimmune condition known as Hashimoto's thyroiditis. ICYMI, an autoimmune condition is when your immune system attacks your body in a way it would a virus or bacteria, and in the case of Hashimoto's, the result is too little thyroid gland to produce thyroid hormone. Hair loss, joint pain, dry skin, constipation, and extreme fatigue are all symptoms we experience when our cells do not get enough of this hormone (see page 194 for a full list of symptoms). While too little thyroid hormone will certainly leave you feeling out of the mood, the accompanying autoimmune response causes a whole lot of desire-stomping inflammation. On its own, inflammation will make you feel achy, cranky, and cause you to retain water. None of that even sounds sexy, amirite? But inflammation takes it to a whole new level by increasing the amount of aromatase, the enzyme that makes your testosterone turn into estrogen. There goes that Marvin Gaye vibe. The increased estrogen levels can contribute to irritability, tender breasts (the *Don't touch me* type), acne, and heavier periods. Inflammation of any kind can do this, not just that caused by autoimmunity, which is why lowering inflammation is going to be key to feeling sexy and actually wanting sex. When inflammation goes up, your adrenal glands are called upon to control the inflammation. Essentially, here comes the cortisol, there goes the progesterone, and buh-bye, libido.

Getting tested is an important step if you suspect you have thyroid disease. You can use https://DrBrighten.com/ITN-resources to help ask your doctor for the right thyroid tests. Working with a provider is important when wrangling the autoimmunity, and there are many nutrition and lifestyle therapies you can employ when seeking treatment. Consuming foods rich in selenium, like Brazil nuts, salmon, and beef, can dampen autoimmunity while also supporting thyroid hormone production. Regular exercise, like walking, biking, and strength training can support the activation of your thyroid hormone. And as you probably guessed, stress reduction can play a big role in removing this potential hurdle to sexual desire. Adding turmeric, ginger, and omega-3-rich fatty fish can support your body in getting inflammation into check, as can optimizing your vitamin D levels. We'll get into more specifics in the 28-day plan for how to create a lifestyle that is hormone harmonizing.

SEX HORMONES AND YOUR LIBIDO

Testosterone is not just for men. Unfortunately, there are still many health care providers who feel it isn't necessary to evaluate women's testosterone because it's a "male hormone" and, therefore, not as important in women's health. This misbelief stems from the biological fact that healthy testicles produce more testosterone than do ovaries. However, while the male counterpart may have more testosterone circulating in their system, you, dear vagina owner, actually have more biologically active testosterone. Your biologically active form is free testosterone, which is not bound to any proteins, so it is free to link up to your cells and perform its job without inhibition.

Free testosterone is what is more important to measure in women, as it has been correlated with sexual desire.[11] Testosterone not only influences your ability to get in the mood, it also plays a role in your ability to have an orgasm.[12]

Of all my patients who have tried testosterone therapy, not one began it only for diminished sexual desire. That might shock you, given how connected it is to our libido. However, the best medical answer is rarely to just give someone testosterone and watch their libido soar. In the cases where there are other symptoms of low testosterone (loss of muscle mass, weight gain, low motivation, prone to crying) and it is verified by lab testing (of free testosterone), this therapy often does aid in improving libido because there was a deficiency to begin with.

Dehydroepiandrosterone (DHEA) is an alternative option to testosterone therapy once you have the diet and lifestyle factors dialed in. This is because DHEA can be converted to testosterone by the body and may result in improvement in low-testosterone symptoms. It isn't without side effects, however. Just like with testosterone, you may develop excess-androgen symptoms like acne, oily skin, hair loss, hirsutism (excessive hair on your body), aggression, an enlarged clitoris, excessive libido, or extra muscle mass. Not exactly fun. A Cochrane database review (the highest-standard research review in evidence-based health care) of DHEA concluded there is evidence of benefits regarding sexual function in women; however, the data is still lacking, and the side effects noted do occur.[13] Additionally, new research suggests the use of DHEA in women taking combined oral contraceptive pills in order to counter the testosterone-lowering effects of the pill.[14] In my patients who are unable to raise their testosterone despite all their best efforts and are suffering from low-testosterone symptoms, DHEA is the option I provide before recommending testosterone. It is important to again keep in mind that data is limited here, and these decisions are very individualized. I would caution anyone thinking they can just replace a hormone without a licensed prescriber's supervision, ongoing monitoring, and important health screening steps to not do so. Please trust me here.

LOW DESIRE WITH SSRIS

Too much serotonin early in your endeavors can lead to anorgasmia, the inability to orgasm or difficulty orgasming. Serotonin is often referred to as the "orgasm brake" for this reason, and it is why SSRIs can mess with sex. Does that mean you need to quit that SSRI stat? While it's well known that these meds can lead to decreased libido and difficulty orgasming, they may very well be a lifesaving measure for you. Options include switching medications, addressing the factors that may be at the root of your depression, meeting with a mental health professional to help you overcome your concerns, and trying some saffron in your routine.

ASK DR. BRIGHTEN:

If I'm turned on, then why am I not getting wet?

Sometimes your brain is totally ready to go, but down there didn't get the memo. This is known as arousal nonconcordance and is totally normal.[15] Because the wet factor is so commonly used to verbalize that we are ready to go—how many times have you heard "I'm so wet right now" in a movie?!?—it has become a metric by which we are all measuring our desire. It can also lead your partner to believe they are doing something wrong, or that you're not that into them, if your body doesn't match your words. But—and this is something to highlight, meme, or put on your fridge—what your words say is more important than what your body says. In a world where research and medicine make men the default, it's easy to see how the confusion arises when men's genital responses match their arousal much more often than women's do.

Arousal nonconcordance can go both ways—your vagina can seem unresponsive to desire that's on point, or it can seem like it's confusingly responsive to something that is sexual but in no way does it for you. Ever scroll through your social media feed and see someone doing a suggestive dance that causes your genitals to wake up, but then you catch yourself being like, *WTF, I'm not into them or this?* That's because your complex inner workings received the memo that read "sex" and decided to jump on board. It doesn't mean something is wrong with you, or that you're suddenly changing sexual orientation. And to touch on this in terms of consent, just because you're wet does not mean you were into it if all the while your brain said *Nope, this isn't for me.* Let me be perfectly clear on this one: if you say no, even when there is a genital response like lubrication, it's a no, and proceeding as if it wasn't is sexual assault.

To drive the point home in a way that the male-centered model of sexuality—cue eye roll here—has helped us all understand, think about the many ways erections have been featured in comedies. The big screen has shown us erections at the most inconvenient of times (even when not thinking about sex), erections that can't be turned off after seeing something sexual and wishing it would go away, and erections that will not happen even when every ounce of their being is willing it into reality. You may take issue with how the entertainment industry has made erections so comical, but the point here is that media has completely normalized arousal nonconcordance, but only for men. There is a caveat here: on screen, the inability to achieve an erection means that there is either something wrong with the guy or he's just not into his partner. (Even guys get sex-shamed sometimes.) The same is true when it comes to women needing lube due to an inability to self-lubricate in that one moment. Nothing is broken or in need of fixing because this is normal. Of course, like everything, there are exceptions to this, which we will discuss in chapter 5.

TL;DR: IS MY LIBIDO NORMAL?

- Your baseline sexual arousal over your lifetime is how to measure it.
- Your libido differs from that of your partner, neighbor, and friend in the same way your energy, mood, and period might.
- What influences your sexual desire is complex and individualized, as is what causes you to become aroused.
- Sexual desire can be spontaneous (like we see in the media) or responsive. Both are normal, and you can experience both in the same relationship.
- Your libido fluctuates with your cycle, can change with life events or medication use, and is dependent on factors such as the health of your relationship.
- Everyone has both a gas pedal and a brake that determine their sexual desire and receptivity to different stimuli. Some of us have more sensitive brakes, and others have less sensitive gas pedals. All of this is normal, and identifying what is true for you can help you gain sexual satisfaction.
- Your adrenal and blood sugar health are the foundation for creating hormone harmony. Addressing these are key to balancing your thyroid, estrogen, progesterone, testosterone, and a healthy libido.
- Testosterone is the hormone most closely associated with libido. Taking steps (like the ones in this chapter) to create healthy testosterone levels can help improve sexual desire, arousal, and orgasms.
- Not self-lubricating when turned on, and self-lubricating when you receive sexual stimuli but aren't turned on, is known as arousal nonconcordance, and it's normal.

CHAPTER 4

ARE MY ORGASMS NORMAL?

PUTTING THE "O" IN OH, UH-OH, AND OMG

If I had to predict which chapter most people would read first, this would be the one. So if you skipped the first three chapters to immediately get your orgasm questions answered—well, congratulations, you're a normal pleasure-seeking human being and you're for sure not alone.

How do I know? Well, I know what my patients ask and what people google. The most googled question in the world about sex in general is "How to make a woman orgasm?" second only to "Where is the G-spot?" which is basically asking the same thing.[1]

Difficulty having an orgasm is the second most common sexual complaint made by women, and if that rings true, you're definitely in good company.[2] (Lack of sexual desire is number one for women across all age groups, so if you did skip those chapters, I highly recommend you go back and read them.)[3] Just about everyone I know has questions about the female orgasm, including how to make it happen, how to know if it's happened, whether it's going to happen, whether it's even possible to make it happen (spoiler alert: yes!), how to have multiple orgasms, if women really "squirt," and whether it's possible to become a squirter if you're not already.

These questions are totally normal. It's really unlikely that you were ever taught anything substantial about female orgasms in sex ed (compared to all we learn about male ejaculation), and our society has historically deprioritized female pleasure. Some of us have even been taught that a man's orgasm is more important than our own, since whether we climax doesn't matter at all in baby-making, or even for the survival of the human race in general, right? Wrong. Biologically, the female body has evolved to orgasm—Mama Nature knew what she was doing with this one. The female orgasm encourages women to have sex and promotes bonding with our partners so that we're more inclined to form a family. Babies aside, having orgasms also has a ton of health benefits, which we'll get into soon.

While female desire and pleasure have come a long way over the past few decades, many still view a woman's sexual pleasure as secondary to a man's. Take, for example, the "scandal" that happened when singer Nicki Minaj told *Cosmopolitan* that she expected to orgasm every time she had sex. "Nicki Minaj demands orgasms" was headline news around the Internet, even appearing in prominent papers like the *New York Post* and *Washington Post*.[4] But let's think about that for a hot second. No one would even blink an eye if a guy declared that he expected to orgasm every time he has sex because that's what society in general already expects, if not guarantees. Case in point: 95 percent of heterosexual men orgasm during sex, compared to only 65 percent of heterosexual women.[5]

Society has also sold us on the myth that the female orgasm is nearly mythical, like seeing a unicorn in the woods or solving a Rubik's Cube in under ten seconds. At the risk of sounding accusatory, this is just a load of patriarchal BS. It comes with an attitude that posits penile-vaginal sex as the norm, which, as you've already learned in chapter 1, it isn't. If you just went into a hard eye roll over the suggestion that patriarchy is to blame for this notion, I'd invite you to slow your roll and allow me to explain that none of us (men included) are really at fault here, because we've all been influenced by the same sociocultural concept of male-centered pleasure. If I had my way, we'd have billboards everywhere exclaiming that the female orgasm isn't as difficult to achieve as we've been told. (CLITORAL STIMULATION, MAKING WOMEN COME SINCE THE DAWN OF TIME.) And to be fair, I think there is a hefty number of men who would like to get in on all this.

In my medical opinion, teaching people about pleasure is one of the most impactful ways that we can increase positive health outcomes, safer sex, and encourage practices that reduce risk. The World Health Organization (WHO) states that pleasure is an important aspect of sexual health to which we all have a right and, as such, the WHO has started the Pleasure Project, which aims to "put the sexy into safer sex."[6] And studies have shown that when pleasure is discussed as part of sexual and reproductive health, knowledge-based attitudes improve, condom use increases, and there is a better understanding of consent.[7] This is all to say that sex ed is most effective when pleasure is a key part of the conversation. If you're wondering how abstinence-only programs stack up—they fail, hard. Unless, of course, you consider the United States ranking first among developed nations with the highest levels of teen pregnancies and STIs a win.[8] If you're mad about these facts, you have every right to be. It's a key reason why we understand so little about our own pleasure, and what fuels the questions I receive.

ASK DR. BRIGHTEN:

What is an orgasm? How do I know if I've had an orgasm? Are orgasms different for men and women?

Ask ten different friends to describe an orgasm, and you'll get ten different answers based on their own experiences. But there tends to be a theme in how all people answer when asked about how they experience orgasms, which includes words and phrases like "release of tension," "pleasure," "satisfaction," and "tingling sensation." I believe the orgasm definition in a paper titled "Women's Orgasm" best captures what most people experience: "peak sensation of intense pleasure, creating an altered state of consciousness" that's usually "accompanied by involuntary, rhythmic contractions of the pelvic striated circumvaginal musculature, often with concomitant uterine and anal contractions."[9] Note the inclusion of the word "usually" instead of "always," since what you feel may be different.

While the physiological changes to genitalia make it easier for researchers to measure and quantify female orgasms, I want to point out that orgasms are primarily neurological events, meaning your brain is the main sexual organ involved. This may explain why many women report immense pleasure without any of that muscle-pumping action just described. No matter how your muscles respond, the net effect of having an orgasm is an acute sensation of sexual pleasure that shifts your mental and emotional well-being. This doesn't mean that all your orgasms have to be the screaming, cataclysmic, "I see fireworks" affairs portrayed in the media.

Knowing when a guy comes is pretty straightforward: he ejaculates. (Side note: some men can have dry orgasms, which happens when they emit little to no semen, but it is rare and usually doesn't occur for extended periods of time.)[10] While some women also produce a thick, creamy ejaculate or even "squirt" when they orgasm, not all do—and among those who do ejaculate or squirt, it's not always noticeable, even to them.

But other than the fluids, are the orgasms between men and women that different? What studies have found is that even the best (s)experts, when blind-reading people's responses, can't tell whether a male or female orgasm is being described.[11] So if our experience is so similar, why is it that the female orgasm seems so elusive? The clitoris, which we're going to talk a whole lot about, is the primary way most vulva owners arrive at an orgasm, and yet so few people are taught about it. While there are orgasm similarities, there's also some special aspects to the female orgasm.

How long do orgasms last?

Stats on this vary, with some published reports claiming the average female orgasm lasts anywhere between thirteen to fifty-one seconds,[12] while others estimate between six and twenty seconds.[13] There's also research suggesting the female orgasm can be as short as three seconds and as long as two minutes.[14] These minute-long orgasms may be a single orgasm, or it is possible they are multiples. Orgasms have a whole lot of variables including stimulation, partner, situation, and your cycle. When it comes to what's normal, a better question is, *What's enjoyable?* Because if it was good for you, then enough said.

Are multiple orgasms a thing?

I don't think I'll ever stop being in awe of just how amazing the female orgasm is. Not only is it just for fun, but you can also experience multiples, which is much more challenging for our male counterparts. How? Women have a shorter refractory period (the time after an orgasm when it is physiologically impossible to have another) than men do, meaning our bodies recover more quickly after climaxing, so we can have multiple Os. Men are usually one-and-done due to their longer refractory period. However, the refractory period limits ejaculation, not orgasms. Some men are able to achieve another orgasm independent of ejaculation and may be able to have multiple orgasms.[15] Women can have up to five orgasms at one time, although some lucky ladies claim to have as many as twenty to even sixty Os in one go. When it comes to the norm, it's a bell-shaped curve, which means some women are having none or one and others are having much more, and others don't even know it is happening.[16] What matters most is, *Are you satisfied?*

Am I normal if I don't moan, groan, or make any noise when I come? Am I the only one faking it?

When it comes to faking orgasms, Sally from the movie *When Harry Met Sally* gave any rom-com viewer pause when she took to moaning and screaming "Yes, yes, yes!" inside a crowded New York City deli before returning calmly to her turkey sandwich. This whole iconic scene was to prove a point: her dining companion, Harry, didn't actually know when his partners orgasmed, despite his confidently saying otherwise, because what he thought was satisfaction was actually a performance. The mismatch between what actually happens and what people think should happen is why I have so many people ask me if it is normal to not make a sound. Totally normal.

Faking it is common, and you're far from the only one if you're doing it, too. Up to 80 percent of women admit to faking their orgasms, according to research conducted mostly on heterosexual females.[17] Researchers have also looked at why women fake it, with the number one reason being "altruistic deceit": women want to make men feel good about their skills in the sack and to boost their ego.[18] Some women also fake it to make sex stop sooner or because doing so actually turns *them* on, according to research.[19] Increasing your own arousal is a great reason to "fake it," in case you're curious. Women also fake orgasms so they seem normal compared to others (who are likely also faking their orgasms). I'm confident you see the problem here. If you're faking it, take a moment to consider how this contributes to the orgasm gap (see the next section) and is depriving you of the pleasure you deserve. No shame in how you roll, but do make sure you're getting yours while you think about your partner's ego.

The Orgasm Gap Is Real

The term describes the abyss in frequency of orgasms between heterosexual men and women, with 95 percent of straight men climaxing during partnered sex compared to only 65 percent of straight women, according to research.[20] That's a 30 percent differential that our society has totally accepted and normalized by perpetuating myths like it's difficult to make women come. Research shows that 86 percent of lesbians climax during partnered sex, meaning the orgasm gap exists only between women and men.

So what's really happening here? One aspect is that women are committed to their partner's pleasure and use it as a measure of their own sexual satisfaction, regardless of the gender of their partner. The thought goes, if it's good for them then it's good for me, even when it really isn't that enjoyable for me. Our poor sex ed also frequently leaves out the clitoris, so if you don't own one, you stand little chance of understanding how to use it to please someone who does (without some guidance).[21] Before you leave this chapter, you will become clit-literate (cliterate)—that is, incredibly knowledgeable about the major pleasure structure that has mystified so many. (Shout-out to Ian Kerner for giving us the terms "cliterate" and "clit-eracy.")[22] For a very long time, society has perpetuated the idea that female pleasure should take a back seat to male pleasure. After all, it isn't necessary for making babies, and a male orgasm is. Well, as it turns out, women are beings deserving of pleasure, and our sole purpose isn't just to crank babies out of our reproductive machinery. Shocker, I know.

If you're inclined to jump on the "it's her, not me" bandwagon that implies women having heterosexual sex are broken and at fault for not climaxing, don't. Penile penetration isn't the golden ticket to orgasm as most men are taught. When women masturbate, they orgasm at a much higher frequency (95 percent report they can orgasm in a solo session[23]) than when they have hetero vaginal sex. Plus in these solo seshes, they can do so in as little as four minutes.[24] So let go that excuse, and embrace the clit.

The Clit Quiz

Answer true or false for the following statements.

_____ **The clitoris is a small pea-size structure.**

_____ **It is nearly impossible to find the clitoris.**

_____ **The clitoris serves no purpose.**

_____ **The clitoris is an unsightly or ugly structure.**

_____ **Vaginal orgasms are more pleasurable than clitoral ones.**

_____ **More pressure or stimulation of the clitoris is better.**

_____ **Everyone knows how to work it.**

_____ **The clitoris is just skin with no blood flow.**

_____ **Women don't get "blue balls."**

_____ **The clitoris is completely unlike any male genitalia.**

Answers to the clit quiz: If you answered false to every single one, congratulations! You are more cliterate than most. Not one of these is true, yet these myths are still alive and circulating everywhere. If you answered true to any of these, keep reading!

Let's Get Cliterate!

If we're going to close that orgasm gap, we all need to get cliterate. In chapter 2 I described the anatomical features of the clitoris, which is worth a revisit because I won't be explaining in as much detail here. The external part of the clitoris, that is, what you can see, lives above the urethra. Stimulating it is *the* chosen path to orgasm for most women. For some, the external part is the size of a pea, for others it is larger or smaller, but for everyone, there's a whole lot more clitoris under the hood (no, literally, there's a clitoral hood). If you don't know your way around your own, you can begin your journey by (A) pulling out a mirror, (B) using a finger or a vibrator to stimulate it; or (C) doing both. (Psst: choose C.) I highly encourage all my patients to be a tourist in their own city and go exploring if they haven't. Take a look at the glans of your clitoris and explore where it resides amid the labia minora, and how much it protrudes from the hood. The amount of the glans that peeks out can change with your cycle and arousal (more on that soon). You can take your finger and feel not only the part that pokes out, but also the cord-like extension of it, by sliding your finger to one side of your labia and wiggling. (If you're not the vulva owner, ask them to show you.) Ninety-one percent of people surveyed reported that they have fantasized about their partner talking dirty to them, so if you're asking for directions, don't be afraid to make it spicy.[25]

A Clitoral Map to Guide You

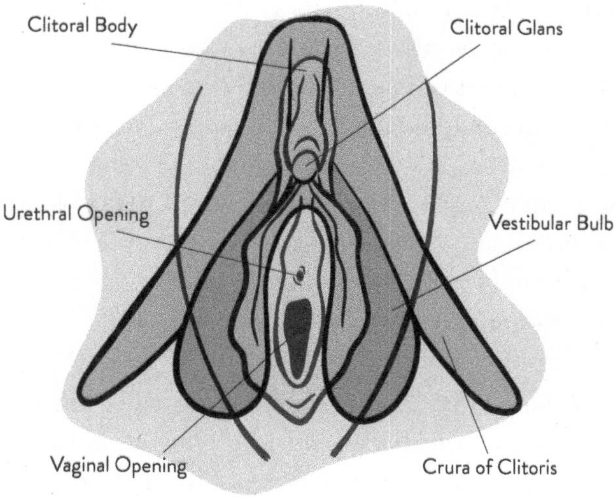

THOSE BLUE BALLS, THO (OR WOULD THAT BE PINK BALLS?)

During arousal, the clitoris becomes engorged with blood just like a penis. And just as a penis that is aroused without release can result in the sensation of blue balls, the same can happen to the clitoris. If you've ever felt an aching or throbbing sensation after being aroused without relief, that's the female equivalent of blue balls (although your tissue tends to turn red or a deeper version of your normal, not blue).

But why the similarity? Well, as we discussed in more detail in chapter 2, early in utero, there is a hormonal surge that makes a baby with XY chromosomes go penis, scrotum, testicles, but the XX doesn't respond to these hormones and, as such, there develops a clitoris, labia, and ovaries. BTW, there are other combinations of chromosomes, but for our purposes here, we're keeping it simple.

So if the clitoris and the penis are the same in origin, why do doctors, researchers, and people altogether think the vaginal orgasm is superior to the clitoral? If you guessed Freud, literally one of the worst things to happen to female sexuality, then you're right. He proclaimed that the clitoral orgasm was infantile, and people have been nodding their heads in agreement ever since. But I submit to you that if we can accept that stimulating the penis is a predominant path to pleasure and orgasm, then the same is true for the clitoris. Because biology.

When it comes to what happens physically when we become aroused, there are shared experiences in how the genitals, and body overall, respond. The four stages of physiological arousal, as defined by William Masters and Virginia Johnson—excitement, plateau, orgasm, and resolution—are a helpful framework for understanding what happens in our body, and make a strong case for how necessary physical stimulation (what people often refer to as foreplay) is for women.[26] Please understand that it is by no means a representation of everyone's experience, so if yours is different, that's normal, too. And remember from chapter 3 that what gets women aroused and ready to go can be much more complicated than what this linear model suggests.

In the excitement stage, you experience a rush of blood to your genitals causing vaginal lubrication—and also clitoral swelling, just as the penis would. It's the rush of blood (thanks to nitric oxide) that causes your vulva to darken in color, so yeah, normal. An increase in dopamine, the "keep going because that feels good" hormone that we'll talk about shortly, keeps you in pursuit of pleasure. The nipples may become erect at this time, and you may experience muscle tension, which can extend to the hands and feet as your body moves into the plateau stage. The vagina and uterus make accommodations in preparation for penetration (you know, just in case). The Bartholin's glands begin to produce additional lubrication, the vagina expands, the uterus moves up, and the clitoral hood retracts to expose more of the glans during the plateau stage. Your heart rate, breath, and blood pressure eventually stabilize (it would be really bad if they kept climbing). With enough of the right stimulation, all the tension that has been building is released, which signifies the orgasm phase. And with that O comes a flood of oxytocin, serotonin, and DHEA, hormones that result in a positive mood and some of the health benefits of orgasms (we'll discuss details soon). Resolution is a return back to baseline, but for women, it is much easier to start the cycle all over again, which lends itself to multiple orgasms.

THE BEST TIME OF THE MONTH TO "O": AKA THE CLITORIS CHANGES WITH YOUR CYCLE

The clitoris fluctuates with your menstrual cycle. In chapter 9 I'm going to get you dialed in on all the changes that happen when your hormones are following their natural rhythm. Around ovulation, the size of your clitoris increases, which correlates to your rise in estrogen. This is part of the reason we are more interested in sex and have better orgasms during that phase of our cycle. We certainly need more research in this arena, but what studies have found correlates with what a lot of women report—increased clitoral sensitivity around ovulation, and less so (comparatively) just before and during their period.[27]

ASK DR. BRIGHTEN:

How much foreplay is normal?

If you watch enough rom-coms, you might think that you should always be able to orgasm within seconds of getting busy with your partner. In these movies, there's rarely attention given to foreplay before an actress is moaning and groaning in pleasure, usually during what is depicted as vaginal sex. But in the real world, outside of Hollywood fantasy, women need an average of fourteen minutes of foreplay before they can climax (that's the excitement and plateau stages combined). Compare this with the five minutes that guys need, on average, to get there during vaginal sex, and you can see another reason why the orgasm gap is so wide.[28]

If you don't have regular Os with your partner, it might be that there's not enough foreplay before you have sex, particularly the kind of foreplay that revolves around your clitoris (rather than the kind that solely features his penis). I tell my patients to expect about twenty minutes of sexual activity, on average, before they're able to climax, and some women may need longer, which is totally normal. Aim to stay present with the pleasure, rather than set off on an internal monologue that things are taking too long, as the latter will make things take too long. And please, ignore all the people on the Internet who will shame you for taking too long or your partner for not going long enough. Every time I talk on social about the need for foreplay, the "pick me" behavior never fails to make an appearance in the comments. The amount of time needed for foreplay will depend on your stress levels, your partner, your type of desire, and so much more. Own your normal and respect what's normal for others.

I also tell my patients to have a conversation with their partners about foreplay. This doesn't have to be an intimidating talk: most partners are more than happy to put in a little prep time in the name of mutual pleasure. And while we're on the topic of foreplay, let's be clear that the acts involved in foreplay are sex themselves. For some people, the word "foreplay" applies unnecessary pressure because it implies that there must be more than what you're doing in order to be satisfied. So if you want to have foreplay with the goal of vaginal sex, go for it. If you want to engage in sexual activity that is satisfying to you and your partner without any expectation of where it'll lead, then that's great, too. In fact, the high-pressure situation that sex-pectations create can be a major turnoff and keep anyone from enjoying themselves. In this situation, it can be helpful for both you and your partner to decide that anything but vaginal sex is on the table, and see where that experience takes you.

All the Different Paths to Have an O, Explained

Every magazine and website looking to sensationalize orgasms, or put a new spin on them, runs headlines telling you all about the latest, greatest way to get one. For many women, the clitoris is the only path to orgasm, but for others it's not. In fact, there are people who can think their way to ecstasy. People with a spinal injury (paraplegics and quadriplegics) can develop increased erotic sensitivity above their injury, and other areas like the nipples, inner thighs, and neck.[29] Heck, some people just need their eyebrows stroked or someone to gently blow on their body hair to get there.[30] All orgasms are healthy and normal, and the best way to arrive there is the way that brings you the most pleasure.

There are dozens of different ways for your brain to register orgasm. I'm only scratching the surface with the nine I've got for you here. As you read through them, know that not one of them is better than the other, there's nothing wrong with you if you can get there only one way, and there is also nothing wrong with you if you can get there any ol' way you choose. If you don't see your favorite or "go-to" O on the list, know that it is due to the fact that I can't fit everything in a single book, and nothing to do with whether your food-gasm, toe-gasm, or fill-in-the-blank-gasm is normal. It is.

Finally, not every way to orgasm on this list might be right or even possible for you. Keep in mind your orgasms can hit differently depending on where you are in your cycle, too, with more intense or explosive climaxes usually happening right around ovulation, so keep it in mind while you give these a try.[31]

Clitoral orgasms are the most common and the easiest for women to achieve. But obviously we're going have to talk about how this is done because hello, orgasm gap! I'm going to give some guidance, but what you like trumps anything I say here. You're the expert on your body and the CEO of its orgasms, in my opinion. So if you and I ever meet in real life and I ask how business is, I sure hope you answer, "Business is good." (This info is complementary to what you will find in chapter 6, which also covers toys and masturbation.)

Work your way to it. Rather than diving straight to stimulating the clitoris, consider stimulating other areas of the vulva to allow the body to become aroused.

Begin gently. When moving to touch the clitoris, start soft and slow. You can always add more pressure or speed, but too much early on can have the opposite of the intended effect.

Try different techniques. Rub, strum, tap, or jiggle the area. You can go up and down, side to side, move in circles, and change directions.

Make it a party. You can use one, two, or three fingers, or the palm of your hand. If you're with a partner, you can have them follow your hand with theirs, or you can invite their fingers to do the walking while you direct.

Add some inside play. The internal portion of the clit is just inside the vagina. If it feels right, you can use an object to penetrate you while simultaneously stimulating the glans of the clitoris.

Vaginal orgasms happen during intercourse. They are not the "go-to" when women masturbate, but as we'll talk about in chapter 5, there are people who enjoy taking this route to orgasm. Some studies have found that women can climax more easily during penetrative sex if there's a shorter distance between their vagina and clitoris,[32] which makes the case for clitoral stimulation being a simultaneous event.[33]

Another million-dollar question is whether there's a difference between vaginal and G-spot orgasms, or if the G-spot even exists in the first place. The G-spot is defined as a specific erogenous point inside the vagina. Recent studies, though, haven't been able to identify or confirm its existence,[34] and many argue that now that we understand just how comprehensive the clitoris is, any G-spot pleasure is really due to the internal clit. The G-spot may be associated with Skene's glands, as well, but since it varies from person to person, it's been difficult to validate how important this area is for all of those with a vagina. No matter which side of the G-spot or vaginal O debate you support, or if it even matters to you, the aim should be finding the stimulation that brings you the most pleasure. For tips on how to climax during vaginal intercourse, see page 97.

Cervical orgasms are another highly debated (or ignored) topic, with some doctors claiming the cervix has no nerve endings so it couldn't possibly be an erogenous zone. I laugh when I hear this–once again, it's a classic patriarchal attitude. While top Google search results might lead you to believe that the cervix has few to no nerve endings, actual research paints a different picture, with studies showing that three nerves–the pelvic, hypogastric, and vagus–all connect the cervix to the brain, and the genital sensory cortex of the brain lights up on MRI when they are stimulated.[35] If you've ever had a penis hit your cervix or an IUD placed, you likely don't need studies to tell you that your cervix can be sensitive–how much so depending on your individual anatomy and personal pain threshold. I learned to appreciate just how sensitive the area can be when I had my IUD placed: The nurse practitioner grasped my cervix to prevent the device from moving. This caused some of the worst pain I've ever experienced. I started to sweat, scream, and then curse like a sailor. Funny enough, she warned me I'd feel just a pinch, but then insisted I couldn't feel any pain because my cervix didn't have nerves. Really.

Since the cervix has nerve endings, it can be an erogenous zone for some women. Women who experience cervical orgasms report they feel pleasure when a penis or toy stimulates the area by sliding above or below rather than hitting their cervix, which can cause pain, bruising, and bleeding if too aggressive. If you want to stimulate your cervix, go slow and start gently. You're totally normal if you find pleasure in this.

Anal orgasms occur when the anus is stimulated by touching, toys, or penetration. The anus is an erogenous zone, packed with sensitive nerves, including the pudendal nerve, which connects the area to the clitoris. If you want to try anal play, one cautionary tip: always use lube, never numb the area, and sober is safer. Unlike the vagina, the anus is not self-lubricating, and penetration without lube can cause rips or tears. Numbing or having sex under the influence will prevent your body from giving you the feedback you need to know how to keep it safe and pleasurable. Also, remember to change condoms or dental dams whenever switching from the anus to the vagina or mouth or vice versa. For more on anal play, see page 136.

Nipple orgasms result from stimulating the nipples. Like the anus, the nipples sit on top a bunch of nerves that, when stimulated, activate what's known as the genital sensory cortex, a region in your brain that maps out sexual stimulation. (BTW this area of the brain can light up whether your body is physically being stimulated or you're just imagining it.)[36] Both men and women can have nipple orgasms, so next time you're getting intimate you can try playing with your partner's or your own nipples to see what feels good, stroking, massaging, pinching, twisting, or licking them. Some people even find that the use of nipple clamps helps boost their orgasm experience (more on toys in chapter 6). Yes, it is normal if find yourself more easily aroused while breastfeeding. You can thank the change in hormones and stimulation of this area for this.

Sleep orgasms are the female equivalent of wet dreams, although women don't wake up with the evidence on our sheets like most guys do. According to a 1986 study–yes, it's super old, but there hasn't been a ton of research on female sleep orgasms since then, unsurprisingly–37 percent of women report climaxing while asleep.[37] When I surveyed my audience on Instagram, 75 percent of the over 47,000 people who participated shared it had happened to them at least once. Even I was surprised by this! Exactly how this happens is still a big question mark, but we do know that sleep orgasms typically occur during REM, when there's more blood flow to the vulva. And sleep Os are different than sexsomnia, when a person engages in sexual acts between sleep phases without any recollection of events. If you want to attempt a sleep O, you can try to fall asleep on your stomach while focusing on erotic fantasies after you turn out the light. You'll also want to get your REM sleep on point by prioritizing the things that foster it, like avoiding alcohol and caffeine later in the day, along with other tips I'll teach you in the 28-day program. If you wake up feeling physically or mentally euphoric–think Cinderella opening up all the windows to sing to the birds–you likely hit an O in your sleep. If you've found the only time you experience this is when you're pregnant, that's normal. There's so much blood flow, hormones, and changes happening down there that it is the perfect combo to get those nighttime Os going.

Coregasms, as *Men's Health* magazine calls them (I warned you about these magazines) are what science recognizes as exercise-induced orgasms–the phenomenon in which engaging the abdominal or pelvic-floor muscles brings about an orgasm.[38] But long before magazines were talking about it, Kinsey noted about 5 percent of women reported exercise-induced orgasms in *Sexual Behavior in the Human Female*. According to published reports, hanging leg raises are the golden ticket for coregasms, although boat pose, running, biking, lifting weights, and other ab exercises can also trigger an unexpected O at the gym. Let's emphasize "unexpected" here, because most women who experience coregasms say they're not thinking about anything sexual when these climaxes occur.[39] When you engage your core properly you are lifting your pelvic floor, and I think by now you are aware that our friend the clitoris is going to get moving when those muscles do.

Peegasm may sound like a trendy new plant-based protein, but it's actually the hilarious expression for when you climax because you held your urine too long. I've had patients tell me that they've woken up in the middle of the night because they've had to pee, then, on their way to the bathroom—*badaboom*, they orgasm. That's great if it happens naturally for you, but no one should intentionally try to hold their urine in hope of hitting an O, since it can cause serious bladder damage and urinary tract infections.

Thinking off is when you have an orgasm just by thinking about sex. Thought-induced orgasms appear to activate the same area of the brain that lights up when women climax from sexual activity, according to research.[40] The even cooler part is that some women can "think off" with calm thoughts, which underscores the role stress (or lack thereof) plays in our ability to orgasm.

DO PEOPLE REALLY HAVE ORGASMS WHEN GIVING BIRTH?

Totally a thing but not totally everyone's thing. The combination of hormones, increase in circulation to your pelvis, and the pressure that small human is creating on your vagina and vulva can be the ticket to an orgasm for some. Unsurprisingly, the OGs of sexual research, Masters and Johnson, recorded orgasmic births as a phenomenon back in the sixties.[41] There's a lot of skepticism about orgasmic births, mostly because it contradicts the birth-is-always-painful story that dominates our society. But orgasms can act as an analgesic, which can ease both pain and anxiety during labor. Midwives have advocated for clitoral and nipple stimulation during birth to help women get natural pain relief and, dare I say, enjoy the fruits of their labor.[42]

Is it normal if I've never had an orgasm or can't orgasm?

Up to 15 percent of all women report they have never orgasmed (what's medically called anorgasmia), according to the National Institutes of Health's Library of Medicine, and it may be due to what is referred to as female orgasmic disorder (FOD).[43] There's two types of FOD: primary, where you have never been able to have an orgasm, despite all phases of arousal being normal; and secondary, where you've had an orgasm but are now struggling to get there again. Your orgasms may have gone on vacation, or are less frequent or intense. There's a strong link to other sexual disorders (see chapter 5 for what causes pain with sex) and anxiety. Other factors that can play a role include nerve damage from injury or surgery (another good reason to consider if that labiaplasty is medically necessary[44]), diabetes, prescription medication, hormone imbalances, and chronic health conditions.

What's the main treatment for FOD? Masturbation. No, seriously. Masturbation has been shown to be an effective first-line therapy for FOD, and there's a whole chapter (starting on page 142) to help you get started.[45] If all other issues have been ruled out and you've addressed underlying causes, this is *the* thing to help you improve or have orgasms.

Beyond the physical, there are two big areas that aren't frequently mentioned regarding women who struggle to reach climax—how comfortable you are with your body, and how cliterate you and your partner are. Everything we discussed in chapter 3 about what pumps the brakes on desire can also take you on a detour when you set off on your journey to orgasm. We have to work on how we see our body and stop negatively spectatoring (focusing on just ourselves) during sex. It's hard, I know—we live in a society predicated on making people feel ashamed and insecure about their bodies, especially when it comes to sex. But it's necessary if you want to have pleasurable sex, and it's OK to get help. To raise your cliteracy, see page 82.

If you've never had an orgasm or stopped having them, this chapter can help you immensely, as can following my 28-day program if you suspect a hormone imbalance. If you suffer from nerve damage, have diabetes, or have been diagnosed with another physical condition, tell your doctor that you're unable to climax. This is important medical information, as an inability to orgasm is a critical symptom that can point to underlying issues. If you have a history of sexual assault, sexual abuse, depression, or negative feelings around sex, try seeing a sex therapist or counselor who can help you work through your trauma or perceptions. And remember: there's a lot that can make sex great, and it doesn't all hinge on having an orgasm.

Can I lose the ability to orgasm if I don't do it enough?

There are plenty of "use it or lose it" functions in the body, and orgasms are one of them. Masturbating can be the CPR your clitoris needs to stay alive. Clitoral atrophy, when the clitoris shrinks and sometimes retreats under the clitoral hood, can develop from lack of stimulation. Clitoral atrophy can also occur with low estrogen and testosterone (see the quiz on page 192), which can be due to a hysterectomy, menopause, or certain medications like the pill. Low testosterone can also be driven by inflammation, stress, and other factors discussed in chapter 8. We'll be employing some key hormone-balancing therapies that can help with these hormone issues during the program discussed in chapter 13. But if the issue is that you're not making enough hormones due to your age or other factors, hormone replacement therapy may be warranted.

ADHD AND BORED WITH SEX

If you've ever found yourself in the middle of a session with your mind focused on just about anything else (*focuses attention on the humming of the refrigerator*), or *This is boring* popped into your mind, that's normal. But that won't stop yourself or others from judging you hard. In one study, 39 percent of male and 43 percent of female ADHD patients were found to have symptoms of a sexual dysfunction.[46] ADHD can be confusing since it can be behind why you struggle to get in the mood or orgasm, but it can also be the drive behind a high sex desire. Does ADHD equal sexual doom and an orgasmless life? Far from it. Instead, this is where the kink bucket is actually a strategy effective for a neurodivergent mind to stay engaged and have a pleasurable experience. Blindfolds, earplugs, dimming or turning off lights, and other ways to decrease sensory input can help amplify your other senses. On the flip side, new positions, new toys, or bringing in things that stimulate the senses, like feathers, can help change things up. Sex that follows the same pattern can become predictable, and predictable can become boring. This doesn't mean you're not into your partner, that you don't still enjoy sex, or that you're losing the feels for that special person. And what's the best remedy for better sex? Communication. If you have ADHD, talk to your partner, and let them know that you have to do things a little differently in life, and that sex is no exception.

Is it normal to cry after I have an orgasm?

It's absolutely normal to cry after climaxing. You might also giggle, yawn, feel chattier, or experience some other kind of emotional release after an O. These reactions are normal and common because sex is emotional and produces powerful neurochemicals that can create many different emotions and mental states. Orgasms can also be cathartic.

What's not normal is to feel sad, depressed, agitated, or angry on a regular basis after consensual sex. Known as postcoital dysphoria (PCD), the condition affects more than 40 percent of all men and women at least once in their lifetime.[47] A one-off doesn't necessitate a call to your provider. But if you consistently experience PCD, meaning it's a frequent occurrence that interrupts your ability to enjoy sex or dissuades you from being intimate in the first place, seek out a trained mental health professional, preferably a sex therapist, who can help you figure out what's triggering your postcoital blues.

Is it normal to have pain when I orgasm? What about pain in my bum?

Simply put, no. Dysorgasmia, the medical term for pain with or following an orgasm, can occur if your pelvic-floor muscles are too tight or you have a medical condition like endometriosis, adenomyosis, fibroids, ovarian cysts, pelvic inflammatory disease (PID), urinary tract infections, inflammatory bowel disease, or pelvic scar tissue. You can also experience dysorgasmia if you've sustained sexual or emotional trauma. Pain in your pelvis, bum, or any other area can be related to the intensity of the muscle contraction. Ever run and get a cramp? It's kind of like that and isn't a cause for concern. But to know for sure, I'd encourage you to find a provider who can help you figure out why your Os aren't bringing the bliss they should be.

WHY ORGASMS ARE SOOOOO-OH-OH-OH GOOD FOR YOU

- Reduces your overall stress and levels of stress-boosting hormones
- Improves your overall immunity[48]
- Increases your blood flow and circulation, especially to your reproductive parts
- Improves your brain activity and may even boost your cognitive function[49]
- Ramps up your sleep quality[50]
- Increases your pain threshold[51]
- May help you live longer[52]
- May help your skin look younger and clearer[53]
- May help you look up to ten years younger[54]
- May help regulate your menstrual cycle[55]
- May alleviate any migraines and headaches[56]
- May reduce severity of menstrual cramps
- Increases bonding with your partner
- Reduces the incidence of infidelity in relationships[57]
- Provides a healthy source of physical, mental, and emotional pleasure
- May boost your mood and improve symptoms of PMS or PMDD (premenstrual dysphoric disorder)
- Releases oxytocin, an anti-aging hormone

HORMONES, BROUGHT TO YOU BY THE INCREDIBLE ORGASM

There's a whole lot of hormone changes that happen with sex and orgasms. The following are some of the most notable shifts we see when we're enjoying ourselves sexually.

Oxytocin

- Reduces stress, promotes a sense of calm, strengthens social bonds
- Counters negative effects of cortisol
- Promotes restful sleep
- Improves brain performance[58]

Dopamine

- Reinforces the pursuit for pleasure (*Good job, do it again*)
- Considered an accelerator in arriving at orgasm

Serotonin

- Improves mood
- Promotes restful sleep

DHEA

- Promotes healthy mood, energy levels, and skin
- Counters aging effects of stress hormones
- Used to make estrogen and testosterone

Prolactin

- May be a measure of how much you enjoyed yourself
- Prolactin rises with masturbation, but the rise following partnered sex is greater by about a magnitude of 400 percent[59]

Testosterone

- Temporarily rises following orgasm[60]
- Improves mood, muscle mass, and sexual desire

Can hormones make you addicted to sex?

Dopamine is associated with gambling and drug use, which is why some people mistakenly classify sexual desire that is above *their* normal as "sex addiction." There's no evidence that sex addiction exists, and there is no medical diagnosis for this alleged condition. Dopamine is also set off by learning something new, or music, but since we don't stigmatize music like we do sex, we don't hear people labeling others as a "music addict" or warning them of the dangers of making too many Spotify playlists.

HOW TO HAVE AN ORGASM DURING VAGINAL INTERCOURSE

Listen, vaginal sex alone may not be the most reliable way to climax—with only 18 percent of ladies able to get there—but that doesn't mean you can't orgasm with intercourse.[61] By simultaneously stimulating the clitoris, you're more likely to orgasm and may even achieve that magical moment where you simultaneously orgasm with your partner like we see in the movies. It's totally normal for one partner to finish first, but I get that you want to try to experience it at the same time. Here are some tips to help you orgasm during vaginal sex:

1. Focus on the dos, not the don'ts. Ask for what you want and focus on positive directions like "Yes, more of that" or "I like it when you do this." This keeps the attention focused on pleasure and can help prevent spectatoring, which is no good for anyone. It's always OK to say ouch if there is pain.
2. If you're in missionary position, instead of an in-and-out jackhammer motion, ask your partner to slow down and position themselves so their body can stimulate your clitoris. Placing a pillow under your hips or using a wedge can help angle your pelvis to make this easier. (See sex furniture in chapter 6.)
3. If you're in cowgirl or doggy style, you can use a toy or hand to stimulate the clitoris. There's lots of positions that can help you achieve this, so try out what works best for you.
4. Use lube. Lubricant is the gateway to great sex. The vulva (where the clitoris lives) and vagina are more receptive to friction-inducing movements when there is lubrication.

5. Increase your foreplay time while also trying to have an orgasm before they even enter your vagina. Some women find "pregame" orgasms lead to more easily achieved orgasms during vaginal sex.

Is squirting during an orgasm normal? Is it just pee?

First, if you've ever tried to google this, then you know that the information is conflicting. I can't imagine why more researchers don't want to explore this. Squirting when you climax may very well be normal for you. When things are super intense, then those muscles may contract your bladder and Skene's glands, too, producing a stream of fluid. Approximately 10 to 54 percent of all women produce measurable amounts of fluid during sexual activity, whether they're squirting or generating female ejaculate.[62] You can also squirt or ejaculate without orgasming, although both are more common during climax.[63]

Some older studies say squirting is simply diluted urine involuntarily released during sex,[64] which is how the "it's just pee" myth was born. But many sexual-health experts argue that squirt is its own unique substance, albeit with a bit of the same stuff that goes into urine mixed in, and female squirters also anecdotally report that the fluid tastes nothing like pee.[65] (And in case the question just entered your mind, tasting your own secretions is normal.) The Skene's glands, the biological equivalent of the prostate in men, secrete a fructose-rich fluid that may be part of the squirt, which would explain the taste.[66]

If you're worried if it's off-putting to your partner, you can ask, but you should also know 90 percent of partners who are intimate with women say that female ejaculation (squirting included) enriches the quality of their sex life.[67] If you're a squirter, you're normal, and you just may find embracing it makes sex even better. If you're not a squirter, that's normal, too. Some women forcibly pee during orgasm to try to mimic squirting, which is a bad idea if you're trying to avoid developing urinary incontinence.

Do I need to orgasm to get pregnant?

According to the upsuck theory, orgasms create a rhythmic contraction of the uterus and help suck the sperm up to meet the egg. One study found that if a woman orgasmed within a minute prior to her partner ejaculating inside her, a greater amount of sperm was retained compared to those who did not orgasm within that minute.[68] The only problem is that there's no way to know how much sperm was actually deposited to begin with. Can orgasms make your cervix the black hole of your reproductive universe, pulling any object that gets near deep inside, never to be seen again? That's not actually how black holes work, and it isn't likely how your uterus works, either. In addition, as I explained, there's a whole lot of heterosexual women not having orgasms. If getting pregnant was dependent on orgasms, I'm pretty sure we'd see a lower pregnancy rate based on how often women report orgasming with a male partner.

There are other theories related to reproduction as to why women orgasm. The big O may have once served as a trigger for ovulation way back in the day, or the fact you can have one more easily due to surging estrogen and testosterone around ovulation makes you more inclined to seek sex. One thing is for certain today: you can have an orgasm when you want, regardless of whether you want a baby or not. While you don't *need* an orgasm to conceive, it couldn't hurt.

Creating the Orgasms That You Want

Nearly everyone can have an orgasm—or have them more frequently, more intensely, or more enthusiastically. Here are thirteen tips to hit the big O as often and as enjoyably as you can. There's no rule saying you must try them all. Use what works for you and leave the rest.

1. **Masturbate.** Learning what you like and how to make yourself cum on your own, without the pressure, shame, expectation, or embarrassment of someone else around, is one of the best ways to eventually orgasm with somebody else. Masturbating on a regular basis allows you to focus on your own pleasure without worrying what someone else is doing, thinking, or feeling. You can also experiment freely with different toys, vibrators, or ways to stimulate your clitoris, giving yourself the opportunity to figure out what you like before asking to introduce new objects or techniques into partnered sex. If you feel comfortable, you can also try masturbating with your partner. In

general, masturbation is so critical to overall sexual health and happiness that I've dedicated an entire chapter to the topic. For more tricks and tips for solo sex, turn to page 142.

2. **Talk it out.** Great sex starts with great communication. Take the time to have an open and honest conversation with your partner about your desires, needs, or concerns when it comes to climaxing. Any person you're having sex with should care enough about you to listen, be receptive, and learn what brings you pleasure. While talking about sex can be embarrassing for some women (and men) because society sees the subject as taboo, let me remind you that you're already sharing fluids, orifices, and intimate activities with this person, so sharing your wants, wishes, and needs should feel safe, too.

3. **Change your position.** According to the *Kama Sutra*, the ancient Indian script on sexuality and eroticism, there are more than one hundred different sex positions.[69] (The book was written with only heterosexuality in mind, but many of the descriptions also apply to same-sex couples.)[70] If you're stuck in missionary or cowgirl (that's you on top), mix it up by trying doggy style, spooning, the wheelbarrow, the butterfly, happy scissors. . . . The list is as endless as the names are amusing.

4. **Explore outside the vagina.** Only 18 percent of women orgasm through vaginal intercourse alone.[71] Vaginal sex is only one type of sex and only one way to stimulate your body. Have your partner explore your external clit, whether through manual stimulation or with their mouth, along with your nipples, anus, and/or any other body part you find erogenous.

5. **Give the clitoris what it wants.** There's more than one way to stim the clit, and what you like can change depending on where you are in your cycle and the context of the situations. If rapid strokes aren't doing it for you, try slowing down, pulsing instead of stroking, or using pressure instead of movement. If you enjoy pressure, try apply-

ing it with your or your partner's full hand. Or if manual stimulation isn't your thing, ask your partner to try using different techniques with their tongue or mouth.

6. **Try a toy or two.** There's nothing wrong with calling in a little help to get your train to O-town out of the station, even if someone else is along for the ride. Fifty-two percent of couples say they use toys during partnered sex, according to research,[72] with studies showing that they help increase desire and orgasm ability for both men and women.[73] And that's just what hetero couples say. You can find a variety of toys, which is discussed in chapter 6.

7. **Get out of your head.** This is a big one. If you're thinking about your to-do list, worrying about your weight or cellulite, constantly wondering what your partner is thinking, or just mulling over what you're going to eat for dinner afterward, you're absolutely normal—but you're not going to have an easy time having an orgasm. Studies show that women who regularly climax during partnered sex are mentally present in the moment.[74] I strongly believe that the ability to orgasm is an act of mindfulness: to climax, we must be present and connected with our bodies, aware of the intimacy, eroticism, and physical and emotional sensations happening in and around us. Apparently, Dr. John Harvey Kellogg (of Kellogg's cereal!) thought so, too, since he declared spicy food would make you too attuned to your senses and would encourage masturbation.[75] (Which is why Kellogg's cereal is bland AF.) While it may seem counterintuitive, meditation and mindfulness practices are among the most effective tools for boosting orgasm ability since they increase the capacity to be present in the moment, whether you're completing a difficult task at work, spending time with family or friends, or trying to hit the big O. It doesn't take much. Eat a spicy or well-seasoned meal and be absolutely present with it—taste, smell, feel, enjoy. Try a walking or seated meditation. And if you do notice your mind wanders with sex, make it spicy (in that other way) and change up positions, add or take away sensory input, or spontaneously kiss your partner. Basically, use the tools that pull *you* back into the moment.

8. **Activate your brain.** Staying mindful during sex doesn't mean you have to think about nothing. Many people need some neurological stimulation to orgasm, usually in the form of erotic thoughts. Whatever images, ideas, or fantasies turn you on, sex is the ideal time to open up the floodgates and let all your kink come in. You can share these, keep them to yourself, or do a combo. And no, thinking about or picturing having sex with someone other than your partner is *not* cheating, but if you find this is the only way you get there, it's a good idea to ask yourself if this is about sex or intimacy, because the former implies it doesn't matter who you're with. A survey of 1,300 people by Lovehoney, the largest online sex toy brand in the UK, found that 46 percent of women admitted to fantasizing about someone other than their partner, while 42 percent of men did.[76] I say "admitted" intentionally, as these surveys are dependent on honesty, so these numbers may likely be higher.

9. **Stream the steam.** I know it's not for everyone, but watching porn may actually help your ability to orgasm. In fact, streaming some steam with your partner may help you both climax more easily while increasing the quality of your relationship, with studies showing that couples who watch porn together are more sexually satisfied and content.[77] But before you cue up your TV or pop open your laptop, talk with your partner and agree on the type of porn you want to watch—if you're into one kind of kink that turns your partner off, you'll have to find common ground. Just be sure to opt for ethical porn, meaning it doesn't feature children, animals, or graphic violence, and that the actors involved (to the best of your knowledge) are treated and paid fairly. And listen, if *at any point* you want to turn it off, you are more than welcome to do that.

10. **Reset your hormones.** As you know from chapter 3, your sex hormones play a role in your libido and ability to orgasm. Lower estrogen levels, for example, can cause vaginal dryness, thin vaginal tissue, and make the clitoris less sensitive, all of which can impair your ability to climax. Too little testosterone, on the other hand, can interfere with arousal and sex drive, while too much progesterone can reduce your

libido, too. Your body's sex hormones also work in concert, so any one irregularity can set off a chain reaction that ultimately impairs your O ability. If you suspect a hormone imbalance, head to page 192 for a quick self-evaluation.

11. **Take away the pain.** You likely won't be able to climax if sex is painful in any way, shape, or form (unless that's the intention and you're into that). Painful sex is *not* normal and is never something you have to accept or tolerate. In most instances, painful sex is treatable. See page 110 for more.

12. **Identify what causes you to hit the brakes.** Our sex drive and ability to be aroused are like driving a car: we all have a gas pedal that we can push to turn ourselves on, and a brake that will stop the action. There are many different individual factors and feelings that can cause everyone, no matter how high sexual desire and arousal may be, to pump the brakes. Identifying what causes you to hit your brakes, and strategizing how to remove those impediments, can help you climax more easily. Some common reasons people hit the brakes when having sex include feeling shame around sex, experiencing relationship issues, constantly feeling stressed or anxious, dealing with body-image issues, feeling obligated to have sex, feeling overwhelmed as a parent, and constantly obsessing over all the things you have to do. If any of these reasons to hit the brakes resonate with you, communicate with your partner about how you can both work together to ease your foot off your brake and apply more gas. For example, if you're a parent and feel "touched out," meaning the amount of touch you already receive from your children is sufficient or overstimulating, then work with your partner to find a way to take a parenting break during the day so that you have the capacity and desire to be intimate.

13. **Call in the medical team.** Many chronic illnesses like hypothyroidism, diabetes, arthritis, and even asthma can interfere with sex drive and the ability to orgasm. Taking certain medications like antidepressants, antihistamines, and high-blood-pressure drugs can also impair your O. If you've been diagnosed with any condition or regularly take

prescription or over-the-counter drugs, talk with your doctor: As a medical provider they need to know if you can't climax, since it's a critical gauge of your overall health. Finally, stress, anxiety, depression, relationship issues, and other mood and emotional problems can all inhibit your orgasm ability. In my opinion, almost everyone can benefit by seeing a mental health specialist, whether you're having O issues or not.

TL;DR: ARE MY ORGASMS NORMAL?

- Can you pass the clit quiz? Just taking it will put you far beyond most others when it cums to your knowledge about the clitoris.
- Women in heterosexual relationships are having far fewer orgasms. It's called the orgasm gap, and the remedy is in this chapter.
- Eighty percent of women fake their orgasms during heterosexual sex.
- While you may have believed the female orgasm to be this impossible feat, it's not, since 95 percent of women can climax on their own with masturbation.
- Orgasms are primarily neurological events, meaning our brain drives a lot of the action.
- It's normal to stay silent or make a lot of noise, have multiple Os or only one, cry afterward, or fall asleep when you're done.
- Orgasms have a ton of health benefits, including the ability to help you live longer and even make your skin look younger and clearer.
- A vaginal orgasm isn't the best or only way to climax—it's just often the easiest one for the penis.

- There are many ways to arrive at orgasm, like stimulating your nipples, working your core, and even thinking off. But not one rivals direct clitoral stimulation in most vulva owners.
- "Squirting" during orgasms is totally normal.
- Women need an average of fourteen minutes of foreplay before they can climax, although it's normal to need as much as forty minutes before being able to come.
- There are lots of tips and tricks to help you orgasm more easily. Needing some help is totally normal.

CHAPTER 5

SEX OF ALL KINDS

GETTING DOWN AND DIRTY WITH VAGINAL, ORAL, ANAL, OUTERCOURSE, AND EVERYTHING IN BETWEEN

"What I really want is to be one of those people who can just have normal sex without struggling to sit for days after, or using every maneuver I can to avoid any type of penetration," Amber desperately shared with me on her first visit. Amber had been struggling with pain during sex as far back as she could remember. She went on to share, through tears, "I thought all my problems started because I was having sex with men when I was so clearly not into them. Being with women makes dodging the penetration part easier, but still, if my girlfriend wants to use a toy or even touches me anywhere but my clitoris, I'm in pain, with an achy, burning vagina for most of the week. I can't even use tampons because it is just too painful."

I wish I could say Amber's conversation surprised me. But as if the orgasm gap I shared with you in chapter 4 wasn't enough of a downer, it's estimated that about three out of four women experience pain with sex at some point in their lifetime.[1] Which means that we can't very well talk about vaginal sex without acknowledging one of the biggest problems vagina owners have with it—pain. Although it was clear there was more than just a lubrication issue at play with Amber, that hadn't stopped her previous providers from presenting lube as the magic solution to her concerns about sex. I was Amber's last stop on a long list of medical providers she had hoped would help her at least *understand* what was causing the pain. "The last gynecologist I saw told me that it's normal for sex to be painful sometimes and that it couldn't be that bad. She said I should try a few glasses of wine to help me relax, and just keep going if it hurt because eventually my body would get used to it."

This, too, wasn't shocking: dismissal of women's pain (especially pain down there) is all too common. (A fair warning that I'm about to throw out some stats that will likely make you mad.) Numerous studies demonstrate that women's pain is often regarded as psychological (a throwback to the days of belief in hysteria), and that women are less likely to receive an accurate diagnosis or adequate therapies to manage their pain.[2] One study found that women were left to wait almost 33 percent longer than men when presenting with severe stomach pain at the emergency room.[3] Another showed that women were seven times more likely than men to be misdiagnosed and sent home while experiencing a heart attack.[4] And if you are a woman of color, the bias is even greater, as a 2016 study showed that doctors' false beliefs that Black Americans have a higher tolerance for pain resulted in disparities in pain assessment and treatment.[5] Heart attacks and ER visits are taken much more seriously in medicine than the inability to have sex, so when I tell you that a gender bias exists in medicine, you better believe that it impacts women's sexual health. When it comes to pain with sex, it's been found that about 60 percent of women who seek care end up seeing three or more doctors, many of whom are unable to provide a diagnosis.[6]

Thankfully, I was able to give Amber the answer to her pain—vulvodynia, a chronic pain condition affecting the vulva, which we'll discuss in the next few pages. It was a relief for her to finally have validation, to know that her pain was real, and that she would have concrete information she could now relay to her partner. As I shared with Amber, context matters for getting in the mood and having pleasurable sex, which we touched on in chapter 3. If you're like Amber—if your experience is that sex is not only scary, but also painful—then there's no number of slow jams or scented candles that are going to help. Conditions that cause pain with sex, like vulvodynia, vaginismus, and endometriosis, are commonly misdiagnosed or reduced to a lubrication issue. It's true, insufficient lube is a leading cause of pain with sex (which we'll discuss in this chapter), but that doesn't get your doctor off the hook. They need to listen to your concerns and provide a thorough investigation, along with treatment options. So when working with Amber, instead of handing her a list of lube recommendations, we took an integrative approach and employed such therapies as a referral to a pelvic-floor physical therapist (PT), an anti-inflammatory diet (like you'll find in the 28-day plan), biofeedback (a body awareness therapy), and having her use topical lidocaine (a numbing agent) on the days she had PT or sex.[7] Amber was eventually able to find relief (along with partnered sex that was pleasurable) through these interventions. But for other people, vaginal sex will never be something painless, much less pleasurable, which is why we're going to discuss sex of all kinds. In this chapter we're going to explore the most-asked questions when it comes to vaginal, oral, anal, outercourse, and everything in between. I'm going to provide you solutions to not just solve the most common issues that can arise, but to understand how to make sex more pleasurable.

ASK DR. BRIGHTEN:

Is pain during sex normal?

What is common often gets mistaken for what is normal, so let me clear up the confusion here: pain with sex is common, pain with sex *is not* normal. And it's not something that you should have to learn to live with. Dyspareunia, the medical term for any genital pain associated with sex, does have a root cause, and contrary to what others (even your doctor) might say, it's not just an "in your head" issue.

How do I know if the discomfort I'm feeling is actually a problem?

If you find yourself feeling anxious or fearful in anticipation of sex, or routinely experiencing pain during or after any sexual activity, then it warrants further investigation. Dyspareunia can present as irritating, aching, throbbing, burning, or stabbing pains, or a sensation of tearing or ripping inside. You can also experience discomfort in the vulvar area, perineum (the area between your vagina and anus), or vestibule (the area around the opening of your vagina). We use the term "superficial dyspareunia" to describe pain at the introitus (the opening of your vagina) and "deep dyspareunia" when you experience discomfort with deep penetration. Some women with dyspareunia can experience pain with arousal (before the genitals are even touched), with tight-fitting clothing, and can even have pain when inserting a tampon.

WHY DOES SEX HURT?

There are dozens of reasons women can experience painful sex—some are physical and others have a psychological component. (But do not take this as a dismissal that your symptoms are just in your head.) Here are some of the leading causes:

- Low arousal
- Vaginal dryness
- Stress or anxiety about sex
- Vaginitis, or inflammation of the vagina
- Vaginismus, or involuntary contractions of the vaginal muscles
- Vulvodynia, or pain around the vulva (the outside)
- Endometriosis
- Adenomyosis (see page 114)
- A tilted uterus, or when the uterus curves backward
- Uterine fibroids
- Pelvic inflammatory disease
- Lichen planus or lichen sclerosus, which are skin disorders that can include the vulva (see page 175)
- Ovarian cysts
- Urinary tract infection (UTI)
- Painful bladder syndrome (commonly known as interstitial cystitis)
- Yeast infection
- Hypertonic pelvic floor, or when the pelvic floor is unable to relax
- Pelvic organ prolapse, or when weak pelvic muscles cause one or more organs to fall

- Certain STIs like herpes, gonorrhea, and trichomoniasis
- Hormonal birth control (which may dry and tighten tissue)
- Low estrogen (which can cause dry, thin, and tightened tissue)
- Being postpartum—especially if you had a difficult labor, vaginal trauma, or episiotomy
- Sexual trauma
- Physical trauma, either from injury or a medical procedure
- Autoimmune disease
- Seminal plasma allergy (allergic reaction to semen)

What should I do if sex is painful?

Because there are so many different reasons for painful sex, addressing and treating it usually requires a trip to your provider and, sometimes, a referral to a specialist. Any provider worth their medical degree should take your concern seriously and work with you to find the root cause and solution. If you're met with a dismissive suggestion along the lines of "just have a glass of wine to loosen up" (hard eye roll), take that for the red flag it is and find a new provider. Painful sex is real and can be an early sign of a serious issue, which means it should be taken seriously. Getting support from the right medical team can make all the difference for your health and your sex life.

Writing down your experience can help you not only advocate for yourself, but also avoid having your concerns be trivialized or dismissed by your provider. Here's the data you can collect now and present to your provider:

- When did the pain start? Was there anything that happened around that time?
- Do you experience pain before, during, or after sex?
- Where does it hurt? Be as specific as possible, whether it's in the vulvar area, at the opening (introitus) or perineum, radiating down your thigh, or deeper inside you.
- What does the pain feel like? Does it throb, burn, feel like a deep ache, or as though something is ripping or tearing?
- How long does the pain last?

- Do you ever have nausea with the pain?
- Do you ever have pain when inserting a tampon, wearing certain clothing, or riding a bike?
- Does it get better or worse during parts of your cycle?
- Can you rate the pain on a scale of 1 to 5, with 5 being the worst? (I know this is a tricky one, but it can help your doctor to understand how serious the issue is for you.)
- What helps? Is there anything that brings you relief?

Four Reasons for Pain with Sex That Your Doctor Might Miss

I wish I didn't have to ask, but has your doctor dismissed your pain? It's common, and when it happens, conditions like the ones below can go undiagnosed, mismanaged, and lead to long-term suffering.

1. **Vulvodynia:** The prevalence of vulvodynia, or localized vulvar pain syndrome, a chronic pain condition affecting the vulva, is largely unknown, as patients either do not seek care or do not receive adequate care, as was the case for Amber. It's estimated that up to 16 percent of all women (that's about 13 million vulvas) may experience vulvodynia.[8] For some the discomfort is constant, while for others it hurts only with penetration, as from a tampon or during penetrative sex. Some women can also feel a burning pain whenever anything touches their vulva, like riding a bike, sitting for too long, or wearing underwear. Not enough is known about vulvodynia, but what we do understand is that inflammation (generally set off by infections like yeast or bacterial vaginosis), nerve dysfunction, and structural issues within the pelvic floor can all play a role in initiating or continuing the pain.

   A diagnosis of vulvodynia requires that your provider ensures there are no other conditions causing your symptoms and performs a pressure point test, commonly called the cotton swab test, to identify where the pain is located. Tracking how long you've had the pain is important since it must present for at least three months to meet the criteria. Eating an anti-inflammatory diet, supporting your vaginal ecology, leveraging mental health support, getting acupuncture, and working with a pelvic-floor specialist can all be beneficial in managing this condition. Some benefit from medications like topical lidocaine or SSRIs, as well as Botox or cortisol injections. There has been some evidence that topical estradiol (a type of estrogen) and testosterone may be helpful, but as with all vulvodynia treatments, the results are individual specific.

2. **Vaginismus:** This condition occurs when your vagina muscles involuntarily spasm or squeeze whenever something enters it, like a penis, toy, speculum, or tampon. This pain can be so bad that nothing can enter. Infections can cause vaginismus, as can a history of anxiety or any type of traumatic experience, including sexual abuse. Some women also develop the condition for reasons that doctors don't understand. There's no test for vaginismus; instead, your provider may feel the muscles tighten up during an exam and use your experience to make the diagnosis. If there is an infection or other condition, like lichen sclerosus (a chronic inflammatory condition that causes an itchy white rash on the genitals), it is important to be treated for that. Mind-body therapies and professional intervention can also help treat vaginismus, including meditation, CBT, trauma recovery, vaginal dilators, vaginal estrogen (if thinning or vaginal dryness is present), and self-massage. Working with a pelvic-floor therapist to relax the muscles around your vagina is an important part of treatment.

3. **Endometriosis:** This inflammatory condition is a common cause of painful sex that nearly no one talks about and not enough research exists on, even though it affects up to 15 percent of all women.[9] This is a big part of why I want you to learn about endometriosis: There's a good chance that if you have it, you'll struggle to get a provider to diagnose it. Six out of ten women with endometriosis are never diagnosed by their provider, and even those patients who do receive a proper diagnosis have to wait an average of four to eleven years to get it.[10] While much of the research is focused on women who were assigned female at birth, endometriosis has been found in cis men,

Endometriosis Symptom Quiz

These symptoms commonly present in those diagnosed with endometriosis. The diagnosis is confirmed via a surgical biopsy procedure known as laparoscopy. However, if you have symptoms that indicate you have endo and you're not planning on pursuing surgical interventions, getting a definitive diagnosis is considered optional.

_____ Without pain medication, my period pain prevents me from going about my normal daily activities.

_____ My period pain can make me nauseous or cause me to vomit.

_____ I often experience lower back or pelvic pain before and during my period that prevents me from going to work, being social, or even doing chores around the house.

_____ I often have pain with bowel movements, especially before and during my period.

_____ I experience pain between my periods that restricts my activities.

_____ It is common for me to experience pain with sex.

_____ I avoid sex because of pain.

_____ I experience persistent pelvic pain after sex or following a pelvic exam.

_____ I experience pain with urination or increased urgency.

If you checked off one or more of these symptoms, it is time to talk with your doctor. Write down your answers and take these to your next doctor's appointment so you can discuss these key areas and get a diagnosis. If you've been struggling to get pregnant and identify with any of these, know that endometriosis can cause infertility.

although believed to be rare.[11] The takeaway: this condition can affect *any* body, but research is seriously lacking.

Endometriosis occurs when tissue that is somewhat like the lining of the uterus (endometrium), yet distinct, grows outside the uterus on structures like the fallopian tubes, ovaries, bladder, or intestines. This tissue responds to hormone stimulation and can build, expand, and bleed, forming painful adhesions. When you have sex, these adhesions can create pressure, pulling, and pain, even if you're fully aroused and lubricated. Along with painful sex, women with endometriosis often experience painful periods and discomfort during ovulation or when urinating or pooping. It's as bad as it sounds, maybe even worse. If you suspect you have endometriosis, find a provider who specializes in it. Endometriosis is diagnosed via laparoscopy, a minimally invasive surgery, during which the painful adhesions may also be removed. Managing this condition, like all chronic conditions, takes an individualized approach–what works for one person may not work for another. While many women can address the condition by changing their diet, taking certain supplements, and making other lifestyle tweaks, removal of adhesions is often a necessary part of treatment. If you're diagnosed with endometriosis, I recommend also working with a mental health expert, as the condition can cause or worsen anxiety and depression.

4. **Adenomyosis:** Struggling with abnormally painful periods, heavy flow, bleeding at irregular times, or feeling like your lower abdomen is growing despite the same diet and exercise habits may be a sign that there are more than the run-of-the-mill period problems happening.

   If endometriosis had a cousin, adenomyosis would be it, as the symptoms are very similar. But rather than painful lesions being outside the uterus, these lesions are embedded in the uterine muscles. Working with a skilled practitioner is the best way to get the right diagnosis and treatment. NSAIDs like ibuprofen, magnesium, and cramp bark tincture can help with pain around your period (see page 384 for specific dosages). Like endometriosis, it needs a comprehensive and individualized treatment approach to get relief. Unlike endo, a hysterectomy (removal of the uterus) may be beneficial for those struggling with significant pain.

Pain with Sex Solutions

Whether it's your first time or you've done it plenty of times, sex can sometimes hurt (even though it shouldn't). Sex should be pleasurable, not unintentionally painful. This list is in no way exhaustive of all the ways you can reduce and manage pain, but it is a good place to start.

Raise your voice and advocate for the care you need. Listen, it should be as easy as making an appointment with a provider and showing up, but sadly, the research shows us it is not. To be heard and get the best treatment, you'll need to advocate for yourself, likely multiple times. Use your answers from the questions on page 110 to communicate the severity of your issues to your provider. If they begin to dismiss you and send you on your way, take the following steps: Ask them what they considered in their differential diagnosis (the conditions they thought it could be) and what they have done to rule those in or out. If you request imaging, testing, or referral and are denied, ask them to document in your chart that you requested them and the reason for their denial. Let them know you'll be requesting a copy of your chart notes to keep a record of this. Ensuring that these steps happen will often prompt a busy doctor to slow down and truly consider the seriousness of your concerns. Finally, always have your symptoms written down. It is much more difficult to be gaslighted when you have your data written down in front of you.

Discuss the deed. Before doing said deed, talk to your partner about what you're interested in, what you're consenting to, and communicate what you need to feel supported. We almost never see this kind of conversation in various media, so it understandably may feel awkward to talk about. But you are about to share an incredibly intimate moment, so having an open dialogue can help alleviate anxiety you may be feeling. If you know you struggle with penetration, tell your partner. It's OK to consent to everything but penetration, too.

Try outercourse instead. Pleasurable and satisfying sex doesn't have to be penetrative. See the section in this chapter on outercourse.

Give yourself adequate warm-up time. Sometimes when we've decided that now is go time, we find ourselves so excited that we jump immediately to the penetration part without enough attention on foreplay. Slow it down, friend! Foreplay can help your body and mind begin to sync up in anticipation of sex.

Bring the lube. Lube is for everyone (I've got a list of what to look for on page 125), and depending on how hydrated you are or the types of medication you're taking (*slow wave at the pill*), you may require support in the lube department. This doesn't mean there is anything wrong with you. Lack of lube is one of the leading reasons for there to be pain anytime there is penetration. The good news is that this is the easiest issue to fix.

Go slow. Slow and steady wins the race when it comes to finding the rhythm that matches you and your partner. You can always speed things up as you get comfortable, but to begin, move at a pace where you can change positions, communicate, and find an enjoyable flow.

Change positions. Speaking of positions, missionary isn't best for everyone. If it hurts, as is the case when penetration is too deep, spice it up and find a new position that suits you both. Anatomy can vary, which means it is normal to need to explore positions to find what's most comfortable and pleasurable for you.

Move more, move right. Sitting for long periods of time can lead to imbalances in your muscles, poor pelvic health, and worsen the issues you're already having. Exercises that support pelvic-floor health (no, the answer isn't just Kegel); your back; and work to lengthen, not just strengthen, can help you create a healthier pelvic floor. Working with a physical (PT) or occupational therapist (OT) can help tremendously. You can also try swapping your chair for an exercise ball, using a standing desk, or setting an alarm every hour to remind yourself to stand up or take a short walk. If you find you can't get out of the building, do a lap around the office or see if your office will get a treadmill desk to help keep you moving. If you find yourself engaging in repetitive motions–running, for example–adding in yoga, Pilates, or strength training can help to create well-balanced physical health. For wheelchair users, a PT or OT can provide exercise modifications, like using a strap for leg stretches, to enable you to address any musculoskeletal issues that can contribute to pain.

Consider mental/emotional support. No, it's not just in your head, but pain can mess with your head. Any type of pain can take a psychological toll on us. It's also important to consider that almost half of all women who experience chronic pelvic pain have a history of trauma—sexual, physical, or emotional.[12] No matter what's causing your dyspareunia, working with a licensed mental health provider, especially one who practices cognitive behavioral therapy (CBT),[13] can help support you on your journey.

Try acupuncture. Seeing a licensed acupuncturist[14] can help mitigate symptoms. Acupuncture has been shown to improve quality of life and reduce pelvic pain without side effects when compared to conventional treatments in women with endometriosis.[15]

Address hormone issues. Having too little estrogen can lead to thin and dry vaginal tissue, while too much can make endometrial lesions worse or contribute to conditions like uterine fibroids, which can cause painful sex. Identify imbalances and support your estrogen naturally with my 28-day plan.

Postpartum rehab. Giving birth is traumatic for your pelvic floor and vagina, no matter how you brought that small human into the world. Some TLC and healing time afterward is a must, but even with the appropriate recovery, pain and pelvic-floor dysfunction can persist for years. The good news is that there are professionals who can help. Seeing a PT or OT who specializes in pelvic-floor conditions can help you address your specific issues, provide you with exercises that can make sex more comfortable, and even give you massage techniques to help with pain related to scar tissue.

Adopt an anti-inflammatory diet. Diet has an undeniable impact on your health, hormones, and pain, but I'm not going to be one of those providers who promises you a diet change will be all you need. It is a foundational piece of addressing your pain that cannot be overlooked, which is why we'll be discussing it in chapter 12.

Practice good hygiene. As in: ditch the synthetic chonies, fragrance-filled cleansers, and moisture-trapping gym shorts, and consider going commando (not wearing underwear) at night. We covered this in chapter 2 and, when it comes to vulvar pain, these steps are nonnegotiable.

ASK DR. BRIGHTEN:

Does size matter?

There are a variety of justifications for the argument that the Goldilocks penis exists for all of us. Yes, it can hurt if it is too big. And yes, it can be less satisfying for certain women if it is too small—although I'll share why that's not always the case. Put simply, size can matter when it comes to penises, but that isn't the end of the story. BTW, when it comes to toys, size definitely matters, and there should be zero hurt feelings if you find yourself saying, "That's not it."

What should I do if my partner's penis is too big?

I once had a patient whose female gynecologist told her to consider having a hysterectomy in order to accommodate her husband's penis. (I wish I was joking.) My patient had seen her doctor because she was experiencing pain when she and her husband attempted doggy style. Your cervix has nerves, and when struck by a penis (or any object), it can hurt. The gynecologist's solution was to remove the patient's normal and healthy anatomy (her uterus) for the sole purpose of allowing her husband the option of this position. Well, the solution to a large penis isn't surgery. And it's not learning to just put up with the pain, either, which is something else I've heard providers recommend. Instead, you have to learn to do things a little differently. In addition to what is listed on page 115 to solve the pain-with-sex dilemma, I'd also encourage you to:

1. Make sure you're fully aroused before any penetration takes place. This allows the vagina to lengthen and the pelvic-floor muscles to relax. In some women, the cervix can move upward. All these changes may make accommodating a larger penis possible.

2. Experiment with positions that put you on top, which allow you to control the movement and depth of penetration.

3. Placing your hand around the shaft of his penis can help provide him stimulation while allowing you to control the depth. Or you can use the Ohnut, which is a condom-compatible, skin-like ring system that helps you control the depth of penetration.

4. Put pillows under your hips to tilt your pelvis upward and relax your pelvic floor, which will help make penetration easier. Put those decorative pillows on your bed to work by placing them under your knees or thighs, depending on the position. The more support you have, the easier it will be for you to release tension in your body.

Does the size of my partner's penis affect whether I can orgasm?

Yes and no. Female orgasm most commonly occurs when the clitoris is stimulated, not with vaginal penetration alone, so for most, size is a non-issue. But size can prevent you from having an O if his penis is too big and causing discomfort. Everyone thinks having a large penis is a good thing, but if a guy is too long or wide, it can hurt—a lot. And if it hurts, you likely won't be able to climax.

What should I do if I think my partner's penis is too small?

Remember: most orgasms happen through clitoral stimulation, which can take place with a hand, tongue, or toy. That being said, women who experience vaginal orgasms have been shown to prefer a larger penis.[16] Keep in mind that the size of his penis may also be small only relative to partners you've had in the past. For reference, the average penis size is about five inches, with a micropenis (exactly what it sounds like) being about three inches.[17] While it's possible his penis isn't enough to help you achieve a vaginal orgasm, know that, regardless of size, most penises aren't going to be enough on their own, since clitoral stimulation through manual or oral means is usually necessary.

What is vaginal dryness and how do I know if I have it?

The vagina is self-lubricating, which means it produces fluids with your cycle to help keep itself clean and healthy. Your vagina also generates arousal fluid whenever you're sexually excited, making it easier for a penis, toy, or finger to penetrate (the details on how all of this works are in chapter 7). But not all vaginas self-lubricate as much or when we want them to. Vaginal dryness is most often felt during penetrative sex, but you can also experience symptoms when you sit, exercise, wear tight clothing, or even walk. Hallmark signs include discomfort, irritation, itching, and burning.

If you think you're too young to have vaginal dryness, think again. The condition affects women of all ages (see below for why). Dryness can also be caused in young women by arousal nonconcordance or where they are in their cycle, in addition to other issues.

What causes vaginal dryness?

Low estrogen is the leading cause of vaginal dryness[18]—which is why as many as three-quarters of postmenopausal women develop it after their bodies stop producing adequate estrogen to sustain their cycles.[19] But estrogen can dip at any age for a number of reasons, including if you exercise too much, lose a lot of weight or are underweight, are depressed or stressed, have a thyroid disorder, give birth, or are still breastfeeding. Low estrogen can also cause a condition called vaginal atrophy, which occurs when your vaginal walls become thin and inflamed, aggravating any dryness. Your ability to self-lubricate is also dependent on where you are in your cycle, your hormone levels, the amount of foreplay, and how into it you really are.

Taking certain drugs like oral contraceptives, antidepressants, and anything that contains antihistamines or decongestants (think cold, allergy, and asthma medications) can also cause dryness. Physical conditions like primary ovarian insufficiency (POI), diabetes, and some immune disorders may also trigger it. Some hygiene habits, like douching, which disrupts your vagina's natural pH, can make you dry down there, too, as can using harsh soaps, detergents, feminine sprays, or other personal-care products that contain chemicals, perfumes, or other irritants.

What should I do if I have vaginal dryness?

Vaginal dryness can sabotage your sex life, in addition to your daily comfort levels. If you suspect vaginal dryness, be sure to talk with your provider. Most women don't bring up the issue with their doctors or even realize that they can, according to research.[20] Why? There's a lot of shame and stigma surrounding the condition, which is why only 4 percent of women, on average, receive the treatment they need.[21] Luckily, vaginal dryness is treatable in most instances, so get the help you need.

Ten Ways to Increase Your Vagina's Lubrication Levels

Whether you have vaginal dryness or not, there's still plenty you can do to increase your natural lubrication levels and make yourself wet when you want. Here are my top ten tips and tricks to increase lubrication levels:

1. **Do my plan for one month.** Even if you don't have an irregularity, working to balance your hormones with my 28-day plan can go a long way to boosting lubrication levels. Regulating hormonal health can also improve your libido, arousal, and overall enjoyment of sex. One caveat: If you're postmenopausal, we won't be able to get your ovaries to restart their estrogen production to counter vaginal dryness. Instead, you may benefit from estrogen or DHEA hormone therapy, vitamin E suppositories, vitamin D supplementation, or vaginal moisturizers.

2. **Drink up, friend.** But not in the way you may be thinking (or maybe your provider recommended). While alcohol may seem like your best bet to get those juices flowing, it actually can lead to dehydration, vaginal dryness, and decreased pleasure—especially when heavily drinking.[22] The "whiskey vagina" phenomenon of decreased sensitivity, struggle to orgasm, and less-satisfying orgasms is real, as alcohol interferes with both your nerves and blood flow to the nether regions.[23] Instead, drink more hydrating beverages like water, sparkling water, herbal teas, and embrace the mocktail. And caffeine? While it

can lead to peeing a lot more, it won't actually dehydrate you since you're also taking in fluid with it.

3. **Try vitamins E and D.** Vitamin E suppositories have been shown to improve vaginal dryness and atrophy.[24] In women undergoing cancer treatment, which can cause severe vaginal dryness, a combination of hyaluronic acid with vitamins E, A, and D as suppositories provided relief.[25]

4. **Try seed cycling.** Flaxseeds and sesame seeds, specifically, contain phytoestrogens, naturally occurring plant compounds that act like estrogen in the body, helping to reduce dryness and increase the vagina's natural lubrication levels, according to research.[26] To seed cycle, include 1 to 2 tablespoons each of flax and pumpkin seeds in your diet from the start of your period until ovulation (the follicular phase). Once you ovulate and enter your luteal phase, eat 1 to 2 tablespoons each of sesame and sunflower seeds daily, switching your seeds at the start of your period. You can also consume phytoestrogens by eating cruciferous veggies like broccoli, and fruits like peaches, strawberries, and raspberries.

5. **Ditch the douche—and anything with fragrance.** Never underestimate the ability of pH-altering and endocrine-disrupting chemicals to cause all sorts of problems, including dryness down there. To alleviate the issue, don't douche or use feminine sprays or wipes, all of which can disrupt your delicate ecology. For the best practices for care of your vagina, see page 49.

6. **Rethink the pill.** For some women, taking the pill can change vaginal tissue and reduce vaginal secretions, which can result in pain with sex. If you're on the pill and dealing with dryness, talk with your prescriber about alternative forms of pregnancy prevention.

7. **Avoid cold and allergy medications.** Decongestants and antihistamines work, in part, by reducing blood flow and dehydrating tissue, which will also dry out your vagina.[27] The good news about colds

is that those viruses don't last long enough for you to stress if you use cold medication. If you have allergies, try natural remedies like nettle tea, neti pots, quercetin, turmeric, bromelain, N-acetyl cysteine (NAC), and acupuncture. If you do need medication, know lube will be your bestie.

8. **Eat more seafood or take a high-quality omega-3 supplement.** High levels of marine omega-3 fatty acids, which are found primarily in seafood, may increase lubrication and combat dryness.[28] To increase your intake, choose fattier fish like salmon or sardines, or opt for a high-quality omega-3 supplement that's been third-party-tested for purity.

9. **Try topical DHEA.** Dehydroepiandrosterone (DHEA) is a hormone made by the adrenal glands that helps the body produce estrogen and testosterone. Studies show that topical DHEA in suppository form can counter vaginal dryness[29] while also helping to tone your pelvic floor and increase the quality of your orgasms.[30] (Wins all around!) Talk with your doctor before using DHEA suppositories, as the hormone can cause unwanted side effects if your estrogen or testosterone levels are already high.

10. **Use vaginal moisturizers.** If you're in menopause, have primary ovarian insufficiency, or have had a hysterectomy, vaginal moisturizers might be your best option to help you fight vaginal dryness. Unlike lube, which is used before or during sex, vaginal moisturizers can be applied whenever you want and will help rehydrate tissue if you use them consistently every few days over time. Look for vaginal moisturizers at pharmacies, and scan labels to avoid those that contain fragrances (natural or synthetic). If you want relief but don't want to deal with label reading, you can apply avocado, sweet almond, or coconut oil to your vulva.

LUBE MYTHS

A lube-free bedroom is where good sex goes to die. For most, the secret to great sex is lube. But the stigma against lube is real: Women think there's something wrong with them if they're not as wet as the movies portray. And even if you are, lube can still transform your sex life in amazing ways. Sometimes in your cycle you're going to be naturally drier—for a reminder of the cyclical nature of lubrication, see chapter 9—and using lube can make sex more enjoyable. But despite all we know to be true, I still get yelled at on social media about how normalizing using lube is "encouraging women to lower their standards, telling people foreplay isn't necessary, and giving men a free pass to just stick it in." None of which is true. So let's do some myth-bustin' and clear some stuff up.

Myth #1: Lube is only for vaginal dryness or older women.

Lube is for everyone, no matter your age, sexual orientation, relationship status, whether you have your period, or if you have vaginal dryness.

Myth #2: Lube stops the action right when it's heating up.

Lube takes two seconds to apply. Keep it by the bedside so it's easily within reach. You can also pre-apply if you're worried about it slowing things down.

Myth #3: Using lube means gross sex sounds.

If you know the Cardi B song "WAP" (Wet-Ass Pussy), then you know the line "Macaroni in a pot," which alludes to the idea that having sex can sound like you're stirring a fresh pot of mac and cheese when you're sufficiently lubricated. While using lube can intensify certain sounds, they're not gross, and it's totally normal.

Myth #4: If I need lube, one of us is doing something wrong.

You know, one of the most common causes of sexual dysfunction is fear of performance. Yes, just being worried that we're doing something wrong can make everything go wrong. If someone needs lube, it doesn't mean anyone is doing things wrong. It could be happening for a variety of reasons—all of which are better discussed outside the bedroom and not in the very moment you need lube.

ASK DR. BRIGHTEN:

What kind of lube should I use?

If you haven't explored the variety of lubes yet, then you may not be aware of all your options. Most products are made from one of three bases: water, silicone, or oil. I recommend experimenting with different brands and bases to see which ones work best for you. For a more extensive lube list of what to avoid and choose go to https://DrBrighten.com/ITN-resources.

Type	Pros	Cons	Latex condom safe
Water-based	• Better for sensitive skin • Won't stain sheets • Easy to wash off • Won't break down silicone toys • Gentle on skin	• Evaporates quickly so you'll need to reapply • Can begin to feel sticky over time • Not water resistant • May contain glycerin, parabens	Yes
Silicone-based	• Hypoallergenic • Lasts longer than water-based • Water resistant • Requires less product • Best for anal sex	• Can stain fabrics • Can be difficult to wash off • May not be safe for silicone toys	Yes
Oil-based	• Long lasting • Water resistant • Can be used with most toys • Can moisturize skin • Can be used as massage oil • May be edible	• Can stain fabrics • Difficult to wash off • Not safe for latex toys	No; may be compatible with polyurethane condoms

Is flavored lube safe?

Licking edible lube off your partner may sound tasty, but the stuff can cause major irritation and disrupt your vagina's pH, increasing the risk of yeast infections and bacterial vaginosis. While flavored lube and food are fair game on a penis, make sure that it's clean before introducing it into the vagina, since sugars and other foods can disrupt microbial health (leading to potential infections) and may be uncomfortable.

Oral Sex: How can I make oral sex better (and safer)?

Oral sex involves using your mouth or tongue to stimulate your partner's genitals. I'll be dedicating this section to cunnilingus, the term for oral sex performed on the vulva, and fellatio, oral sex performed on a penis. (You'll find anal-related information in a little bit.)

Will eating pineapple change the way I taste?

Listen, as a Latina, I'm a big fan of all things pineapple (mmm . . . tacos al pastor). And as a hormone expert, I also know that the fruit is fantastic for hormonal health, helping to ease period pain, reduce bloating, and even boost libido, thanks to its concentration of bromelain found in the core, an anti-inflammatory enzyme shown to increase testosterone.[31] Seriously, pineapples are awesome all-around.

But no matter how much pineapple you eat or drink, your vagina will likely never smell or taste like a piña colada, despite what trending TikToks tell you. For years now, social media posts and blogs have gone viral with claims that pineapple, on its own or mixed with other ingredients like cranberry juice, can turn your vagina into a tasty tropical treat. You may have heard the same myth about semen—that if he consumes enough pineapple, his semen will go down as smoothly as an Aloha smoothie from Jamba Juice.

I hate to be the bearer of bad news to anyone who's spent days loading up on pineapple before a big date, but there's no scientific evidence to support that the fruit—or any other sweet food—can transform your discharge or his ejaculate into a Cold Stone Creamery. Yes, we are lacking data in the "eat fruit and taste test" arena, and we might come to find, in the future, that there's a sweet spot for fruit consumption in shifting flavor profiles.

Regardless, you should never be made to feel ashamed for how you smell or taste when it's normal. While some foods can shift the smell of urine (think asparagus) and sweat (if you've ever caught the pungent whiff of something not right during your workout the day after drinking too much), the body doesn't use our vaginas to detoxify, like urine or skin. If you or your partner feels the odor or taste of your vaginal secretions is off, that may warrant a trip to the doctor. Head over to chapter 7 to learn what does change your discharge and what to do about it.

HOW WHAT YOU EAT *DOES* AFFECT YOUR VAGINA'S SMELL AND TASTE

While pineapple won't turn your vagina into a fruit smoothie, what you eat can still affect the smell and taste of your genitalia by influencing the kinds of critters that live in your vaginal microbiome. Eating a healthy diet high in fiber—and the beneficial bacteria known as probiotics, found in fermented foods like kimchi and sauerkraut—can help support your vagina's good microbes, preventing an overgrowth of the microorganisms that can lead to infection.[32] Consuming too much sugar, on the other hand, along with alcohol and processed foods, can trigger the growth of unhealthy microbes, boosting the potential for pH imbalances, infections, and funky discharge. In diabetics, a high-sugar diet can leave the vagina susceptible to yeast infections.

How do I make it so I don't smell down there? Will douching help?

Genitals have an odor. If there is something seriously off, like we talk about in chapter 7, then it should definitely be addressed. Outside of that, the basic hygiene for vulvas we covered in chapter 2 should be enough if you feel the need to clean. Everyone can have more of an odor after a long day, following a workout, or if they've skipped their daily shower. While it is common (and exhaustingly acceptable) for vulvas to be shamed for having an odor, everyone will generate an odor if they do not practice adequate hygiene. It's all normal.

Try one of these tips before receiving oral sex if you're concerned about odor:

- Wash the area with warm water and mild soap (remember: soap is optional for the vulva, but you may want to use it for surrounding areas).
- Use an unscented baby wipe–which will be free of harsh chemicals and is made for delicate skin–to gently remove oils, dead skin, and sweat.
- Wear cotton or moisture-wicking clothing to allow the area to breathe throughout the day.
- Shower shortly after your workout or any activity where you work up a sweat.

What *can* change the smell and taste of your vaginal secretions—and not in a good way—is douching, using scented intimate wipes, or relying on those relatively new vaginal moisturizing melts that are featured all over social media and marketed in flavors like chocolate, strawberry, and vanilla, making it seem like the vagina should be an ice cream sundae.[33] All these products, though, can disrupt the delicate ecology of your vaginal microbiome, which contains billions of beneficial microorganisms, increasing your risk of itching, burning, infection, and foul-smelling, bad-tasting discharge. Yeah, not good. While you may be tempted to spritz some perfume or cologne, or apply a scented lotion down there, know that those may not only contain endocrine-disrupting chemicals, but may also taste terrible.

The even bigger problem with many so-called feminine hygiene products is that they reinforce what women have been led to think for centuries: that our vaginas are somehow dirty, smelly, and gross, and that we need to cover their natural odor and taste in order to avoid the shame ascribed to a vagina in the wild. This is complete and utter nonsense—there is absolutely *nothing* wrong with how a healthy vagina smells or tastes. In fact, your vagina has its own signature scent, made up of natural chemicals called pheromones.[34] You've likely heard about underwear fetishes, where people find themselves aroused by the odor that a well-worn pair of underwear can carry—and often, the more used, the better. Beyond fetish, both men[35] and women[36] report being turned on by the smell and taste of their partner, making a case for leaving things be if the goal is to get it on.

Is it that I don't enjoy receiving oral or is my partner just awful at it?

We all have our personal preferences, and whenever I receive this question, I always think, *One thing is for sure: You don't enjoy the way it's being performed currently.* So how can we make it better? First off, communication is key. (Through the page, I can see your eye roll at having to read this phrase for the zillionth time, but that doesn't change the fact that it still is true.) When it comes to receiving oral that brings you pleasure, you're going to need to be as clear with the directions as air traffic control is with a plane. Trust that your partner is doing this because they want to provide you pleasure, and that your direction should be welcomed. And remember: as we talked about in chapter 4, the clitoris is where it's at when it comes to the utmost pleasure. Inviting your partner to switch things up by treating the vulva like an ice cream cone, or flicking their tongue solely on the clitoris, can help you both explore what feels best. Sometimes guidance is needed here to help your partner get acquainted with your terrain.

Is oral sex completely safe, since I can't get pregnant?

The short answer is no. What prevents pregnancy doesn't always prevent STIs. It is possible to both transmit and contract an STI during oral sex, which means the need for regular screening still applies. Because human papillomavirus (HPV) is associated with the development of head and neck cancer, regular dental exams (at least once a year) should be part of your safe sex plan. You'll find more on HPV in chapter 7. In addition, dental dams (or Lorals, which are FDA-approved latex underwear that don't need to be held in place, unlike a dental dam) and condoms should be used to prevent the transmission of infection. While I've told you that flavored lubes are a no-no for the vagina, flavored dental dams and condoms for oral sex are a different story. Not only do some people find that these make the need for a barrier more pleasurable, but there is a very low risk of any significant amounts of chemicals disrupting your flora or pH. Are they going to have endocrine disruptors? Possibly, but it is highly unlikely this source is going to have a significant impact on your health.

Is it OK to have oral sex on my period or if I'm pregnant?

If you both consent, yes. Blood has a metallic taste, which means your partner may notice things are different down there when it's that time of the month. You can give them a heads-up on what to expect and discuss using a dental dam if it would make you both more comfortable.

Have you ever heard that you should never blow air into a pregnant woman's vagina because it could lead to death? While it sounds like an urban legend, it is actually true. In very rare cases, air introduced into the vagina can make its way into the bloodstream, resulting in an air embolism that can harm both the person who is pregnant and the baby.[37] This doesn't make oral sex dangerous, but it does mean you shouldn't treat the vagina like a balloon. Pregnancy complications can create special circumstances when it comes to sex, so when in doubt, ask your provider about what you should be aware of.

Should I be concerned if my partner's penis isn't circumcised?

In the United States, an uncircumcised penis is a rare find, with estimates showing about 58 to 71 percent are circumcised, compared to the global estimate of roughly 38 percent.[38] Uncircumcised penises are normal and, in fact, the ancient Greeks (who were said to be big fans of fellatio, as evidenced by their art[39]) considered the unaltered penis to be the perfect specimen.[40] Foreskin is an unsung hero in male pleasure. Because it is filled with nerves that detect both light touch and heat, similar to our lips or fingertips, it is highly sensitive. Some people believe that an uncircumcised penis is dirtier than a circumcised one, but if basic hygiene (think cleaning a vulva) is practiced, then this isn't an issue. It's a myth not unsimilar to that of vaginas smelling bad. There have been studies that show lower incidence of contracting HIV or STIs in circumcised men; however, it is debatable if this procedure is necessary, and it doesn't negate the need for a condom.[41] I recognize there are a lot of reasons people choose circumcision, some deeply rooted in religious belief. Please do not misconstrue my statement that there's nothing wrong with an uncircumcised penis as implying that there is something wrong with a circumcised one. Just like all vulvas are unique and beautiful, so are penises.

If you've never encountered an uncircumcised penis before, it can be understandably intimidating the first time it happens. Here are the tips I share with my patients:

Oral sex. Retracting the foreskin exposes the head of the penis, which can make oral sex much more pleasurable. It shouldn't hurt to retract the foreskin, but you should always ask your partner if it is OK to do so.

Hand jobs. When it comes to hand jobs, an intact penis may be more sensitive than penises you've experienced in the past. As such, you can ask your partner to place their hand over yours to show you how much pressure, or how long of a stroke, is their preference.

Condoms. If you're the one placing a condom, it is generally done by first retracting the foreskin. If it is your first time, ask your partner for feedback to ensure you've placed it in a way that is comfortable for you both, and effective.

Something a little different. Some people enjoy a well-lubricated finger placed between the penis and foreskin–just be careful of fingernails.

What's normal, what's not, when it comes to semen and sperm?

Remember that *Sex and the City* episode when Samantha brings up "funky spunk" over brunch with the girls? Specifically, she wants to know why her new guy has semen that tastes like "asparagus gone bad." IMO it's awesome to be curious like Samantha (maybe for other reasons, though) about what's normal and not normal when it comes to semen. Just like our discharge, there's normal or not-so-normal when talking about a guy's spunk, and if you're interacting with it, it helps to know the facts and warning signs. Let's go through some of the most common questions I get from patients and followers on social media.

How much semen is normal?

Despite what buddy comedies might say (looking at you, *Step Brothers*), the average man produces between 1⁄4 teaspoon and 1 teaspoon of ejaculate when he orgasms, which can be less if he's older, uses nicotine, eats a poor diet, or has a health condition.[42] The average ejaculate contains between 15 million to over 200 million sperm per milliliter,[43] which can live in the vagina for up to five days.[44] The notion that the fastest sperm wins the race and, therefore, gets to fertilize the egg is wrong. Newer science has shown us that vaginal discharge plays a large role in the process, and that the egg actually chooses the sperm.[45]

Is there less risk of pregnancy if he pulls out before he comes in me?

Pre-ejaculate, also known as pre-cum, is produced with arousal, before orgasm, and can contain live sperm that are "ready to mingle" with your egg. Meaning you can get pregnant (or an STI) if you're using the pull-out method without a condom or other protection.[46] While he can tell when he's about to have an orgasm, he can't tell if and when he's about to pre-ejaculate, so don't buy it if he says he'll pull out before any pre-cum is produced.[47] This is, in part, what contributes to the 1 in 5 pregnancy rate when couples use the pull-out method alone.

Is semen supposed to be thick or watery?

Normal semen should be thick and viscous, similar to an egg white consistency. (Sound familiar?) Funny how women get the not-so-fun-sounding term "cervical mucus," but penile mucus gets not one, but two special terms—"ejaculate" and "semen," even though it has a mucus consistency. If semen looks watery or curdled, though, it could be an indication of low sperm count or an infection.

Healthy semen should also be white or slightly gray, although taking some supplements or medications, eating certain foods high in sulfur or other plant compounds, using nicotine, needing to pee, or not ejaculating for days can give it a yellowish appearance.[48] Yellow-ejaculate, semen that looks greenish or contains blood, however, can be also a sign of an STI, especially if he has other symptoms.[49] If you see semen that's a dark yellow or green, he most likely has an STI such as gonorrhea.[50]

Is it normal if it smells like bleach?

Healthy semen shouldn't have any off-putting smell, either. If you get a whiff of ammonia, bleach, or bathroom cleaner, that's normal and all thanks to the chloride content. Semen has a pH of about 7.2 to 7.4, which is alkaline, or basic. (Did I just call semen basic? Yes I did. It is. But not like that.) This contributes to a bit of an odor and is necessary for sperm to survive the acidic vagina. If you're smelling something fishy or foul, he could have an STI, and you should definitely step away from the penis until he's been tested.

What happens when you swallow sperm? Will I be less likely to get an STI?

First, semen and sperm aren't the same thing. If you're swallowing, you're ingesting both, but let's break it down. Semen, also called ejaculate, is the whitish substance that comes out of a penis with orgasm. Sperm, on the other hand, are those squiggly little cells that can fertilize an egg. Semen helps carry sperm into the vagina and is full of protein, sugar, vitamins, and minerals to help nourish them as they make the trip. It also carries unwanted cells, like the kind that cause STIs. Now, I've had many patients under the impression that their stomach acid will kill all invaders, and while I like this sophisticated thinking, your mouth, throat, tonsils, and everything before your stomach is susceptible. We'll talk more about STIs in chapter 7, but gonorrhea, herpes, chlamydia, HPV, and the whole lot of them don't care which orifice it is—they are always down to invade and cause an infection. Let's normalize having conversations about testing and using barriers for oral sex, OK? (See the information beginning on page 178 about how to use barriers to prevent STIs.)

How nutritious is semen?

Contrary to popular belief, it is not a great source of protein . . . unless you drink, like, a gallon of it. Let's be real, no one is doing that. If you've ever had someone try to persuade you to swallow by citing nutrition facts, know it is not as nutritious as many people believe.[51] But let's say each set of testicles came with a nutrition label; what might it say? Semen contains 5 to 25 calories, depending on how much is produced. When it comes to nutrients, you'll find traces of calcium, magnesium, zinc, selenium, phosphorous, and vitamin C, as well as sodium and potassium. Make no mistake, we're not even edging close to the recommended daily allowance (RDA) here for it to be a meal replacement. While it does contain sugar, like female discharge, the amount is negligible and won't ruin your keto diet or break your intermittent fasting routine.

Will swallowing semen make me happy?

Well, almost certainty it will make *him* happy. *Ba-dum ching.* All joking aside, it may in fact be a mood booster.[52] Semen contains the hormones progesterone, estrone (a type of estrogen), serotonin, and oxytocin, all of which elicit a positive effect on mood. It also contains thyrotropin-releasing hormone, which is involved in thyroid hormone production. In addition to some of the nutrients discussed, semen, when coupled with these hormones, may have mood-benefiting properties. But you may not need to swallow it. Remember from chapter 2 that your vagina is a mucus membrane that shares the same tissue as your mouth? Well, it just may be that it's worth potentially disrupting your pH, as it may boost your mood. Please note that semen is not a substitute for medication, and that STIs are bad for your mood, so be wise.

Why do I feel so sleepy after he comes in me?

OK, so the act alone or an orgasm can set off a hormone cascade that helps you get to sleep faster, and maybe even get more quality sleep. Is it just the semen? Hard to say, but it does contain melatonin, so maybe there's something to that.

Will adding semen to my skin care routine improve my skin?

Maybe you saw the TikToks circulating with women showing us their nightly skin care routine that included applying their partner's ejaculate to their face. As of now, the science on the spunk is bunk when it comes to anti-aging. While it is a source of antioxidants like glutathione, superoxide dismutase, and vitamin E, it's not even close to the amounts you can get in an over-the-counter product that can actually help your skin. In addition, as we talk about on page 176, some people are allergic, so keep that in mind.

Is semen supposed to be salty?

How semen tastes and smells varies, and has a lot to do with who is tasting and smelling it. Just like none of us taste or smell a strawberry the same way, the same applies here. Some would describe the taste as sweet, while others describe it as more bitter or salty, all of which is totally normal and may be reflective of him or your taste receptors. But there are some things that make for some funky spunk. A man's ejaculate can vary if he smokes, drinks a lot of alcohol, eats a lot of garlic, or is dehydrated—all of which can make it far from desirable.

Cum Quiz

Evaluate your ejaculate expertise with this true-or-false quiz. The answers are below. Read the "What's Normal for Semen and Sperm" section for more details.

1. Semen is high in protein. _____
2. Semen contains calcium. _____
3. Semen applied to the skin can reverse the effects of aging. _____
4. Semen contains progesterone. _____
5. Semen can boost your mood. _____
6. There's no risk of STI if you swallow. _____
7. About a cup of ejaculate is released with each orgasm. _____
8. There's no risk of pregnancy if he pulls out before he ejaculates. _____
9. Semen should be watery. _____
10. Semen that smells like bleach means he has an infection. _____
11. Green semen can mean he has an STI. _____
12. The fastest sperm fertilizes the egg. _____
13. Semen is alkaline. _____
14. The taste of semen is always salty. _____
15. Smoking can make his semen taste bad. _____

1. False 2. True 3. False 4. True 5. True 6. False 7. False 8. False 9. False
10. False 11. True 12. False 13. True 14. False 15. True

5 WAYS FOR HIM TO FIX THE FUNKY SPUNK

- Stop smoking.
- Avoid heavy alcohol use.
- Drink plenty of water.
- Avoid asparagus, lots of garlic, and other strong-odor foods.
- Try wheatgrass.

Anal Sex: Is it normal to be interested in anal sex and what should I know about it?

"Anal play" is the umbrella term for all sexual activity involving the anus, including anal intercourse, anilingus (giving or receiving oral sex around the anus), and manually stimulating the anus. And in the 2020s, there seems to be more openness about anal. According to PornHub, online searches for anal sex jumped by 120 percent in recent years.[53] Major media brands like *Men's Health* and *Glamour* are also running articles targeted mostly to heterosexual readers on why and how to try anal play. This all comes after years of stigma around anal sex, and horrific sodomy laws that criminalized anal intercourse for both heterosexual and homosexual people (FYI, the US Supreme Court declared sodomy laws unconstitutional in 2003, although a few states still force those "caught" having anal sex to register as sex offenders).[54] Today, around 40 percent of straight women and men have tried anal intercourse, and even more have tried anal play by using a finger, toy, or tongue to stimulate the area.[55]

Why do people want to have anal sex?

The anus is an erogenous zone, packed with nerves, including the pudendal nerve, which connects to the clitoris. Both women and men can feel a great amount of pleasure from anal play. I've also had patients ask me if it's weird that they're able to orgasm more easily when their partner stimulates their anus while they're having vaginal sex. It's not. At the same time, anal play isn't for everyone, and if you never want to try it, that's totally normal and just fine.

Is anal sex dangerous?

Anal play isn't dangerous if you use lube, wear protection, and change condoms before proceeding to any other area of the body.

Unlike the vagina, the anus is not self-lubricating, and trauma can occur when there isn't sufficient lube. While bowel perforation—when there is a rupture in the wall of your colon—is rare, without lube you can develop microtears, which can cause bleeding and pain and increase the risk of infection, including STI transmission. Silicone-based lube is best for anal sex, since it lasts longer than water-based lube.

In addition, you should always consider wearing a condom, dental dam, or finger condom, even if you and your partner have been tested for STIs, as the bacteria that live back there can cause infections elsewhere. All these barriers are single use, meaning if you use them for the anus, they should be tossed after and not used again for the vagina. No matter how well someone washes or whether you do an enema beforehand, poop can still exist in and around the anus and spread to your partner's penis, tongue, or finger, putting you at risk for a possible infection. Washing anything that comes into contact with the anus is a must, especially before returning to the vagina. Covering a toy with a condom is another way to cut down on the risk of transferring organisms to other parts of the body.

Is it supposed to hurt?

It can if you're not relaxed and well lubricated. Just like the vagina, the anus also has muscles that need to relax for it to feel pleasurable. Since it can be difficult to relax when trying anything for the first time, it's best to go slow and communicate with your partner. It may be helpful to work your way up to anal intercourse, starting with manual or oral stimulation outside the anus. When you feel comfortable, try inserting a finger, then eventually a toy or your partner's penis. As always, good communication is critical.

Is bleeding normal?

A small amount of blood isn't abnormal, especially if you've had a vigorous sesh or haven't applied enough lube. If you find a small amount of blood on your toilet paper, in your stool, or in the toilet, monitor it, but don't panic.

If the toilet water contains a lot of blood, your stool is completely covered in blood, it saturates your underwear, or it is continuous, see your doctor. Also, any bleeding other than a spot or two that occurs during the act is a red light to stop what you're doing.

Is it possible to get pregnant with anal sex?

You can't get pregnant in most cases. In extremely rare cases, this has happened due to an anal fistula, which is an abnormal opening between the anus and vagina. But again, it's super rare, and if you have an anal fistula, you'd also have a lot of other issues that would already have you in a doctor's office.

Can anal sex cause hemorrhoids or incontinence?

Anal sex shouldn't affect your ability to poop or cause things to become so loose that you have to worry about it leaking out. If you already have hemorrhoids, though, anal sex can irritate them.

How do you clean up after anal sex?

While it's hard to hit pause when things are hot and heavy, it's really important to wash anything that touches the anus *before* it touches anything else. Anal play can spread bacteria and viruses to other areas, including your bed, bedroom furniture, cell phone, and other objects you might touch after sex. If you're using condoms or dental dams, trash them after anal sex and use new protection to keep going. Even if you're not using condoms or dental dams, go to the bathroom immediately after anal play and wash hands and penises with warm water and soap, or rinse your mouth with water or mouthwash. (FYI, the jury is out on whether brushing teeth after anilingus is a good thing since it may cause tiny tears in the gums, potentially allowing bacteria to enter.) The take-home is we need to wash up afterward, and unlike the vagina, this area does need soap.

Is it normal for my anus to be darker than my cheeks?

Whatever the natural color your anus is, that's normal. The anus is darker than the rest of your body due to the concentration of melanocytes (pigment cells). While the rumors on the Internet may lead you to believe your body should be one uniform color, I want to assure you that's not true; in fact, that's called Photoshop. If you find it is deviating from its normal color (e.g., red, dark blue, white and scaly) or there are lumps, bumps, or tears, then it's time to see your provider. Human papillomavirus (HPV) can cause warts, which can show up as small bumps and grow to have a cauliflower appearance. While rare, melanoma, a form of skin cancer, can develop on your anus, so if you see changes that look suspicious, go to the doctor, not the aesthetician. I know—new fear unlocked. But you've gotta know this stuff.

Anal bleaching, a cosmetic treatment that lightens skin around the anus, can cause burns, discomfort, and even permanent scarring and discoloration. You can also develop fissures in your rectum that will cause major pooping problems for the rest of your life. BTW, butt hair is normal, too, and if you want to remove it, that's OK, but please first jump to page 38 to get in the know on that one.

Outercourse: Is it normal if I enjoy (and even orgasm) with everything but intercourse?

Many people can remember a time where kissing or, heck, holding hands was the most thrilling experience. But somewhere in the journey sex became a penetrative act, and for some (many, if you're one of the hetero women lost in the abyss of the orgasm gap we talked about in chapter 4), far less exciting and satisfying. But for many of my patients, sexual activity that's satisfying and pleasurable involves "outercourse." For many people, outercourse refers to everything that isn't penile-vaginal sex. It's a problematic definition when you consider that it centers vaginal sex as the norm. Not only is there a wide variety of sexual acts to choose from—a buffet, if you will—but this definition also creates a perception of what should be the standard, and anything that can't meet that standard is somehow defective. Amber, like the millions of other women struggling with pain with sex, couldn't tolerate, let alone enjoy, penetration. Yes, oral sex performed on a woman is considered outercourse by many definitions because it is nonpenetrative, but there's many other ways people find pleasure that are normal, healthy, and satisfying.

If you're thinking outercourse sounds like some high school BS, I would challenge you to reexamine your views on sex and consider that the following are technically considered outercourse. In addition, the nostalgia of reengaging in acts that were once incredibly exciting can have the effect of enhancing sexual pleasure.

- Oral sex
- Kissing (not just on the mouth)
- Frottage (dry humping)
- Tribadism (scissoring)
- Erotic touch or massage
- External toys, like vibrators
- Mutual masturbation
- Nipple play
- BDSM acts like spanking
- Voyeurism (pleasure from watching someone naked or engaging in sexual behavior, or in being so watched)

Why would someone choose outercourse?

Other than pain with sex, which we've discussed, some people choose outercourse to avoid STIs or pregnancy, or while healing from a medical condition or procedure, or because it is something highly exciting and pleasurable for them. While outercourse may sound like a risk-free alternative to intercourse, it's not—HPV, herpes, and other STIs can still be contracted depending on what acts you're engaging in. Some people use outercourse as a way to spice things up in their relationship or revisit acts that in the past have been immensely pleasurable, and it is sometimes incorporated into role-playing. Beyond healing from trauma or avoiding acts that cause pain, outercourse can be a way to deepen communication and explore other erogenous zones that bring you both pleasure.

What's the difference between outercourse and foreplay?

Foreplay implies that what you're doing is in preparation for penetration. With outercourse, you're engaging in and enjoying what you're doing with no expectation or anticipation that penetration will follow.

TL;DR: SEX OF ALL KINDS

- Painful sex is common, but it's not normal: it can and should be treated.
- Vaginal dryness is a common cause of pain with sex, and the solution is simple—use lube.
- Endometriosis, vaginismus, vulvodynia, and adenomyosis are commonly missed conditions that can cause pain with sex.
- No, drinking wine won't solve your sex problems, no matter how many doctors say so.
- You can increase how wet you get naturally with a few very easy tips and tricks.
- Different types of lubes are better for certain uses (e.g., shower sex, anal sex, sex with condoms, etc.) than others.
- Size does matter, but not in the way you think.
- Flavored lubes are for a penis during oral sex, but should be washed off before switching to vaginal sex.
- Barriers are intended to be used in one area and then thrown away.
- Great communication is essential to having pleasurable vaginal, oral, and anal sex.
- Most penises aren't circumcised, and that's normal.
- Anal sex is normal, safe to practice, and doesn't result in hemorrhoids or incontinence.
- Outercourse isn't just an alternative to painful sex; it could spice up your love life.
- There's a cum quiz. Seriously, go take it.

CHAPTER 6

IS MASTURBATION NORMAL?

WHY PARTIES OF ONE ARE FUN AND GOOD FOR YOU

I never set out to be one of those people whose vibrator went off in the TSA line, let alone rolling with a bag of them through the airport. Turns out that no amount of double-checking that every off switch was in the correct position, or removal of all the batteries, could save me from that mortifying moment.

Several years ago, I was in LA for the annual Biohacking conference and was making guest appearances on several podcasts, including *Sex with Emily* with the astoundingly knowledgeable and playful host, Dr. Emily Morse (if you haven't heard of her, she's the Dr. Ruth of the 2020s; check her out). So it should come as no surprise when I tell you that this woman took my sex toy knowledge (and collection) to the next level. Her parting gift to me was a trip to a well-organized closet of adult goodies, including dildos, vibrators, lubes, and more. She excitedly asked what I would like, as I stood there with my eyes wide and jaw hanging slightly open. I had so. Many. Thoughts. I was excited. I wanted to choose wisely, like I was Indiana Jones presented with the Holy Grail, or a kid at Willy Wonka's factory. Because what does it say about me if I tell her I want this item, and don't choose another? Excitement ultimately won, with each of us swapping stories while Emily placed one toy after another in my hands—I'd seriously gotten the Golden Ticket here—until, like a small baby, my arms were holding a trove of toys. The crew managed to find me a tote, but that could hold only so many. Cue the image of me climbing into an Uber with toys spilling across the back seat. Wait for it—it gets even more awkward.

As I arrived at my hotel before my evening flight, I had to cross the lobby filled with colleagues, including people who had come to the conference just to see me, and my brain reminded me that in the age of social media, yes, everyone does have a phone. I made it to my hotel room undetected. Phew! "OMG, why did I have to take the Magic Wand?" I sighed exasperatedly as I tried to fit the monstrous beast of pleasure into my bag. I pressed on, trying different configurations, double-checking that each item was going to be cool and that none would go popping off as we went through airport security. Fortunately, my Tetris skills were on lock that day and everyone, including my cute shoes, made it in the bag.

At LAX the next day, I found myself unjustifiably confident that getting through security was going to be more than fine. Without a hitch, I made my way through the airport and placed my bag on the conveyor belt. *You got this*, I thought, giving myself an inner wink. Then my bag stopped, reversed, then moved forward again. Nope. Stopped. Back it up. OK, here it goes. Nope. I can only imagine what I looked like watching my bag go back and forth, until it came to a halt and the TSA agent gave me a glance. He called yet another agent to his side. I felt the knots in my stomach begin to build and twist. Then I saw the giggles. *Wait, they're laughing? OMG, this is funny to them.* I watched their eyes dart from the X-ray to me. Then it hit me: I was wearing faux leather leggings with black thigh-high boots and a leopard blouse, had bright red lips, and had a bag full of sex toys. No, I had not in fact thought this through. As their eyes made their way to me, I decided to embrace the awkward. "Listen," I called to the agents, "I have a suitcase full of sex toys. I'm more than happy to open it up and show you them and answer any questions you might have." Their eyes quickly met the floor, faces turning red. Then one gave me a short "That's OK" as my bag was spat out onto the conveyor. As I grabbed my bag, one female agent asked me, "OK, so what is it that you do?" I laughed and said, "Would you believe I'm a doctor?" She raised one brow and said, "I think I need a doctor like you." We shared a laugh and I made it to my plane just in time to grab my seat.

I share this story with you because it highlights three important things:

One, everyone has their awkward sex-related stories (trust, that's not my only one); two, everyone is curious about topics society has put the hush on; and three, sex is humorous, so it's OK to laugh (just not at the expense of other people). And let me be clear: sex toys are allowed by TSA in carry-on luggage.[1]

There's an interesting dichotomy where we find ourselves simultaneously fascinated by and wary of sex toys since they're so strongly associated with masturbation. (Psst: partnered sex can use toys, too.) And no matter your gender, you will not dodge the masturbation myths and attempts at shame that pervade our culture in this lifetime. Allow me to ruin Halloween for you, because those witches you see riding brooms are born out of seventeenth-century England, a time when banned sex toys inspired creativity and women crafted their own from broomsticks. This also doubled to deliver otherwise purge-inducing herbs in a more tolerable way—soaking the broomsticks in the herbs and inserting them into the vagina, hence, witches riding the broom.[2] Suppositories sure have come a long way. BTW, if you're not catching on to the negative vibes around masturbation, "witches" were tortured and killed. This underscores not just shame, but a real level of fear that surrounds masturbation. If you're wondering what myths are true, if masturbation can really hurt you, and if there is any medical benefit to it, this chapter is going to give you the science behind all of it.

ASK DR. BRIGHTEN:

Are the myths about masturbation true?

OK, so I know I said Freud was the worst, but Jean-Étienne Esquirol is a close second. Way back in 1816, this French psychiatrist wrote with certainty that "masturbation is recognized in all countries as a common cause of insanity."[3] The only thing insane here is that it took until 1968 for masturbation to be removed from the *Diagnostic and Statistical Manual of Mental Disorders* (DSM) as a diagnosable condition. Look who caught up in 1972: the American Medical Association publicly states masturbation is normal.[4] And since we're keeping tabs here, hysteria (Hippocrates, the father of modern medicine, proposed our uterus wandered our body, making us crazy) wasn't removed from the DSM until 1980.[5] Fast-forward to 1994 when US surgeon general Joycelyn Elders is fired for suggesting masturbation be taught as part of sex ed to prevent the spread of AIDS.[6] If you feel your views of masturbation are in any way messed up—you're not messed up, our history is messed up, and I'm here to set the record straight.

MYTH #1: MASTURBATION HAS NO BENEFITS AND ONLY CAUSES HARM.

Masturbation doesn't cause harm, full stop. At the same time, solo sex has numerous health benefits. I'll name just a few biggies here: it can help reduce stress, improve how long and how well you sleep, boost your mood, increase your self-esteem, improve your body image, ease menstrual cramps, relieve headaches, decrease pain, and strengthen the muscles in and around your pelvic floor.[7] Masturbation is an important medical treatment for female orgasmic disorder and as part of rehabilitation for spinal cord injuries.[8] In addition, while erectile dysfunction gets a lot of play in our culture, finishing too early is actually the biggest complaint men have. Masturbating in anticipation of partnered sex may delay ejaculation due to the refractory period and prolactin hormone discussed in chapter 4. Everyone's refractory period is different, it may be minutes to hours, so this will have to be dialed in to your needs.

All the health benefits of having orgasms—see page 95 for a reminder of these—are true if you climax during solo sex, but without the risk of pregnancy or an STI.

MYTH #2: MASTURBATION DAMAGES YOUR GENITALS OR CAUSES INFECTIONS.

Sure, should you choose to go at it lube free, there's going to be problems. If solo sex is ever irritating or chafing, then, just like other sex, you likely need a little lube. You won't be putting yourself at risk for STIs, but depending on hygiene (clean your toys! See page 154) and the lube, you could throw off your pH and encourage overgrowth of organisms that already live in your vagina. But these risks are the same, if not more, when you're with a partner, since other people's flora, friction, and the presence of semen can disrupt your microbiome and pH (see chapter 7 for more on this). Important to note is in one study, over 70 percent of those who use a vibrator reported never having any negative side effects, and those who did noted that they were temporary and self-resolved.[9] On the other hand, not all objects are designed for pleasure, and retained objects (we'll talk about how to avoid this in the section on sex toys on page 153) pose one of the greatest risks, solo or partnered.[10]

MYTH #3: IF YOU MASTURBATE, YOU HAVE A MENTAL HEALTH ISSUE, ARE ADDICTED, OR AT RISK OF DEVELOPING A MENTAL ILLNESS.

You can feel compelled to masturbate, but there is no scientific evidence to support the idea of masturbation as sex addiction. Masturbation can present a problem if it becomes distracting or distressing, undermines relationships, or is carried out in public, but on its own it is not a mental health issue. The much more common and larger issue we see with masturbation is guilt and shame, which can seriously chip away at mental health. *The stigma around masturbation is more damaging than the act of masturbation.*[11] If you're struggling with this, meet with a certified sex therapist or counselor to help you heal. I'd also recommend the book *The Myth of Sex Addiction* by Dr. David J. Ley.

MYTH #4: MASTURBATION WILL PREVENT YOU FROM BEING ABLE TO ORGASM WITH A PARTNER AND ENJOY VAGINAL SEX.

The opposite is true, since it may improve your ability to climax by helping you know and locate your pleasure points, increase your natural lubrication levels, tone your pelvic floor, and reduce any pain or discomfort you might feel during sex. And once again, you can enjoy all these benefits without *any* of the risks that come with partnered sex.

MYTH #5: MASTURBATION WILL NUMB YOUR CLITORIS.

Hear me now: masturbation just may save your clitoris! (Need a refresher? We covered clitoral atrophy in chapter 4, which is when the clitoris shrinks with too little stimulation.) Concerned about vibrators? A small study showed (and many of my patients report) no issues with numbing or damaging the clitoris.[12] Truth be told, spin classes or horseback riding can be more traumatic to your clit than most sex toys (although it still won't permanently numb your clitoris).

MYTH #6: MASTURBATION WILL PREVENT YOU FROM HAVING A RELATIONSHIP.

There's this huge misconception that if you masturbate regularly for long enough, you won't want to find a partner or be able to be turned on by anyone else other than your own hand or sex toy. Which is totally false. Quite the opposite is true: masturbation may even raise your libido and arousal levels, increasing your appetite for and enjoyment of partnered sex. When it comes to vibrator use, studies have shown a positive relationship between desire, arousal, lubrication, and the ability to orgasm and experience less pain.[13]

MYTH #7: IF YOU'RE MASTURBATING IN A RELATIONSHIP, THERE'S SOMETHING WRONG WITH YOUR RELATIONSHIP OR YOU'RE CHEATING.

Some people think women have a limited amount of sexual energy, and that masturbation threatens to use it up. True, there is a refractory period (discussed in chapter 4) that can impact when a man can ejaculate again, but when it comes to sexual desire, masturbation for either sex will not make the well run dry. In fact, studies have shown that when sexual frequency goes up in a relationship, women masturbate more.[14] For men, if frequency goes down then they might masturbate more, but only if they are unsatisfied by the decline in frequency. Masturbation is never an indicator that you, your partner, or your relationship isn't "enough" or is unsatisfying in some way. And it's never cheating.

MYTH #8: MASTURBATION CAUSES INFERTILITY.

Nope, definitely not true. On the contrary, climaxing during masturbation (and partnered sex) can help balance and optimize hormones while increasing immune function, all of which can boost your ability to conceive. See chapter 4 for more.

MYTH #9: MASTURBATION CAUSES HAIR TO GROW ON YOUR HANDS AND WILL MAKE YOU GO BLIND.

If these tall tales were true, we'd see hairy palms everywhere. These myths likely have Victorian origins, with hair on the palms being a sign of laziness, something heavily associated with masturbation. The original stories of Dracula alluded to him being a chronic masturbator, describing his palms as having hair.[15] Yes, masturbation was just that scary. Benjamin Rush, a physician who also signed his name on the Declaration of Independence, is credited with the myth that you could go blind. In reality, it was more likely undiagnosed STIs or other infections that were behind the loss of sight. BTW, he also thought leeches were the solution for treating masturbation, nymphomania (sex excess in women), and satyrism (sex excess in men). There's no real condition of excess sex, and leeches on the genitals won't keep your brain from desiring it.

MYTH #10: MASTURBATION CAUSES ACNE OR IS BAD FOR YOUR SKIN.

Some people think that masturbation increases testosterone, which, in turn, makes your skin break out. It's true, as we discussed in chapter 4, that an orgasm can bump your testosterone levels, but it is temporary. Judging teens with acne is lame, and placing blame on them, as if masturbating is causing their skin struggles, is worse. If anything, the oxytocin, DHEA, and increased blood flow that accompanies orgasms could have anti-aging effects and benefit your skin greatly.

How often is it normal to masturbate?

If you masturbate daily, weekly, monthly, or even yearly, that's all normal. According to one survey, 22 percent of women masturbate several times per month, 20 percent do it at least once a week, 19 percent do it a few times a week, and 6 percent do it daily.[16] However, surveys are highly dependent on people being honest about masturbation habits, and some have shown nearly 30 percent lie about solo sex at some point in their lives.[17] Other research has found that sex surveys in general are often inaccurate, since participants can be dishonest or uncomfortable about sharing their personal proclivities, even when their identities are kept anonymous.[18] As we've already discussed, shame and stigma added to the mix means there's no way we're getting accurate data. So how often is it normal to masturbate? In most cases, as often as you feel stirred to do so.

Is it normal if I never masturbate?

If you're not down to get down with yourself, that's totally fine. If you do want to masturbate, but you're struggling with feeling shame or like something is wrong with you, you're not alone.

While hand-to-genitals is the type of masturbation we most commonly see represented in the media, it's not fully representative. Lack of masturbation can be due to difficulty or inability to self-stimulate, especially when you consider most pleasure devices are designed for able bodies. In chapter 4 we discussed the orgasm gap, but there is a little-known pleasure gap in the disabled community. In one small survey, 56 percent of disabled people reported difficulty self-pleasuring, with 63 percent citing hand limitations as a primary challenge.[19] While the World Health Organization (WHO) classifies sexual pleasure as a human right, we aren't seeing changes in health care that enable everyone to achieve such pleasure. What's worse, research has shown that following spinal cord injuries, pleasure isn't even part of most rehab plans.[20] Disabilities aren't limited to what we see on the outside, as the millions of women diagnosed with autoimmune disease can attest. It's normal to mourn the sex you had before your disability, especially when it is rare for a provider to discuss this aspect of managing your health when you're handed a life-changing diagnosis. The good news is that there's hope. I'll highlight in the sex toy section on page 150 some items that are working to close the pleasure gap. One resource I recommend is *Pleasure ABLE*, a medical manual on how to adapt toys and leverage furniture to help those with medical disabilities. *The Bump'n Book of Love, Lust & Disability* is another sex-positive resource for those with disabilities and the Bump'n company is working to market the Joystick, a toy designed by and for disabled people.

What if I used to masturbate but have now lost interest altogether?

When some people get stressed or tired, they don't have the mental or physical bandwidth for solo sex, which can be normal. But if you find that your libido takes a nosedive alongside your masturbation habits, I'd say it's time to make an appointment to see your provider, as it could indicate an underlying medical condition or that stress is taking a serious toll on your health. Hormonal changes from pregnancy, being postpartum, or from menopause can also change your masturbation habits, which is normal. But if you're not satisfied or you're concerned, try out what you learn in this book and get support when needed.

Is it masturbation even if I don't have an orgasm?

There's that pressure to orgasm coming back at us. A pleasurable sexual experience is more than just an orgasm. If you're engaging in erotic self-touch, you're masturbating. If you don't orgasm, but you feel satisfied, then that's all that matters.

Is it safe to masturbate on my period?

Totally safe and maybe even helpful. As we'll discuss in chapter 9, orgasms and period sex have menstrual benefits—masturbation is no exception.

How *should* women masturbate? How do I know if how I masturbate is normal?

There's no one best way to masturbate. Some choose to stimulate themselves externally (most common), internally, or both, using their hands or objects, like toys. And similar to intercourse, there is no "normal" position you have to be in to masturbate. Just remember not to put anything up your vagina that doesn't belong there—see page 47 for a reminder.

Is it normal to use sex toys?

If you too became the proud owner of a new gadget with the onset of the COVID-19 pandemic, you're not alone. Sex toy sales boomed and rivaled hand sanitizer sales as people took their self-care (and isolation coping skills) to the next level.[21] And it wasn't just because oxytocin is great for the immune system and masturbation may improve immune function.[22] In fact, it may very well have been because 80 percent of people in the US view masturbation as a form of self-care and used it as a way to manage the stress of the pandemic.[23]

Sex toys have been around since the dawn of civilization, with evidence of ancient Greeks constructing them out of brass, leather, and old loaves of bread.[24] Cleopatra allegedly attempted the first vibrator by filling a gourd full of live bees. (Kind of brilliant, if you ask me, unless one gets out. Ouch!) The Han dynasty had some of the OGs of kink, with jade butt plugs (although these may have been reserved for spiritual practice) and bronze strap-ons reserved for the upper class of society.[25] Oh to be on these archeological digs! The evolution of sex toys has brought us next-level advances that our ancestors could only dream of. Basically, if you can think of a way to stimulate your genitalia, there's a sex toy out there to do it for you. But despite the shift in some people's perspective, shame and stigma are still a major factor in why women feel inhibited and intimidated in obtaining a toy. Again: thanks, Freud, for ruining a good time.

Here are some popular categories of sex toys:

Vibrators stimulate the clitoris, vagina, or anus by using pulses or vibrations that can be constant or intermittent in frequency. Some are designed to stimulate your external clit; others can penetrate your vagina, anus, or both at the same time; others mimic cunnilingus. There are vibrators to stimulate penises as cuffs or during intercourse, in case your partner feels left out. Vibrators can take on many shapes and forms. A few examples: they can look like a penis, a tongue, a clitoris-sucking squirrel, an elephant with a changeable trunk, or nothing at all. There are also wearable devices that double as an accessory, like Crave's Vesper necklace, which will make you feel like a secret agent of solo sex. Seriously, Q from James Bond couldn't make a gadget so clever. Some are hands free while others can be controlled by a remote or Bluetooth, which can allow you to control the settings from any position or put your partner in charge. You can also find vibrators that cover just your fingertips; and vibrating panties, which you can wear and operate from your smartphone. More toys are being made with the disabled community in mind, which is why I love Dame's Fin, which comes with a finger strap for extended reach.

Dildos are essentially artificial penises that come in many different materials. Some are flexible, while others, like those made from break-resistant glass and metal, are firm. You can find thrusting dildos, which expand and retract inside you, or custom-molding kits that you can use to make a casting of your partner's penis. There are also strap-on dildos, which are worn with a harness and are typically used during partnered sex.

Pumps are devices that create suction around your clitoris, vulva, or vagina. Some are hand-operated while others are battery-powered. Pumps increase blood flow to the vagina and may help strengthen your pelvic floor and improve lubrication levels. They can also help with female orgasmic disorder (discussed in chapter 4) and help maintain the health of your clitoris. This is why the Eros clitoral therapy device is FDA-approved to help treat reduced sensation, lubrication, and ability to achieve orgasm.[26]

Butt plugs are meant to be placed inside your anus to stimulate the sensitive nerves that some report can make for a fant-ass-tic time. If you've never tried anal play, butt plugs can help train your sphincter muscles to relax during anal penetration. All butt plugs should have a flared base so that they can't slip and get lodged up your rectum. If this happens, you'll have to see a doctor to get it removed, which I know is a visit no one wants to schedule, but it is definitely necessary.

Anal beads are a stimulating series of bulbs on a cord that resemble a beaded necklace. They are designed for the inside of the anus, with a safety handle or loop so they do not enter the land of no return (which is when you need to see a doctor). There's also vibrating anal beads. Anal beads used for the anus stay in the anal play-only arena. Do not take those beads to the vagina. You can get a different set for that.

Nipple clamps cinch your nipples, causing pressure or even slight pain while stimulating the nerves there with or without vibration. Some clamps include chains that you or your partner can tug or pull or that connect to a **clit clamp**, which is designed to be attached to your external clitoris and stimulate the nerves there. If you want to use a nipple or clit clamp, experiment first by putting the device on a less sensitive body part, like your finger or toe. When using clamps, some choose to remove them before they climax, which will create a rush of sensation that can increase the orgasmic experience. As with anything that can cut off blood flow, check on the health of the tissue—extensive use or too much impingement can cause nerve damage.

Ben Wa balls are weighted balls designed to go inside your vagina and stay there. Ben Wa balls, sometimes called Kegel balls, are primarily used to strengthen the muscles in and around the vagina and pelvic floor, but can also create pleasure for some women. If you're using them for therapy, make sure you're working with an expert because, without supervision, it could make issues like pain and incontinence worse.

Sex furniture is exactly what it sounds like: stuff you use solo or with a partner for having sex that's not the typical bed, couch, or kitchen counter. Sex furniture includes items like sex swings, chairs, hammocks, wedges (similar to yoga blocks, helping you to assume certain positions), elastic balls, saddles, benches, and racks, some of which are constructed with vibrators or dildos for solo sex fun. For example, the Magic Ball looks and feels like a Swiss ball but has a dildo and two handles to allow penetration and bouncing at the same time. The Perfect Pleasure Cushion, designed by someone with a disability, allows you to get into more positions, use toys hands free, and makes pleasure possible for all bodies.

What kind of sex toys are best? Is there anything I should avoid?

Durable, nonporous, and actually built for sex are best when getting it on, as opposed to items you find around the house. While these, like the "red light" list on page 47, may sound tempting, I assure you that it's all fun and games until you're dealing with a genital injury or hanging out in the ER waiting for someone to retrieve an object. The sex toy industry isn't regulated by the Food and Drug Administration (FDA) or by any other consumer agency, and many items include toxic materials that can disrupt hormone production and cause other health concerns. You wouldn't put phthalates in your mouth (they are banned, at least, in pacifiers) because they can mess with your hormones, so don't go putting them directly in the area where you make those hormones.[27] The squishier the toy, the higher the probability it has phthalates, even if it says phthalate-free. (Because who is going to check? The manufacturer knows the answer is: no one.) In general, the safest sex toys are made from break-resistant glass, stainless steel, and medical-grade silicone.

Porous toys, like those made from rubber, jelly, PVC, vinyl, and silicone blends, can harbor microorganisms that can fester and infect you on next use, even if you clean them thoroughly. If you choose to use porous toys, always cover them with a condom, even if using them alone or with an exclusive partner who's been STI tested. Porous toys can also hang on to microscopic amounts of any soap or detergent you use to clean toys, which can irritate sensitive skin when you use them again.

Not all lubes are compatible with toys. For a list of which lubes are safe for sex toys, see page 125.

Where should I buy my toys?

Well, it depends on where you live. If you reside in Alabama, you can own a sex toy, but you may not purchase it. In Texas you can own only six dildos, which means you can have more guns than sex toys. Laws and restrictions like these can drive people to seedy Internet sites or questionable locations just to get their hands on a vibrator. When it comes to down there, make sure what you're using is legit. Buying your toys from legitimate stores and websites can help ensure quality, safe products. If you have access to a high-end sex toy or adult entertainment store, I recommend shopping in person so that staff can help recommend safe toys based on your preferences or intended uses, plus show you how to clean and store them. If you feel embarrassed to shop in person, keep in mind that these people chose to work there, and it's very unlikely you'll be sharing anything that they haven't heard before.

If you're shopping online, look for discreet shipping practices. Many sellers will ship your package so your mail delivery person won't be able to tell.

How to clean and store sex toys

Safe sex is the best kind of sex, always. Learning how to properly clean and store your toys is the only way to make sure things stay safe. Here's how:

1. With clean hands, wash toys with warm water and mild soap (the same kind you'd use on your vulva) or toy cleaner. If they've made their way to the anus, give them a three-plus-minute wash.

2. Never submerge those that contain batteries in water unless the manufacturer specifies it's safe to do so. Opt for a washcloth soaked in warm soapy water instead, and wipe them down. This wipe-down works for porous toys, too.

3. Some nonporous, nonmechanical toys can be boiled or can go in the dishwasher if the manufacturer specifies they're dishwasher safe.

4. Never use household cleaners, essential oils, or anything other than mild soap or all-natural detergent to wash toys.

5. Remove all batteries before storing toys so that they can't leak any battery acid, which can damage sensitive tissue or skin on your next use.

6. Dry toys thoroughly in a drying rack or with a clean towel after washing and before storing, to prevent mold and other bacterial and viral growth.

7. Store toys individually inside a lint-free fabric bag, or a zip-top case. You can also purchase boxes made specifically for sex toy storage that sterilize products at the same time, or just go with that glass lunch container. Never store porous toys anywhere humid, like your bathroom or under the kitchen sink, to avoid potential mold contamination. Jelly and other soft (nonsilicone) toys can melt together, so store separately.

8. Don't store sex toys in a nightstand unless they're sealed in a protective case. I've heard too many stories from patients who've experienced irritation from toys because they threw them in their nightstand without a case, allowing them to encounter lube, medication, money, chargers, or any of the other things people keep beside their beds.

TL;DR: IS MASTURBATION NORMAL?

- Masturbation is normal, healthy, and can't harm you in any way.
- Masturbation doesn't ruin women for relationships, doesn't desensitize your vagina or clitoris, and won't make it more difficult for you to climax during partnered sex.
- Masturbation can help you orgasm by teaching you more about your body and pleasure points.
- Masturbation has significant health benefits, like helping to improve sleep, balance hormones, relieve stress, boost immunity, and clear skin.
- There's no right or wrong way to masturbate—anything that's pleasurable, safe, and doesn't include animals or children is a great way to get off.
- Most women masturbate at least several times per month, if not more frequently.

- Masturbating with a partner can improve your relationship by helping you learn what the other likes, spicing up your routine, and adding another option when you can't have penetrative sex for some reason.
- Using sex toys for any kind of solo or partnered sex is normal, healthy, and fun.
- There are many different sex toys, and if you can think of a way to stimulate your clitoris, vagina, anus, or nipples, there's likely a toy to do it for you.
- Sex toys made from break-resistant glass, stainless steel, and medical-grade silicone are safest, and are least likely to lead to an infection, irritation, or STI.
- Properly cleaning and storing sex toys can prevent infection and other health concerns.

CHAPTER 7

IS MY DISCHARGE NORMAL?

THE GOOD, THE GREEN, THE GOOEY

"They told me not to take it the wrong way and then told me I smell like tacos down there. I don't know if this is a Latinx thing, or if they just think that is the smell because I'm Mexican, but how are you going to tell me I smell like a taco after going down on me and me not take it the wrong way?" Sofia said, visibly annoyed by the conversation she'd had just the day prior. She had made a visit because she feared she had contracted an STI. While her discharge, sexual health, and vulva were free of any other symptoms, the taco talk had her in a panic.

While being told you smell like something does make for an awkward conversation, I carefully explained to Sofia that her partner did her a solid in bringing it up, and a partner that kindly communicates concern is acting in your best interest. After a series of additional questions and running an STI panel—necessary since this was a new partner—we found there was absolutely nothing wrong. *Phew!* But tacos?

There are many reasons our vaginal odor can shift. Some are totally benign, and others warrant an investigation. Odor, itching, burning, pain, and discharge down there rightly give anyone a cause for concern, which is why I'm going to give you the DL we all should have had when the hormone changes of puberty sparked the fluid changes of your nether regions. Because what you see in your underwear is important; it is a daily indicator of your vaginal health, plus it can help you predict when you're most fertile in your cycle. Discharge is the umbrella term for the fluids that come out of the vagina. But it's not just fluid; bacteria, yeast, your own cells, and whatever else may have made its way in there (nod to your partner) are all exiting with your secretions. There's a lot at play here. So buckle up, as we'll be decoding discharge in this chapter, so you understand which discharge is normal and which requires a visit to your medical provider.

ASK DR. BRIGHTEN:

Is it normal to have vaginal discharge? What if I don't have any?

Not only is vaginal discharge totally normal, it's also a sign that your vagina, cervix, and hormones are healthy and happy. Secretions are made by cells in your vagina and cervix (also called cervical fluid) and fluctuate throughout your cycle, change based on sexual activity, and may dry up when there are problems with your hormones. Other habits like douching, smoking, taking oral contraceptives, dehydration, and using chemical-based soaps, detergents, and other personal-care products can also reduce your vaginal secretions.[1] Reduced vaginal discharge and vaginal dryness can arise as we enter menopause, or with conditions that cause us to lose our period due to a reduction in hormone production. See chapter 5 for vaginal dryness solutions.

What should my discharge smell like?

Vaginal odor can change with what you eat, where you're at in your cycle, when you've got too much or the wrong kind of organisms growing in there, or when there's a serious issue. If you experience a change in odor, especially with unpleasant symptoms like burning, itching, or generally feeling unwell, see a medical provider to get tested and the right treatment. Odor alone isn't a reliable way to diagnose what is going on. Here's how to tell what's normal and what's not:

Fermented-smelling discharge, like bread is rising, can sometimes indicate a yeast infection, which is commonly accompanied by itching, thick white discharge, and redness of the tissue (depending on the color of your skin).

Tangy or sour may be due to healthy bacteria called lactobacillus, which produce acid that maintains a healthy vaginal pH of 3.8 to 4.5 by making an environment ideal for the good stuff and far from ideal for the organisms you don't want there. These are the same organisms that help ferment yogurt.

Sweet can be a normal shift in the organisms that are meant to grow there. Your vaginal cells contain a bit of sugar (known as glycogen), which is used to support the growth of the lactobacilli bacteria. A super sugary sweet scent may point to diabetes, especially if accompanied by yeast infections that just won't quit.[2] Although if you're struggling with diabetes and yeast infections, odds are you're going to have more of the classic yeast symptoms talked about on page 169. Elevation in blood sugar can cause a drop in the pH of your vagina, making you so much more susceptible to yeast overgrowth.[3] This is why metabolic health is pivotal in vaginal health.

Ammonia-like discharge can be a sign of bacterial vaginosis (BV), an infection caused by an overgrowth of certain strains of bacteria in the vagina–see page 172 for more. Urine can also have an ammonia scent, especially if you're dehydrated, so if you smell something like household cleaners down there, make note of other symptoms you may have. Pee when you sneeze, jump, or cough? That's stress incontinence, and a pelvic-floor physical therapist can help. Got thin, gray discharge with an itch? That may be BV.

Fishy odors are never normal, and it isn't you–it's the bacteria producing amines. If you notice it's worse after unprotected sex with a male partner, you can thank his alkaline semen for messing with your pH. If you notice a fishy smell, you may have BV or another infection, like trichomoniasis (an STI). More on this soon.

Metallic odor, like a penny, is a sign that blood is present, since iron (the main mineral of red blood cells) gives discharge a metallic scent. This can happen on or around your period or if you've had bleeding with sex. It's not generally a cause for concern, unless you have significant bleeding when you shouldn't, experience pain, or have signs of infection like a fever.

Slightly skunky discharge that has a whiff of sweat, body odor, or cannabis is also normal. If you're already sweating or have a distinct body odor that others notice, your genital area will likely emanate the same odor. I once had a patient tell me her partner said she smelled like bong water when he'd perform oral sex on her following her bicycle ride home from work. "It's not your vagina," I explained. Instead, apocrine glands, a type of sweat gland concentrated in the armpits and genitals, can emit an odor that people have described as similar to cannabis when stressed, but also during sex. Researchers believe that may be related to consuming foods that contain certain plant compounds called terpenes.[4] Terpenes are found in so many plants that I wouldn't dream of telling you to cut them out because the health benefits are numerous.

Rotten- or foul-smelling discharge can mean a lost condom or forgotten tampon. See page 270 for how to retrieve these. If you've recently put something else in your vagina like jade eggs, or any other item that has been forgotten, the foul odor you smell is likely due to bacteria, and it's most definitely a time to see a doctor.

WHY DOES MY TACO SMELL LIKE A TACO?

Twaco, as it is called by Urban Dictionary, is a phenomenon where people describe the scent of the vulva as giving taco-meat or fajita notes. Do you eat the ingredients of taco seasoning? Onions, garlic, chiles, and herbs? These can enter your sweat and vaginal secretions (although to a much lesser extent) giving off an odor that may make your partner crave Taco Bell. More likely, the bacteria inhabiting your groin (yes, that's normal) are munching on the sweat secretions and producing thioalcohols, which smell similar to onions or meat. This concern has also come up among my patients who use coconut oil as lube, so maybe there's a correlation with the lube you use. I know this is shocking, but labia laden with the scent of taco seasoning hasn't been prioritized in the research. As long as there is no itching, burning, or abnormal discharge, this is totally normal. I've yet to have a concerned patient report that their partner found this offensive.

In fact, several have said their partner enjoys it. No need to douche, but showering may help. In terms of the foods? I'm a Latina, so I'm not about to tell anyone to cut these healthy foods from their diet. (You'll have to pry my salsa from my cold dead hands.)

Is the color of my discharge normal?

Depending on where you are in your cycle, discharge can be milky white, clear, or have a tinge of blood (normal when around ovulation or just before your period). See page 167 for a chart on how your discharge changes throughout your cycle. If you see any of the following changes in color, especially if you have other symptoms like pain, discomfort, itching, or generally feeling unwell, it's time to see your provider:

Green or yellow discharge is almost always a sign of sexually transmitted infections (STIs) like trichomoniasis, gonorrhea, or chlamydia. See page 164 for more information.

Gray discharge accompanied by other symptoms like a fishy odor, mild discomfort, or painful urination is most likely BV.

Brown discharge is common at the beginning or end of your period, as old, oxidized blood leaves your uterus. Brownish-reddish discharge can also be a sign of implantation bleeding, which occurs when a fertilized egg attaches to the uterine lining in the early stages of pregnancy–if this happens to you and you don't have your period and have recently had sexual intercourse, I'd recommend taking a pregnancy test. If you've just had a baby, brown secretions are likely lochia, which is normal discharge that occurs after childbirth and is normal.

Is the texture of my discharge normal?

Discharge texture varies with your cycle and can help you get dialed in on when your ovaries are about to release an egg (hello, fertile window) and when you're least likely to get pregnant. Although if you're not cycling due to hormonal birth control, medical conditions, or menopause, you won't see these changes. Here's what's normal and when it's time to meet with your provider:

Sticky discharge can bookend ovulation, showing up as you approach it or just passed it. This may feel a bit confusing, which is why more details are on their way.

Creamy or lotion-like discharge is a sign that your fertile window (nearing ovulation) is approaching—be careful if you have unprotected sex now, unless you want a baby. While the egg hasn't been released yet, those sperm can be waiting in the wings for their moment to shine. More on this on page 165. Thick, creamy discharge can also occur when you get pregnant, so get a test if you're concerned.

Slippery or stretchy discharge that's clear, copious, and often looks and feels like raw egg whites is fertile cervical mucus. Fertile cervical mucus occurs with ovulation when you're most fertile. It has the important role of ushering the best sperm to the egg in hope of conception. If you see this stuff, along with a spike in basal body temperature (the temp you take first thing in the morning), and your libido is up—it's go time for creating a small human. If making babies isn't on the to-do list, use a condom, try any other types of sex from chapter 5, or abstain (your hormones laugh at this last one because they know how good they're making those orgasms). If you don't have a sperm-producing partner, proceed with care to the wind regarding pregnancy risk.

Cottage cheese-like discharge that's white or a pale yellow is usually a sign of a yeast infection—see page 169 for more signs to look for and what to do about it.

Clumpy discharge might indicate a yeast infection, but if it looks more like pus than cottage cheese, or has a green or yellowish hue, you may have an STI or different condition that warrants attention. Head straight to a clinic that can test you for STIs.

Is it normal if the amount of discharge changes?

How much discharge you produce varies with your cycle. You will likely notice your underwear is more wet around ovulation when you produce cervical mucus, then dry, sticky, or watery at other times of the month. You may also notice more discharge after exercising, jumping, or dancing, since these activities engage the pelvic floor and other muscles, fast-tracking secretions out of the vagina.[5] When you're sexually aroused, you may also produce more discharge, which is known as arousal fluid. Some women also have measurable secretions when they orgasm, which we'll cover at length on page 175.

WHY DOES MY VAGINA BLEACH MY UNDERWEAR?

If you've ever found yourself muttering "WTF" as you examine the bleached spots on your favorite black underwear while doing laundry, you're not alone. It's totally normal for your vagina to bleach your favorite panties, which happens when the naturally acidic pH of your secretions causes underwear dye to separate from fabric. Water then removes this dye completely when you do laundry, leaving you with colorless blotches in your panties. What to do about this? Nothing. Bleach spots are actually a sign of healthy vaginal pH. While wearing synthetic underwear can reduce the likelihood of bleaching, doing so may also increase your risk of vaginal infections. And on the flip side, if you've never seen this, that's also normal.

What makes it so we get wet when aroused?

When you are sexually aroused, blood flows to your vagina (see chapter 4 for the phases of arousal) causing fluid to pass through the walls of your vagina. As the stimulation persists, the Bartholin's glands (located just inside the vaginal opening on either side) and the Skene's glands (located on either side of the urethra) begin to secrete fluid to add to the lubrication.

Is WAP a medical condition?

"WAP," a term popularized by Cardi B that stands for "wet-ass pussy," opened the conversation about whether this phenomenon is normal. There were numerous people who took to the Internet to exclaim that WAP is a medical condition that would necessitate a doctor's visit. The problem here is that none of these folks were actual medical experts, and every one of them a hater of Cardi B's music. It was nothing short of body shaming and once again pathologizing a normal bodily function, which left women questioning if something was wrong with them. Listen, your vagina and its secretions don't care about what's on your Spotify playlist, your personal ideologies, or who you vote for, for that matter. Your body is gonna do what bodies do.

The days leading up to ovulation, and ovulation itself, are the most "wet" times of our cycle. And are completely normal. The need for a bucket and a mop when aroused by your partner because your genitals respond with *I'm into this*? Normal. By the way, you can think of a panty liner as pretty much a portable mop. WAP does not require medical care. . . . It may require a different kind of care, but that's outside my scope.

Trigger warning: sexual assault. There may be times when, consciously, you are thinking *I am not into this* and *I am definitely not turned on*, but still

DECODING DISCHARGE

Your discharge can provide insights into what might be going on in your body, but if you suspect an infection, testing is the most definitive way to make sure you're getting the care you need.

DISCHARGE TYPE	WHAT IT COULD BE
White, thick, clumpy, cottage cheese-like	Yeast infection
Gray, thin, thick, fishlike odor	Bacterial vaginosis
Green, yellow, thick, pudding-like, foul smell	Gonorrhea, chlamydia, other STI
Brown	Beginning or end of period, sign of bleeding
Pink	Ovulation, implantation, early period

find that you are producing arousal fluid. When our brain recognizes something—anything, really—as sexual, it can set off the physiological cascade that causes vaginal lubrication. In some cases of sexual assault, the vagina self-lubricates, which can leave the victim questioning and confused. Worse, it can make the aggressor feel justified in the assault. Lubrication is not consent. No matter what your body does, only your words matter. If consent was never explicitly and enthusiastically given, it is assault, and not one moment of it was your fault.

Discharge Across Your Cycle

I still remember when I got a call in my office from my patient Shiloh, who was panicked by the discharge she saw in her underwear. "It's like my vagina is sick! There is all this mucus and it's thick and stringy." The thirty-two-year-old had recently stopped taking birth control pills, which she'd used since age twelve. There was nothing wrong with her discharge, though. In fact, she was experiencing fertile cervical mucus, a healthy sign that her ovulation had returned, and her period would soon follow. For the first time in decades, Shiloh was ovulating—something she hadn't experienced in her adult life, so the appearance of this slimy substance was foreign.

Never heard much about cervical mucus? Very few of us learn about cervical mucus in sex ed, and often it isn't until we struggle to conceive that we discover this knowledge. I've had many patients share that because they were taught that it's "impolite" or "disgusting" to speak about female-related subjects such as vaginal discharge, even when talking to your doctor, they've felt intimidated when looking for support. There's nothing disgusting about cervical mucus, and anyone who tries to shame you about it hasn't a clue how your body works. All of this can make the sudden appearance of a big snot-like wad of secretions in your underpants particularly alarming, which is why I want to break down everything you need to know about it, along with the other types of discharge you can expect to experience at different times of the month.

AROUND OVULATION

If you're not using a form of hormonal birth control that stops ovulation, your body will produce a clear, slippery, stretchy discharge, known as fertile cervical mucus, every month around ovulation. It most closely resembles raw egg whites. The whole point of fertile cervical mucus is to provide a superhighway for selected sperm (it helps filter out those that don't quite make the cut), making it easier for you to conceive. For some, it can be heavy enough that they feel the need to wear a panty liner, which is normal. You may also notice your desire for sex increases around this time, since your estrogen spikes right around ovulation and testosterone rises at this part of your cycle. All that estrogen adds to your ability to self-lubricate. But remember: the reason your body makes cervical mucus in the first place is to try to get you pregnant, so if you don't want to have a baby, be sure to use protection.

AFTER OVULATION

After ovulation, your body begins producing progesterone, which shifts production of cervical mucus, with it eventually becoming lighter and stickier. For most, the fluid will become more noticeably sticky within a couple of days, but the sperm-blocking properties of the discharge have already taken effect well before we notice the change. Your discharge will likely stay light and sticky to the touch and eventually may become absent, leaving you with a sense of dryness in the days before your period, when your body starts to produce even fewer natural secretions. This is the key time in your cycle where lube becomes your bestie, so be sure to keep some on hand.

DURING YOUR PERIOD

During menstruation, you bleed as your body sheds its uterine lining, which makes it difficult to discern any kind of discharge. While some women are afraid to have sex during menstruation due to rampant misinformation that it's dangerous or gross, it's neither (see chapter 10 for more info on period sex).

END OF YOUR PERIOD, BEFORE YOU REACH OVULATION

When your period ends, your discharge will still likely be on the dry side as you await estrogen's grand return. You'll likely need lube if you engage in sexual activity, and it is once again totally normal. This dryness doesn't last long, though: as your estrogen levels begin to rise during the follicular phase (period until ovulation), it triggers your body to start producing more discharge, which can be thick, white, and creamy, like lotion, before once again turning into the more wet and clear fluid as you approach ovulation. Just like cervical mucus, this lotion-like discharge helps provide lubrication for sexual activity.

ASK DR. BRIGHTEN:

What if I'm on the pill?

If you take the pill or any form of birth control that stops ovulation, your discharge-lubrication levels won't follow this cycle, since the medication's job is to prevent ovulation (a major way they're effective in preventing pregnancy) and suppress production of estrogen and other hormones. As a result, your discharge might stay dry or light, sticky, and tacky to the touch for most of your cycle—all of which is normal. This is one reason why it is said the pill more closely mimics menopause, when the ovaries don't produce hormones and vaginal dryness can be an issue, than it does pregnancy, a time when we are bathing in higher amounts of hormones and vaginal dryness is almost never an issue. Women on the pill can experience vaginal dryness and pain during sex, even though you can still produce arousal fluid.[6] This doesn't mean there's anything wrong with you, but this is a medication side effect. If you're using these forms of contraceptives, now is the time to experiment in finding your favorite lubes—your sex life will thank you for it.

Time of Cycle	Cervical Mucus
Period	Undiscernible due to bleeding
Immediately Following Your Period	Dry, absent
Leading Up to Ovulation	Lotion-like, white, sticky
Days Prior to Ovulation	Wet, clear, thin
Ovulation	Clear, thick, stretchy
Following Ovulation	Sticky, dry

BUSTED: THREE DISCHARGE MYTHS THAT ARE JUST PLAIN WRONG

1. **Discharge is just your uterus trying to detox. FALSE.** The popular myth that a woman's discharge is full of uterine toxins comes with the age-old sociocultural, patriarchal construct that the vagina is inherently dirty. In reality, vaginal secretions are normal, healthy, and necessary to keep your vagina happy. Without them, you'd experience deterioration in vaginal health, an increase in infections, and difficulty conceiving.
2. **Most women self-lubricate easily, all the time. FALSE.** Just like your period is cyclical, so are your secretions and your ability to easily self-lubricate. Despite what some may claim, no vagina is super wet all the time. Sometimes you can produce a lot of arousal fluid, while other times you may need a little help—and there's nothing wrong with needing some lube. If you routinely suffer from vaginal dryness, you may have a hormonal issue and should talk with a provider. There are also ways to increase your natural lubrication levels—see page 121 for more.
3. **If you don't have a lot of cervical mucus, you're definitely infertile. FALSE.** Your individual amount of cervical mucus isn't a definitive gauge of your fertility. If you produce a lot of cervical mucus, you can still experience fertility problems, while a woman who routinely sees only one day per month of light cervical mucus could still get pregnant just as easily as someone else. Some women may not feel or notice their cervical mucus, either, for a number of different reasons. However, the presence of no cervical mucus (if you're not using hormonal birth control) could point to an issue. But we never diagnose based on cervical mucus alone, so if you're concerned, have a conversation with your provider.

Why do I keep getting yeast infections and what can I do about it?

Three-quarters of women experience yeast infections, so if you read "discharge" and your mind bounced immediately to yeast, you're among the majority who've dealt with this.[7] I have no doubt your polyester pants are on fleek, but they are not letting your vulva breathe. Many everyday habits like wearing moisture-trapping/promoting clothing, taking the pill or antibiotics, hanging out in a wet bathing suit or sweaty workout apparel, douching, and using tampons or pads can leave your vagina vulnerable to yeast overgrowth.[8] Stress, poorly managed diabetes, and certain immune conditions can also make you susceptible. Both period blood and semen can change the pH of your vagina and alter your vaginal microbiome, which can give yeast the opportunity to multiply. Hormonal changes triggered by pregnancy, menopause, your cycle, hormone replacement therapy, and vaginal progesterone suppositories can also increase the risk.

The yeast that causes yeast infections sure does make you feel bad down there, but the organism itself is not bad. The same goes for the bacteria that causes BV. Both of these organisms call your vagina home, but given the opportunity (everything we just talked about), they will get rowdy and wreck the place. While many of these factors aren't within your control, there's lots of lifestyle habits that can make a difference when it comes to keeping yeast in check.

Think it might be yeast? Jump to the Decoding Discharge (page 164) chart to look for the signs. In addition to changes in discharge, you may also experience itching, burning, swelling, pain during urination or sex, or redness around the vulva. Note that the more melanin you have the less your tissue will appear red, so don't put a whole lot of weight into that one.

Yeast Infection Treatment Options

If you suspect a yeast overgrowth, it's a good idea to see your doctor for a diagnosis and to discuss treatment options. Sometimes yeast infections self-resolve, but most of the time, you'll need some level of intervention to clear them. If you choose to use a medication and are worried that your yeast troubles may come back, know there are steps you can take to help prevent them.

Fluconazole (brand name Diflucan) is a single-dose prescription drug that often clears yeast infections in several days. Side effects to be aware of with fluconazole are headaches, gastrointestinal issues, dizziness, and rashes. If you think you might be pregnant, don't take this drug.

Topical miconazole (brand name Monistat) is a common over-the-counter medication that can effectively clear most yeast infections within a week. Monistat usually takes longer to work than fluconazole, can be messy, and is a known endocrine disruptor, meaning it contains chemicals that can cause hormone imbalances. If used infrequently, the drug shouldn't lead to significant hormone issues, but if you find yourself relying on Monistat every month, talk with your provider.

Boric acid suppositories are available by prescription and over the counter. Both contain boric acid, a natural antifungal and antiseptic that helps restore normal vaginal acidity.[9] Research shows that boric acid suppositories can successfully resolve both yeast infections and BV,[10] with some studies suggesting it is just as effective as fluconazole in combating vaginal yeast overgrowth.[11] In addition, boric acid has been shown to be effective against both *Candida albicans* and the more resistant *Candida glabrata* strains of yeast.[12] But know that boric acid is a vagina-only medication: taking boric acid as an oral supplement can be fatal. And while natural, the chemical is also an endocrine disruptor, so if you're using boric acid suppositories routinely, speak with your doctor.[13] Boric acid suppositories can be used alongside medications to treat yeast.

Coconut oil is an age-old antifungal that recent research shows can help to kill yeast.[14] Applying it to your vulvar area can also soothe itchy, swollen skin, although it's unlikely to be enough to resolve an acute yeast infection.

Apple cider vinegar diluted in a warm bath can help kill yeast,[15] and may be used as an adjunct therapy, meaning it's best used with another primary treatment. Some women report this reduces itching and temporarily eases symptoms. Be cautious when using it, and never douche with vinegar or apply it directly to skin, which can aggravate your condition. Always dilute vinegar in water to avoid irritation.

Plain yogurt has long been touted as a remedy for resolving yeast infections, and you may be surprised to know there is some research to back this up. In one study, a mixture of yogurt and honey applied vaginally was found to be more effective than clotrimazole in relieving some of the symptoms of yeast overgrowth.[16] Other studies have shown that eating plain yogurt (the fruit-on-the-bottom, or sugar-added of any kind, won't help here) is also beneficial for gut and vaginal health.[17] This mostly comes down to supporting vaginal growth of lactobacillus, which is an organism that produces lactic acid to maintain the pH in the vagina. In my opinion, though, taking a probiotic, eating probiotic-rich foods, and leveraging some of the other therapies here is a better way to go than placing yogurt in the vagina.

Tea tree oil has been used for centuries as an antifungal and antibacterial, and some studies suggest it can treat yeast infections[18] and BV.[19] But that doesn't mean you should buy tea tree oil over the counter and apply it directly to your vulva: Doing so can damage the delicate tissue and may even worsen symptoms. It's a risk I don't advise anyone to take. You can get a prescription for compounded tea tree suppositories, which is a better way to go if you're really interested in trying this therapy.

CAN TAMPONS OR PADS CAUSE A YEAST INFECTION?

When do you use a tampon or pad regularly? On your period. Period blood shifts the pH in the vagina, which leaves you susceptible to yeast infections. Because tampons and pads can keep things moist and allow for yeast to proliferate, there is a chance they can make you even more susceptible to a yeast infection if not changed regularly. The solution? Change your tampon every four to six hours, and your pad anytime it's saturated. Even on your lighter days, be sure to change these products regularly, especially if you struggle with yeast infections.

Why do I have a fishy odor down there?

I encourage all my patients who struggle with bacterial vaginosis (BV) to ask themselves, before having unprotected sex with a new male partner: Is he really worth disrupting your pH? Seriously, because the risk of BV (or yeast, for that matter) is real when you introduce a new partner, semen, lube, or anything new to your vagina. And honestly, if you're not into it, or you don't think it'll be good, or you're feeling obligated, you should just save your vagina the trouble. BV is the most common cause of abnormal discharge in premenopausal women.[20] While many people incorrectly believe BV is an STI, you can develop the infection even in the absence of sex. All the discharge and discomfort without the fun—lame. BV is the result of an imbalance of vaginal organisms that allows for the overgrowth of bacteria like *Gardnerella vaginalis* and others. Sexual activity does increase the risk of developing BV, but that still doesn't make it an STI.

One of BV's hallmark symptoms is fishy-smelling discharge, which can intensify in odor after sex or during your period. To be clear, that odor isn't you—it's the bacteria producing a chemical compound called an amine. Yes, all the people who make jokes about how all vaginas smell like fish have no idea how vaginas work. Other symptoms include gray discharge and, less frequently, vulvar swelling and itching. Up to 84 percent of all women with BV, however, don't experience any symptoms.[21]

While you may be able to clear the infection on your own or at home with natural remedies, it's important to get an accurate diagnosis and make sure that you properly address the ailment—if left untreated, BV can cause pelvic infections, increase the risk of contracting an STI, and trigger miscarriage and other problems if you're pregnant.

The standard treatments for BV are the prescription antibiotics metronidazole and clindamycin, both of which can be taken orally or administered topically. In pill form, both antibiotics have a greater risk of side effects, including possible nausea, digestive troubles, and diarrhea. Also be forewarned that you should not consume alcohol if you take metronidazole in any form. Topical creams and gels may make latex condoms ineffective, meaning you should use backup protection if you're sexually active. There's no perfect treatment for BV (as in, there are tradeoffs), which is why working with your provider is best, and doing all you can to prevent it is even better. If you think you might be pregnant, tell your provider, as antibiotics can affect your baby's health.

Bacterial Vaginosis Treatment Options

If it's not your first rodeo with BV, you may already know exactly what you're dealing with and the remedies that can help. If not, be sure to check in with your provider, who can take a vaginal swab and tell you exactly what is causing those vaginal woes.

Boric acid suppositories have been shown to be an effective treatment for BV. (See the yeast infections treatment section on page 170.)

Lactobacillus probiotics that are taken orally can be both a short- and long-term strategy. The organisms that cause BV thrive in an alkaline environment. If you remember, it is lactobacilli that produce acid and keep the vagina in the optimal pH range of 3.8 to 4.5. When the pH creeps to 7 and above, BV symptoms typically occur. Clinical trials have shown *Lactobacillus acidophilus* and *rhamnosus* to be effective in reducing unfavorable bacteria and discharge.[22]

Vitamin C suppositories are one of the most overlooked yet effective natural treatments for BV, in my opinion. They're low-cost and available over the counter, which is why they were my go-to BV treatment when I worked at a homeless-youth clinic. Studies show that vitamin C suppositories can work as well as the prescription antibiotic metronidazole for BV.[23]

Hydrogen peroxide is pretty effective, but it can be a little too aggressive in how it affects your flora, and can leave you susceptible to other infections. It has been shown to decrease odor and eliminate symptoms of BV.[24] However, there isn't really enough evidence to recommend this, and there are better methods available.

Is It Yeast or BV?

Yeast	Bacterial Vaginosis
Caused by fungal overgrowth	Caused by bacterial overgrowth
No odor	No odor or fishlike odor
White discharge	Gray or white discharge
Thin to thick and clumpy discharge	Thin or watery discharge
Red, swollen, itchy tissue	Tissue is usually normal
Normal pH	Increased pH
Treated with antifungal	Treated with antibiotics

WHEN TREATMENTS FAIL, CONSIDER OPTION C

If your doctor is treating for the usual suspects (yeast or BV), but nothing is getting better, it may be time to look at other causes. Vaginitis is the umbrella term used to describe any inflammation of the vagina that can result in discharge and pain. It applies to a number of conditions, including yeast infections, BV, and these more rare conditions:

DESQUAMATIVE INFLAMMATORY VAGINITIS

Desquamative inflammatory vaginitis (DIV) is a relatively rare inflammatory skin condition (not an infection) that typically affects perimenopausal women, although it can also occur postmenopause.[25] In one study, symptoms of DIV were pus-like discharge, pain with sex, and vaginal inflammation in 70 to 90 percent of people.[26] Other symptoms include yellow or gray discharge, itching, burning, and pain in the area.[27] In patients diagnosed with DIV, many report having received unsuccessful treatments for other conditions prior. At this time, topical antibiotics and/or steroids are the best course of treatment.

LICHEN PLANUS

Lichen planus is another inflammatory skin condition. It causes your immune system to attack normal skin, causing patches of thickened tissue, ulcerations, and pain. If you develop lichen planus, your vaginal discharge may increase and be irritating.[28] You may also experience redness, burning, or raw skin that bleeds with sex. This discharge and discomfort are unresponsive to typical therapies used for vaginitis. A doctor can diagnose lichen planus, and treatment usually involves different ointments that help heal skin and prohibit your body's antibody response. Working with a naturopathic or functional medicine physician can also help you get to the root of your immune issues and employ diet and lifestyle therapies.

What About Sex and Your Discharge?

I first want to clear up a common cause of post-sex scaries for women: If your partner ejaculates inside you during vaginal intercourse, you will experience "discharge." But all that stuff dripping out of you after sex isn't entirely your secretions—his deposits (and maybe some lube, too) are also being evicted by the ever-fastidious cleaning machine that is your vagina. Almost all of us have had to do that awkward walk to the bathroom, cupping our hands between our legs to prevent semen from falling onto the floor. Let's normalize it. Pro tip: keep some tissues on the nightstand to do a quick cleanup.

It's also normal for your vagina to continue to remove ejaculate over the next couple of days. While I've seen some people claim on social media that a woman should be able to absorb all of a "man's essence," that's not biologically possible. Semen will exit your body. And if you don't want to deal with the post-doing-it drip, pregnancy risk, or are looking to reduce the risk of infection of any kind (staring down those STIs), opt for a condom (saving women from awkward bathroom walks since 1855).

There are many other ways, too, that sex can change your secretions. Whenever you have sex with someone new, it can introduce you to the bacteria, yeast, and other organisms that ride along with your partner. These critters, whether they're coming from saliva, semen, or body parts, can, in some cases, alter the consistency, smell, and color of your discharge. Couple that with the alkalinizing semen (remember from chapter 5 that your vagina needs to be acidic) and you may find yourself experiencing a case of BV or yeast vaginitis. While having sex with someone new doesn't automatically set you up for an infection, it's helpful to monitor your discharge afterward, paying attention to any shifts in color, consistency, or odor.

An infection is unlikely to manifest in symptoms in the first few hours after sex (although it can), and any itching you may experience down there soon after can be due to exposure to chemicals you've encountered, vaginal dryness, latex allergy, or the rare issue of semen allergy (more on this soon). Mild itching isn't necessarily concerning and may be as simple as changing lube—unless it becomes more severe, persists more than a couple of days, or is accompanied by other symptoms like changes to your discharge, redness, pain with urination, or odor.

If you've ruled out lube, condoms, and other irritants, but still experience mild itching after sex, I recommend taking a shower after, and using water only to wash your vulva (that's the outside—remember that you should never wash your vagina). If you don't want to ruin an intimate moment by jumping in the shower, you can opt for a quick rinse using a travel bidet or portable peri bottle, which can travel with you in a purse or be stored under the bathroom sink. If you're inclined to reach for the adult equivalent of scented baby wipes, don't. It can make itching worse. Instead, opt for unscented baby wipes, which are designed for delicate skin and aren't loaded with hormone-hating chemicals under the guise of making you smell more feminine. Avoid douching, which can intensify your itching and further disrupt your natural vaginal ecology.

IS IT NORMAL FOR SEMEN TO CAUSE BURNING OR ITCHING?

It is possible to be allergic to semen, which can cause itching, burning, redness, and swelling after sex, usually showing up within an hour of contact with semen.[29] These symptoms can show up anywhere on your body that comes into contact with semen. If you notice your chest, abdomen, thighs, or other nongenital regions are hot, red, swollen, and itchy after semen has landed on them, then that may point toward an allergy. Women with a semen allergy, known as seminal plasma hypersensitivity, may experience symptoms the first time they have sex, later down the line, or with only some men. It's also possible to develop the condition after months or years with the same partner. While the allergy is rare, it's frequently misdiagnosed as vaginitis (inflammation of the vagina) or a vaginal infection. The best way to discern a possible semen allergy is to try using condoms with your partner, which should prevent symptoms. If removing contact with semen does the trick (and you've ruled out everything else in this chapter), it may very well be that you have a semen allergy. Talk with your medical provider about this, as in some rare instances, a semen allergy can lead to anaphylaxis. A semen allergy won't directly affect your fertility, but the discomfort may inhibit you from wanting to have unprotected sex. Some women with the condition may choose to use artificial insemination or in vitro fertilization to become pregnant.[30]

ASK DR. BRIGHTEN:

How common are sexually transmitted infections (STIs)?

While no one wants to think about it, we all think about STIs, especially when engaging in sex that might put us at higher risk. If you remember from chapter 3, the thought of contracting an STI can not only keep you from getting in the mood, it can also derail your arousal no matter how into it you are. So we're going to talk about it, because part of creating great sex is ensuring it is safe sex.

First things first: it's an infection, not a disease, which is why we dropped that *D* (formerly STD) and all the stigma that came with it. When it comes to sex, preventing STIs may be the arena you feel you're an expert in, at least if you've been living in the US most of your life. That's because most parents, teachers, and doctors in the US tend to focus on the dangers and risks of sex. Conversations about mutual trust, pleasure, and responsibility take a back seat to telling women they're at threat of pregnancy or disease when sexually active. As I shared with you in chapter 4, the approach we've been taking in the US just ain't it, especially when you consider 1 in 5 have an STI and half of those are people ages 15 to 24.[31] I'm going to give you the facts on STIs, but keeping in line with the WHO and many other countries employing successful sex ed (by the measure of lower STI and unplanned pregnancies), I have also provided you plenty of pleasure-based education in other chapters.

When we assign a narrow definition to sex—the standard penile-vaginal intercourse—sex gets less safe because people are less inclined to think oral, anal, or anything else requires protection and, sometimes, even consent (see chapter 5 for all the other kinds of sex). If you're engaging in any kind of sexual activity that results in the swapping of fluids, barriers and STI prevention should be considered.

How can I prevent getting or spreading an STI?

Barriers, frequent testing, and honest communication with your partner are key. Barriers have been covered extensively in chapter 5, but as a reminder, condoms (even when you can't get pregnant), dental dams, and finger cots can all help reduce the spread of these organisms. If you're starting a relationship, going to have sex with someone for the first time, or your partner has been diagnosed (or you suspect) with an STI, then it's time to test. Several STIs can take years to show up and many are symptomless, so screening is best. Be honest if you have an STI. Even if it is one of the ones that ride with you for life without always making a visible appearance, you need to tell your partner. If you get an STI, tell the people you've been in contact with. I have some tips on this on page 179.

What if we just do it one time without a condom?

The number of women I've had ask me this after their male partner tries to tell them that "one time is fine" has me seriously questioning the education and the ethics of these men. Because no, one time is all it takes for y'all to receive some contaminated fluids and wind up with an STI.

Why does my doctor insist on screening me for STIs?

Simply put, you can have an STI with big consequences despite having no symptoms. Untreated STIs can lead to infertility, chronic pelvic pain, cervical cancer, and infections of your fallopian tubes or uterus. In addition, many STIs can be passed to a fetus, resulting in infection, miscarriage, or stillbirth. But with treatment, we can prevent many of the "big scaries" of STIs. Part of how we catch infections, even when there are no symptoms, is with regular screening.

Do I really have to call that one-night stand if I find out I have an STI?

When it comes to most STIs, you're going to need to make that call to people you've encountered sexually. I know that people shame and blame people for these infections. And yeah, it can feel really intimidating to make this call. But listen, humans get infections. We get the flu, cold viruses, and heck, we can get hepatitis A eating at a restaurant (new fear unlocked). And we can spread it to others. You should always tell your partner if you have an STI before having sex, and you should always feel comfortable asking your partner if they have one or have been screened. If your partner is offended or declines to discuss their STI status, then, girl, don't do it, it's not worth it.

HOW DO I TELL MY PARTNER I HAVE AN STI?

Getting tested ideally happens before you engage in sex with a new partner and should happen periodically if not in a monogamous relationship. Most STIs are silent, meaning lurking without symptoms, and others (like HIV) can take months or more to detect. Even though there should be zero shame here, we've all gotten plenty of messages from society that make it near impossible to not feel at least a bit uncomfortable sharing this info. Here's some tips to tell your partner you have an STI:

1. **Know what's next for you and your partner.** Ask your provider if your partner can be given a prescription or will require testing. In some instances, as with chlamydia and gonorrhea, your provider can give your partner a prescription as well.[32] Most people want to know what they need to do when they are told they might have an STI, and having that information can help alleviate anxiety and tension in the conversation.

2. **Decide how you want to communicate.** A phone call or text message is more than fine. Face-to-face might work, but it might also put you in an unsafe situation. Be sure you always have an exit if having this conversation in person, and consider a public place, where other people are present, but not in earshot. You can also bring a friend.
3. **Understand their sexual history.** Ideally, we'd do this before having sex, but life isn't perfect. To help you figure out if they are who you contracted it from, ask if they know if they have an STI and if they always use protection. Treat it like a data-gathering session and opportunity for communication, not an open invitation to place blame. Other ways people contract STIs can be via tattoos, piercings, using IV drugs, or sharing toothbrushes or razors.
4. **Know what's safe while you treat.** While outercourse may be fine, other acts may be totally off-limits. If you have a cold sore on your lip (herpes), for example, then oral sex is a no, as should be kissing. Talk to your provider about what is safe and what isn't, and let your partner know.
5. **Honor your efforts.** Congratulate yourself on a job well done because these conversations aren't easy, and most people want to dodge them. Even though you're a rock star for making it happen, you may also need some extra support. Phone a friend or talk with a counselor if you need support processing.

STIs: Who's Trying to Hitch a Ride in Your Body?

There's over a dozen organisms to be aware of, which can certainly sound like a lot. But when you understand that medicine is very good at testing and treating them, plus you've got tools to take steps to avoid them, things get a lot less scary.

Chlamydia and gonorrhea are bacteria that infect your genitals, cervix, urethra, eyes, and throat (making a very good case for barriers during oral sex). They both can take a free ride in your body undetected, meaning you may not have symptoms. If you do have symptoms, there may be pain with sex, pelvic pain, pain with urination, and discharge that is a thick yellow or green. You may also have bleeding between periods or after sex. Discharge may smell pretty foul as well. Antibiotics can help you eradicate these organisms, but you can't have sex until seven days after starting your treatment, and your partner can reinfect you, so they need treatment, too (which is true of all STIs, if your partner has them).

Trichomoniasis, or trich, as it is commonly called, is a major cause of vaginitis. While it can be asymptomatic, foul discharge, pain with urination, and itching can accompany a trich infection. There is a correlation with HIV, either putting you at higher risk of contracting HIV or higher incidences of trichomoniasis if you have HIV, so your provider may want to screen you for HIV as well if you're positive for trich.[33] It needs to be treated with a round of antibiotics.

Syphilis, left untreated, can cause serious problems for your brain and heart, which is why treating these bacteria with antibiotics as soon as it is detected is a must. Although less common than trich, syphilis is also associated with HIV transmission.[34] If you notice a painless sore or multiple sores on or around your genitals, get it checked out. This can be an early sign of syphilis. If syphilis is left untreated, fever, rashes, swollen glands, sore throat, muscle aches, headaches, and weight loss can occur over time.

Genital herpes can be caused by HSV-1 or HSV-2, whereas oral herpes is caused only by HSV-1. Yes, herpes on your lips can spread to your other lips (or vulva altogether) and other genitals. It's really common, with about 572,000 new cases in the US alone in 2018 being reported.[35] The thing about herpes is that you can spread it even if you don't have a visible sore, which is why you *must* communicate this to your partner even if you don't have an active lesion. Unlike the STIs we've discussed so far, there is no cure for herpes. If you have it, you can take a medication, like Valacyclovir, when prodrome symptoms (burning or tingling) arise to keep outbreaks in check. If you do have an outbreak, it will appear as a single blister or a few that can be accompanied by fever and feeling unwell. These blisters can take a week or more to resolve and are very contagious.

Hepatitis A, B, and C are all viruses that can impact the liver and cause chronic disease. Hepatitis A is spread from fecal contamination, which is why you should wear a condom or a use a barrier with any anal play. Sharing razors, toothbrushes, needles, or anything that exposes someone to semen, vaginal fluids, or blood when you have hep B or C can put them at risk. There are vaccines available to help prevent these. If you do contract them, your provider will recommend treatments that include medication, diet, and lifestyle interventions.

HIV (human immunodeficiency virus) is the virus that causes AIDS (acquired immunodeficiency syndrome), causing impairment of your immune system and putting you at risk of becoming very ill even with the mildest versions of other infections. This virus is another one that is with you for life, but the invention of several pharmaceuticals has made improvements in managing the disease and quality of life. Sex, contamination with blood or infected fluids into open wounds, IV drug use, tattoos, and piercings are all ways in which this is spread. Hugging, sharing drinks, holding hands, cuddling, or even a heavy makeout session won't put you at risk of contracting HIV. HIV can take years to show symptoms and, even when it does, they aren't always that telling–for example, a yeast infection you can't kick. It's best to be screened if you have had unprotected sex, your partner has been diagnosed, you've shared needles or a common cup when filling your syringe with drugs, have had a piercing or tattoo with a potentially contaminated needle, or you've just found out you're pregnant.

Pubic lice, scabies, and molluscum contagiosum can all be spread by contact. Up until this point, none of the STIs we talked about can be spread by hugging, cuddling, or spooning. This crew is an exception.

Pubic lice (aka crabs) aren't dangerous and don't make you dirty, but damn can they make you itch. These little critters are most commonly spread when pubic hairs unite, but they can also catch a ride on fabrics, make their way to chest hair, and even end up in facial hair. You can get checked for pubic lice, but a lot of the time, people aren't wrong when they see evidence of them. There's medication available at the drugstore to evict these freeloaders from your fun parts.

Scabies–while I respect their tenacity for survival, I really hate these guys. That's because while I can easily prescribe meds for my patients to treat them, I also have to inform them that everything they've come into contact with (bedding, clothing, towels) needs to be washed and dried at high heat. Anything that can't be washed needs to be sealed in a bag for three days, and you must vacuum like your in-laws (or maybe landlord) are paying a visit. As if that wasn't bad enough, the itching is downright maddening, and worse at night or with hot showers. Even two to three weeks after treating, the itching can persist. These parasites burrow under your skin, causing bumps and little lines as they make their journey within your body. Yes, you can get them from sex, but also by sharing towels, bedding, or close contact with someone who has them.

Molluscum contagiosum is a virus picked up by having contact with the skin of someone who is infected, or something they've touched. Adults usually get it from sex and kids get it from, well, doing what kids do–touching everything from toys, clothes, and play equipment. Excuse me while I ruin donuts for you, because that is exactly what these hard, flesh-colored bumps look like with their dip in the middle. Treating this is similar to treating warts–you can put medicine on them or have a doctor remove them.

What Is HPV? Can I Prevent HPV? How Can I Keep My Cervix Healthy?

Human papillomavirus is an STI that can infect your mouth, throat, or genitals, and can lead to cancer. HPV isn't just one virus. In fact, there are nearly 150 known strains of HPV. The thing about HPV, unlike other sexually transmitted infections, is that it is super common. HPV is so prevalent that nearly all sexually active adults have at least one strain. It's highly likely that you or someone you know has HPV, so it's silly to try to stigmatize this one (or any of them).

"Papilloma" means "wart" in medicine, but not every strain of HPV actually causes warts you can see. There are two types of HPV: low-risk and high-risk strains. Low risk generally causes genital warts or no symptoms. HPV 6 and HPV 11 are responsible for about 90 percent of genital warts. If you have visible warts, it's likely you're carrying the low-risk HPV 6 or 11.[36] The type of HPV that causes warts has not been found to cause cancer. High risk can cause cervical cancer. HPV 16 and 18 cause nearly 66 percent of cervical cancers in the US. That's right. HPV can seriously and dramatically harm your cervical, sexual, and overall health.

ASK DR. BRIGHTEN:

What are the symptoms of HPV? How do I know I have it?

Because there generally aren't symptoms, the majority of people with HPV realize they have it only once a lab test comes back positive. Your gynecologist, nurse practitioner, naturopathic physician, or other provider who performs gynecological exams can test for HPV at the same time as your Pap smear, which is typically standard after age thirty. HPV is typically only tested for in women under thirty following an abnormal Pap. Testing earlier has led to more invasive and unnecessary procedures, which is why we don't do it. It's important to note that new HPV infections often occur close to the time a woman begins having intercourse. So it's common for women to contract HPV before age twenty-five. But before you start to worry, know that most women will be able to clear the virus at this age, with the majority of new infections testing negative six to twelve months later. If you do test positive for HPV, your doctor will be able to counsel you about next steps based on the strain of the virus and the results of your Pap, which reveal the health of your cervical cells.

How can I prevent HPV?

While barrier methods may help, not all types of HPV can be prevented this way. When it comes to the ones that cause cervical cancer, there is a vaccine available. I recommend talking to your provider about the best options for you.

Do I need a Pap smear if I'm a virgin?

The guidelines about Paps vary between associations. The American College of Obstetricians and Gynecologists recommends that a patient initiate cancer screening at age twenty-one regardless of sexual activity. For the American Cancer Society, the age is twenty-five. The incidence of cervical cancer is low at these ages, but it is worth discussing with your doctor, if you're over twenty-one, about what is right for you. You always have the right to refuse a Pap smear.

Are urinary tract infections (UTIs) or bladder infections considered STIs? Why do I always get one after sex?

While some of the organisms that are considered STIs could be causing urinary symptoms, odds are your UTI is from another culprit—E. coli. UTIs are frequent after sex because the friction, combined with what you're doing, can spread organisms and force them into the urethra. Most people generally know they have a UTI because they experience pain with urination, an increase in how often they need to go, a feeling like it's urgent, and an achy feeling in their lower abdomen, and there may even be a bit of blood in their urine. While there's no large study showing definitively that peeing after sex can prevent a UTI, it is something many women report finding helpful. That's because urinating helps flush the urethra (how the organisms gain access to your bladder) and, in theory, would push these organisms out.

While most UTIs are easily treated (and annoying), some can progress into a kidney infection, which is a serious situation. If you have any of the following symptoms you must seek immediate medical treatment and will likely be prescribed antibiotics. I know no one likes to jump on a round of antibiotics (especially with the threat of a yeast infection), but your kidneys are really important—like, can't-live-without important. Fever, chills, significant fatigue, or pain in your lower back, or on one side of your body, can point to a kidney infection.

TL;DR: IS MY DISCHARGE NORMAL?

- Discharge is normal and changes with your cycle. You can use it, along with other signs and symptoms, to tell when you're most fertile.
- Fishlike, foul, and yeast-like odors down there warrant a trip to your doctor. As does cottage cheese–like gray, thick yellow, or green discharge.
- Semen is alkaline. The vagina is acidic. Put them together and your pH may be thrown off enough to land you with a case of bacterial vaginosis.
- Bacterial vaginosis is the most common vaginal infection among women of premenopausal age, but it's not an STI. It (not you) produces a fishlike odor and needs to be treated.
- There is no such thing as being too wet.
- Yeast infections are common, uncomfortable, and have a variety of treatment options.
- STIs don't always have symptoms, which means regular screening is a must. They should always be treated promptly to avoid serious complications, like pelvic inflammatory disease and infertility. Yes, if your doctor says you need antibiotics, you absolutely need antibiotics.
- UTIs aren't the same as an STI, although they are more common after sex.

Part 2

YOUR CYCLICAL SELF

CHAPTER 8

ARE MY HORMONES NORMAL?

STRESS, PMS, AND OTHER NOT FUN THINGS

Reece sat rigidly in the chair, her arms crossed defensively as she began to explain why she had scheduled a visit with me. "I'm just so tired all the time, my periods are becoming more unpredictable, and I just keep gaining weight for no good reason," she said with a huff. "Please don't be one of those doctors who just tells me to stop eating so much and exercise more, because that's not it. And I don't need the pill. I tried it. It just makes me incredibly depressed, and I already feel sad enough as it is. Oh, and so you know, I googled 'perimenopause' and I'm thirty-four years old, which isn't old, so please don't give me that speech, either," Reece said, speaking rapidly and sounding more agitated with every word.

I'd have to tread carefully. "I can hear you're frustrated by these symptoms and that the previous solutions you've been offered haven't worked, which probably made you more frustrated. I want to help you find the right solution. So how about we start with when was the last time you felt like yourself, and you explain to me what that looks like. Then you can walk me through how these symptoms began, and we'll decide on the best lab testing," I said empathetically.

"You mean you'll actually test my hormones? And you won't just tell me everything is normal, and to put down my fork between bites and get a gym membership?" she said with hopeful excitement. I responded with a smile. "Based on the brief information you just provided, we absolutely need to test your hormones, and if you're telling me that the 'eat less and move more' mantra that should have been banished from women's medicine before it even got a chance to creep in isn't working for you, I believe you."

Reece's experience is like so many of my patients'—she had classic symptoms of hypothyroidism, but her doctor's focus was primarily on managing her weight and "regulating" her period with the pill. That provider didn't look at the whole picture. Reece's experience surrounding her weight had felt so traumatic that she was reluctant to step on the scale at my office, so I invited her to skip it, and let her know we could revisit that data point in the future if we felt it was necessary. The anti-fat attitude of her doctor, something that is unsettlingly pervasive in health care, led to her mistrust of medicine, and her doctor's bias was a barrier to her getting the care she needed.[1] Her previous provider had also refused to do any hormone testing, telling her that hormones are wildly unpredictable and that there's no such thing as a hormone imbalance—a common statement I see parroted across the Internet. Which is wrongly simplistic.

If you're living in a body today, you don't need me or any other doctor to tell you a hormone imbalance is real—you've already felt it. Hormone imbalance is a broad term used to describe the many symptoms that can arise when there's too much or too little of a hormone. As a board-certified naturopathic endocrinologist, it's my job to take this general complaint that patients express and find out the exact cause. Because hormone imbalance can be a lot of different things. It might refer to insulin resistance (often too much insulin present, but the cells are unable to use it); hyperandrogenism (too much testosterone); hypothyroidism (too little thyroid hormone), as was the case with Reece; or a myriad of other conditions and issues. The key to addressing it is to home in on which hormones are causing symptoms and address those appropriately. Remember the hormone pyramid we discussed on page 69? Building from the bottom up is a strategy I employ with my patients to get them the results they seek and make them stick. I'm going to help you do the same, but first, we need to figure out what hormones are driving your symptoms. The Hormone Symptom Check on page 192 will help you get clear on the primary hormone imbalances you're experiencing. I've included it this early on so you can keep your hormone symptoms in mind as you continue reading this chapter. You'll also want to take it again when you've completed the 28-day program, and use it as a tool for future issues that may arise. I've also provided a list of labs at https://DrBrighten.com/ITN-resources to help you communicate to your provider what you want to investigate. Hormones do fluctuate—Reece's doc was right about that—which is why the time of day and timing of your cycle matters greatly in getting the right data. If your doctor isn't advising you on timing, there's a pretty good chance your labs won't reflect accurate data, and you'll be met with "Everything is normal."

There are two things you should know about hormone imbalances. First off, there's rarely just one hormone that's an issue because as one moves out of balance, the others will shift to compensate. Which is why you may find that you have a high score on more than one hormone in the checklist on the next page. That's totally normal when the system is out of balance. For example, it is common to see excess-estrogen and low-progesterone symptoms go together. You may also find you have high- and low-cortisol symptoms, but with the high showing up in the evening and the low showing up in the morning—the opposite of what it should be.

Second, hormones share commonalities in the things that will throw them out of balance and the things you need to do to recalibrate the system. In the page that follows, I'll discuss the most common causes of hormone issues, and I'll provide you tips on what to do about it. Outside this list, there are other, rarer causes, which include: tumors, medications (like chemotherapy or certain antidepressants), and injuries (like traumatic brain injury). All of these require working one-on-one with a medical provider. Real talk, though, I could write an entire book on just hormones, so rather than hitting you with a fire hydrant of information, I'm aiming to give you just what you need to eliminate those unwanted hormone symptoms.

Hormone Symptom Check

These are the questions I use to assess my patients to understand the source(s) of the imbalance. It guides what we test and how we address those issues they're struggling with. I've provided you an online version at https://DrBrighten.com/ITN-resources to help you track changes as you implement the strategies you'll find in this book. (And because I personally hate ever writing in a book.) Check the symptoms that you've had in the past month. Aim to choose the most important symptoms you would discuss with your doctor, rather than checking every symptom you have ever had in your lifetime.

HIGH CORTISOL

- ☐ Life feels like a constant state of high stress
- ☐ Stress is overwhelming
- ☐ Feeling burnout or exhausted
- ☐ Easily distracted, especially when stressed
- ☐ Memory issues
- ☐ Feeling on edge and easy to anger
- ☐ Difficulty falling asleep, staying asleep, or insomnia
- ☐ Often experience headaches in the morning
- ☐ Feeling tired, but mind is wired at bedtime
- ☐ Weight gain, or difficulty losing weight around my midsection
- ☐ Ovulation or periods are irregular
- ☐ Irritable, anxious, or meltdowns
- ☐ Crave salty or sweet
- ☐ Frequent colds or illness
- ☐ More wrinkles than match your age
- ☐ Low or no sexual desire (libido)

LOW CORTISOL

- ☐ Wake feeling tired despite a full night's sleep
- ☐ Can't get going without coffee
- ☐ Energy crashes in the afternoon
- ☐ Need stimulation in the afternoon (coffee, chocolate, etc.)
- ☐ Periods leave me depleted
- ☐ Feel the need to nap most days
- ☐ Craving salty or sweet
- ☐ Dizzy when standing too quickly
- ☐ Any amount of stress feels like too much
- ☐ Muscle weakness
- ☐ I get sick often and/or have a difficult time getting over infections
- ☐ I have low-blood-sugar issues

INSULIN/BLOOD SUGAR DYSREGULATION

- ☐ Elevated blood sugar
- ☐ Diagnosed with diabetes, metabolic syndrome, insulin resistance
- ☐ Dark, velvety skin on neck, armpits, groin
- ☐ Skin tags
- ☐ Shaky if going too long between meals
- ☐ Tired after eating
- ☐ Tired all the time
- ☐ Weight gain or inability to lose weight around midsection
- ☐ Extreme thirst
- ☐ Extreme hunger

- [ ] Frequently urinating
- [ ] High cholesterol
- [ ] Acne, cystic acne
- [ ] History of gestational diabetes
- [ ] Hair thinning or loss
- [ ] Low sexual desire (libido) or arousal
- [ ] Decreased clitoral sensation

HIGH THYROID

- [ ] Missing or irregular periods
- [ ] Racing heart
- [ ] Difficulty sleeping
- [ ] Anxious, panicking, sense-of-dread feeling
- [ ] Sweaty often
- [ ] Loose stools or diarrhea
- [ ] Weight loss without effort
- [ ] Hand tremor or feeling shaky
- [ ] Heat intolerance, feeling flushed
- [ ] Swelling at the front of the neck
- [ ] Bulging, swollen eyes

LOW THYROID

- [ ] Irregular, missing periods
- [ ] Fatigue, exhaustion, extremely tired
- [ ] Difficulty concentrating
- [ ] Brain fog, memory issues
- [ ] Dry skin, scaling

- ☐ Losing hair on head, body, outer third of eyebrows
- ☐ Brittle, splitting nails
- ☐ Joint pain, muscle aches
- ☐ Slow heart rate, palpitations
- ☐ Anxiety or depression
- ☐ Hair is dry, tangles easily
- ☐ Constipation, need stimulants to have a bowel movement
- ☐ Feeling cold all the time, cold hands and feet
- ☐ Difficulty getting pregnant (trying for six months or more)
- ☐ History of miscarriage
- ☐ Postpartum depression or postpartum thyroiditis
- ☐ Low milk supply when breastfeeding

HIGH ESTROGEN

- ☐ Periods are seven days or longer
- ☐ Heavy periods
- ☐ Large clots in menstrual blood
- ☐ Bloating, puffiness, fluid retention
- ☐ Cranky, irritable, mood swings
- ☐ Breast tenderness, swelling, cysts
- ☐ Acne, acne rosacea
- ☐ Weight gain or difficulty losing weight on hips, butt, thighs
- ☐ Hair loss
- ☐ Cyclical migraines, period headaches
- ☐ Uterine fibroids
- ☐ Gallbladder issues, difficulty digesting fats

LOW ESTROGEN

- ☐ Irregular or missing periods
- ☐ Period is a day or two of spotting
- ☐ Periods are light
- ☐ Breasts feel less full
- ☐ Anxiety, depression
- ☐ Difficulty concentrating
- ☐ Brain fog
- ☐ Thinning skin, more fine lines and wrinkles
- ☐ Bone loss
- ☐ Frequent urinary tract infections (UTIs)
- ☐ Urinary leakage
- ☐ Difficulty sleeping, night waking
- ☐ Joint pain, prone to joint injury
- ☐ Night sweats, hot flashes
- ☐ Sun damage is more noticeable
- ☐ Low sexual desire (libido)
- ☐ Difficulty self-lubricating with sex
- ☐ Vaginal dryness
- ☐ Pain with sex

LOW PROGESTERONE

- ☐ Irregular or frequent periods
- ☐ Heavy periods
- ☐ Difficulty sleeping, especially before period
- ☐ PMS seven to ten days before period

- ☐ Short luteal phase (ovulation to period is fewer than twelve days)
- ☐ Spotting several days before period
- ☐ Anxiety, depression
- ☐ Migraines, headaches
- ☐ Agitated, weepy, sad before period
- ☐ Recurrent miscarriage
- ☐ Difficulty getting pregnant (trying for six months or more)
- ☐ Low or no signs of ovulation (cervical fluid, basal body temperature)
- ☐ Weight gain

HIGH TESTOSTERONE

- ☐ Irregular periods
- ☐ Missing periods for several months
- ☐ Thick, dark hair growth on face, chest, and/or abdomen
- ☐ Acne, cystic acne
- ☐ Oily skin, hair
- ☐ Thinning hair, hair loss on head
- ☐ Strong body odor
- ☐ Diagnosed with PCOS
- ☐ Difficulty getting pregnant (trying for six months or more)
- ☐ Mood swings, rage

LOW TESTOSTERONE

- ☐ Lack of motivation
- ☐ Depression, anxiety, panic attacks
- ☐ Fatigue, low energy

- [ ] Low sexual desire, difficulty staying in the mood
- [ ] Difficulty achieving orgasm
- [ ] Loss of sexual fantasies
- [ ] Cry easily
- [ ] Losing muscle, unable to gain muscle
- [ ] Bone loss
- [ ] Urinary incontinence
- [ ] Cardiovascular symptoms, heart disease
- [ ] Weight gain

ANSWER KEY:

Checking four or more boxes in any one of these ten groups points to a hormone imbalance in that area. If you check eight or more symptoms, then that is an area in need of attention, and you may have a significant imbalance. If you checked three or fewer, this is not likely to be your problem area. The 28-day program can help you address many of these symptoms and issues, and in chapter 8 you'll find a list of what commonly causes these issues, and guidance on what can help.

Hormone imbalances often go together. For example, high-estrogen and low-progesterone symptoms often accompany each other in the luteal phase and can manifest as symptoms of PMS (more on this in chapter 9). We also often see insulin dysregulation and high testosterone, especially in cases of polycystic ovary syndrome (PCOS). If you're scoring high in both too much and too little cortisol, don't freak. This is actually normal for adrenals that have been struggling with too much stress for too long. It is often a sign that you're spiking cortisol at the wrong time of the day (evening) and not getting enough of it when you need it most (morning).

Why is there no high progesterone on the symptom check? Well, unless you're using a progesterone replacement therapy, it is incredibly rare to see high progesterone causing significant symptoms. Progesterone replace-

ment therapy is most commonly used in perimenopause, postmenopause, and pregnancy. When your provider prescribes it, they should counsel you on the possibility you may experience dizziness, bloating, increased frequency of yeast infections, tender breasts, and feeling groggy when you wake. It is also possible to have symptoms of low estrogen if you're using progesterone replacement therapy. It is important to note that birth control does not contain any progesterone but, rather, has progestin. Progestin has a different set of side effects associated with it. So if you're on a form of birth control that stops ovulation, like the pill, your estrogen and progesterone symptoms may not be accurate on this symptom check. All the other hormones, however, can be gauged using this symptom check while on birth control. And yeah, we are not at all surprised if your testosterone is too low while on the pill (see chapter 3 for more on that).

ASK DR. BRIGHTEN:

What causes hormone imbalances?

I'm going to walk you through the largest contributors to hormone imbalances and provide you tools on how to mitigate them along the way. And I want to warn you against falling into the "If I just did this one thing or took this one supplement then all my symptoms would magically go away" mindset. I wish it was like that, but the reality is the combination of dietary and lifestyle practices can push you in or out of balance. If you picture a scale (the old-school kind, with trays balancing on either side), we've got optimal on one side and less optimal on the other. Daily we want to be contributing to the optimal side in some capacity, because life generally hands us plenty of less optimal items. I can hear you already: *But wait, wouldn't that throw the scales out of balance if all I did was just push for optimal all the time?* Um, yeah, and that manifests as a boring AF life. No, but seriously, perfection isn't the goal and striving for that can actually throw a whole lot onto the less optimal side, like being anxious about everything you eat, engaging in negative self-talk when you skip your workout, or pondering if it is your fault that you're not in the mood because of something you did wrong. Yeah, none of that is optimal and none of that is good for your health. The point is, I want you to nourish your body, move in the best way for you, get amazing restorative sleep, but also, eat the freakin' cake, take a full day to lounge on the sofa every now and again, and stay up late catching up with a good friend, dancing your heart out, or lovemaking with that new partner. I know I'm a heretic in the wellness world in saying all of that, but you get one life and you were not put this earth to abide by rigid rules that keep you from living it—so we're going to have our cake and balanced hormones, too!

Endocrine Disruptors: The Environmental Chemicals That Mess with Hormones

Oh, right. She says all that about living life and then dives headfirst into criticizing my favorite blush. Yeah, I'm gonna go there because every human on this planet is being affected by environmental chemicals, and they are seriously messing with our hormones. Endocrine-disrupting chemicals (EDCs) are a group of chemicals that mimic and stimulate your hormone receptors, block your body from making hormones, or keep you from using the ones you make. When it comes to your sex life, EDCs are the ultimate cockblock (aka blocking you from having sex). Phthalates, found in many personal-care products, have been associated with lower testosterone levels in both men and women and have been shown to block our ability to use testosterone (buh-bye, sexual desire).[2] EDCs are also linked to primary ovarian insufficiency (POI), when those ovaries quit too soon in life.[3] POI comes with a whole host of symptoms described on page 235, including vaginal dryness, thinning of the vaginal tissue, and pain with sex. Chemicals like bisphenol (found in most food storage plastics, including BPA-free plastics), phthalates, parabens, and PCBs are also linked to fertility issues and accelerate ovarian aging.[4] Yes, sometimes the stuff in your anti-aging face cream is prematurely aging your ovaries. If that ain't some bullshit.

Beyond fighting the urge to want to get it on and enjoy sex, these chemicals are also linked to an increased incidence of endometriosis, with some chemicals being found in higher amounts in those diagnosed with the condition.[5] It is very difficult to conduct a study that shows definitively that one EDC caused a disease, but what we do know is that they are linked with several hormonal conditions like PCOS[6] and fibroids.[7] This is a good time to remind you that you did not cause your endometriosis, PCOS, or other hormone condition by choosing to use a certain perfume or get your nails done. While we don't know the cause of endo or PCOS, I highly doubt we're going to have a groundbreaking study that points to only your lotion. Endo and PCOS predate the ubiquitous use and environmental overwhelm we are currently experiencing. But when it comes to effectively managing these conditions, EDCs cannot be ignored, and their contribution to keeping you unwell is undeniable.

Bisphenols are a group of EDCs we all need to be aware of. Structurally they are similar enough to estrogen that they can lock on to the cell's receptors and stimulate it—in all the wrong ways. This can lead to symptoms of excess estrogen in some, which shows up as PMS, heavy periods, and fibroids.[8] They can also prevent androgens, like testosterone and dihydrotestosterone (DHT), the more potent form of testosterone, from doing their jobs, like supporting immunity, muscle mass, energy, and better moods.[9] Bisphenols disrupt thyroid hormone[10] and play a role in the development of autoimmunity, which primarily affects women.[11] And they are associated with infertility, endometriosis, obesity, breast cancer, and birth defects.[12] If we could avoid all plastics, that would be my number one personal choice and recommendation, but we can't. But what you can do is minimize your exposure by drinking from glass or stainless-steel water bottles, rather than disposable plastic. I seriously just use mason jars and have been spotted drinking out of recycled pasta sauce jars—no shame when it comes to protecting my hormones. Avoiding canned food lined with BPA, thermal receipt papers (I tell all my patients who touch receipts for a living to wear gloves), and food heated up in plastic containers can also reduce bisphenol exposure. Because the topic of EDCs is so big, I've made a chart for you to easily identify the common offenders (beyond bisphenols), where they are found, and how to avoid them. You can download it at https://DrBrighten.com/ITN-resources.

Detoxing All Day, Every Day: Your Liver Health

One of your liver's many jobs is to package up what needs to be eliminated from the body—hormones, environmental toxins, metabolic waste—so that it can be excreted. Your liver is doing this all day, every day, and requires specific nutrients to do its job. In fact, there are ways you can support your liver to make healthier estrogen metabolites that can help reduce breast tenderness, heavy periods, and the risk of certain cancers.[18] See the image on page 203 for the nutrients that support the liver. You'll see in that image that once your liver has neutralized and prepared the hormones (and other waste) your body no longer needs, they are then removed from the body via the kidneys and gut. You probably guessed that if you need urine to get estrogen and waste out, then you're going to need to drink water (we'll discuss that in the program), which will also support the bowels (and obviously your kidneys).

THE ESTROGEN BREAKDOWN

Estrogen must be broken down in order to be removed from the body, so we don't end up with a state of excess. Once your body is done with the estrogen you no longer need, it's up to your liver to package it up and move it out. In the first phase of liver detoxification, your estrogens are turned into these three metabolites: 2OH-E1, 4OH-E1, and 16OH-E1. We want to help the liver favor making the 2OH because that's the least cancer-causing of the bunch. Hello, cruciferous vegetables! But know you will have some 4 and 16 floating around, which has benefits like supporting bone health. Balance is key! Your liver then moves these metabolites through phase 2, and eventually they go into the gut and kidneys to be removed from the body.

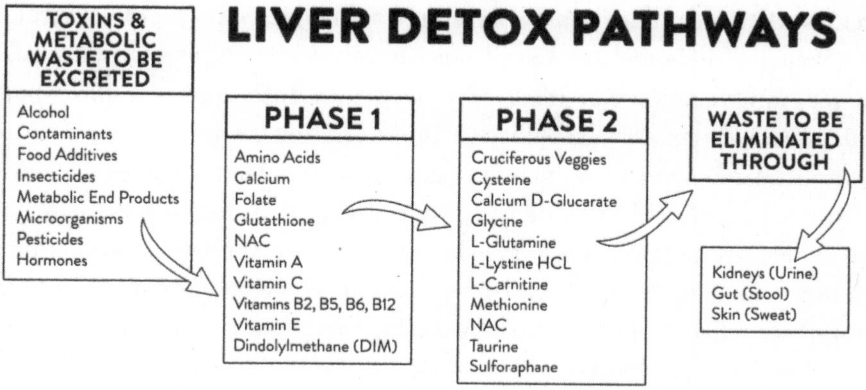

Gut Health: Where Pooping Problems and Period Problems Collide

If you want to get that estrogen out of the bowels, you gotta poop it out (you pee it out too, which is why water is so important). But hold up: through what is called the estrobolome (the microorganisms and enzymes that interact with your estrogen), estrogen can be reactivated and recycled, allowing it to stimulate tissues.[14] These organisms create an enzyme called beta-glucuronidase and when these critters get out of balance, in what is called dysbiosis, there can be an excess of beta-glucuronidase, which ultimately leads to some of your estrogen being recycled rather than removed in your poop.[15] Yes, all that work your liver does can be undone by the enzyme beta-glucuronidase being produced by bacteria in your gut. Imbalances in gut flora have been linked to issues such as endometriosis,[16] PCOS,[17] and certain cancers like breast cancer.[18] We, of course, want to deal with the root cause of the dysbiosis, but if beta-glucuronidase is the cause of your estrogen woes, I recommend supplementing with calcium D-glucarate, 400 to 1,000 mg daily. Constipation, diarrhea, gas, bloating, and seeing undigested food in your stool are just a few signs that things aren't right in your gut and that it's time to see a provider. Unfortunately, it is possible to have zero symptoms and still have estrogen issues stemming from the gut. But it's not just your gut that affects estrogen; in fact, throughout the menstrual cycle (as estrogen fluctuates), it influences the gut microbiome composition, as well as what does and doesn't get through the single-cell layer of your gut.[19]

Your gut is home to most of your immune system, and as we've discussed, inflammation can affect your hormones. Infections can upregulate inflammation, impact your ability to digest and absorb nutrients, and cause a whole host of symptoms, including digestive complaints. And problematic digestive practices like not chewing your food well, eating in a stressful environment, eating foods you know don't agree with you (lactose intolerance calling your name?), drinking heavy amounts of alcohol, or using certain medications like ibuprofen can also impact your gut's ability to maintain microbial balance and get your body the nutrients it needs.

Your liver and gut are the tag team duo of moving out waste, and work together in a lot of ways to support your hormones, from getting rid of estrogen you don't need to activating thyroid hormone. It's a huge topic we could talk much more about, but the key thing to understand is that if they ain't happy, then none of your hormones will be happy. They are two areas I always address in all my patients, which is why we'll be setting up nutrition and lifestyle practices to help you optimize the function of these two key organs as part of your 28-day hormone plan.

COULD YOUR GUT CAUSE VAGINAL PROBLEMS?

Got yeast infections that won't quit, or BV that keeps coming back like we talked about in chapter 7? The estrobolome, how your microbiome and estrogen interact, also affects the microbiome of the vagina and the health of the tissues there. Your estrogen is connected to the vaginal glycogen (sugar) levels that feed the good guys, like lactobacilli, which create the acid that maintains your vagina's optimal pH.[20] In addition, what grows in your gut can also set up home in your vagina, which is why what you put in your mouth—food, prebiotics, probiotics, medications, and more—can influence your gut and vaginal health. We need to care for our gut to care for our hormones and vagina. Plus, as you've learned, happy hormones and a healthy vagina lend themselves to more pleasurable sex.

Suboptimal Nutrition

Aside from the fact that the average doctor has barely, if any, training in nutrition, it's a major problem that they tend to look only for signs of major deficiency. Listen, there are absolutely real diseases caused by malnutrition, like rickets (vitamin D deficiency) and pellagra (niacin or tryptophan deficiency), but these are more rare in developed countries. So unless you're a pirate sailing the seas for months on end, living on only what you can catch, you're not likely going to develop scurvy from lack of vitamin C in your diet. But when I tell you that you can't make vitamin C (unlike other animals) and that the adrenal glands' tissues have one of the body's highest concentrations of C because they depend on it, it almost goes without saying that we want optimal vitamin C so they can do their job, and shouldn't wait until our gums are bleeding (a sign of major deficiency) to supplement it.

There is indeed such a thing as a sex diet, and no, I don't mean an orgasm fast. Our brain, the major sexual organ and master hormone orchestrator; the hormones involved in sexual desire and arousal; and the blood vessels that supply our clitoris, vulva, and vagina all rely on optimal nutrition. Underfueling and overfueling are both problematic for our hormones, but while everyone is debating calories in and calories out (which is an outdated way of approaching weight loss), or whether you should or shouldn't eat carbs and fat (you need both, but your individual needs will vary), what gets almost no play in these conversations is how much we depend on certain nutrients for optimal hormones. Now, I don't play the good food/bad food game—it's rarely helpful. Instead what we want to focus on is providing our system with what it needs to do its job.

In my practice, we focus on food first and supplements second. Supplements can be beneficial for filling in where your diet is lacking, and for helping correct your hormone symptoms much faster when part of a solid lifestyle and nutrition plan. (On page 369 you'll find a chart listing individual nutrients, where you can include them in your diet, how they help your hormones, and the signs you aren't getting optimal amounts.)

WHICH ORAL PROBIOTICS CAN HELP?

What grows in the gut definitely influences the vagina—for better or worse. In addition to eating a fiber-rich diet, adding a probiotic to your supplement routine can help support digestion, estrobolome function, and balance inflammatory chemicals. *Lactobacillus acidophilis* and *Lactobacillus rhamnosus* are the two strains you want to look for in a probiotic. That's because these two hold it down in your vagina by producing acid and other antimicrobial agents that keep everyone in check. They're like the bouncer at the club making sure no one gets too rowdy, but everyone has a good time (that includes in the bedroom, too). In one fifteen-day clinical trial it was found that women who consumed both strains showed improvement in their vaginal microbiome, plus they had a reduction in itching and discharge.[21] Not too shabby for such little organisms. Other studies on these organisms have found similar benefits, along with women reporting improved quality of life.[22]

There are three strains in particular, *Bacillus subtilis*, *B. coagulans*, and *B. clausii*, which act like managers of the microbiome, influencing microbial diversity, the health of the gut lining, and estrogen levels. *B. subtilis* in particular has been shown to reduce two inflammatory cytokines (IL-6 and TNF-alpha),[23] which have been implicated in vaginal atrophy (shrinking tissue)[24] and produce substances that work against E. coli (one of the primary culprits in UTIs).[25]

While probiotics are great at "seeding" the soil, you need to make sure you're adding fertilizer (aka prebiotics). Prebiotics are a type of fiber that feeds the good-for-you organisms that keep your gut healthy and your hormones in check. Some quality probiotics will include prebiotics, and you can also get them into your diet by eating berries, oats, leeks, garlic, dandelion greens, and asparagus.

Inflammation: Ovulation Blocking, Orgasm Sabotaging, and Hormonal Chaos Culprit

If you're sick, cut your finger, or need to fight off a foreign invader (virus, bacteria, parasite, splinter, or the like) then inflammation is your ally. The trouble is, for some of us, the body brings the heat and it just won't quit. Chronic inflammation can occur due to unresolved infections anywhere in the body, eating foods that don't agree with *your* body, autoimmune disease (when your immune system attacks the body), poor gut health, mold exposure, obesity,[26] dental infections, environmental toxicants, and heavy metals, as a few examples.

When inflammation is up, there are immune-system chemical messengers called cytokines going around the body and telling everyone what they should do. Short term, these cytokines are the best; long term, the worst, because they mess with your hormones by disrupting your brain's hormone signaling.[27] If your brain hormones ain't right, your sex, adrenal, thyroid, insulin, or, um, any hormones won't be right. But inflammation takes it to the next level by also preventing your mitochondria from doing their job. You might remember from high school biology class that mitochondria are the powerhouse of your cells (no, I don't actually expect you to remember that, but props if you do). On top of making energy, they also make your hormones. Cortisol, the adrenal hormone that squashes inflammation that we talked about in chapter 3, and the sex hormones we talked about earlier in this chapter, are made in the mitochondria. But girl, inflammation is messing with your brain and your ability to make hormones, so how are we not gonna talk about this when the goal is to optimize your hormones, get you feeling your best, and get your sexual desire and orgasms where you want them to be?

If you're not ovulating, you have a hormone imbalance. Inflammation can absolutely disrupt ovulation, leading to irregular cycles, missing periods, and difficulty getting pregnant. Inflammation can be a chronic stressor and, as you've learned, chronic stress chips away at the foundation of your hormone health. Buh-bye to healthy adrenal function, hello to blood sugar imbalances, and farewell to energy, feeling chill, like, ever, having clear skin, or having periods that don't suck. Sigh. And to make things worse, when there is chronic low-grade inflammation, as we see in obesity, an enzyme called aromatase takes your testosterone and turns it into estrogen.[28] Now we've got more estrogen circulating, leading to more inflammation, stimulating fat cells to grow, and causing plenty of hormone symptoms like irritability, PMS, heavy periods, and headaches. Let's be clear: there are lean people whose labs reveal major metabolic issues and have the same hormone-wrecking inflammation we're talking about. On the flip, there are absolutely metabolically healthy people who fit into the overweight or obese category.[29] You can't just look at someone and know their inflammation status, which is why testing a C-reactive protein (inflammatory marker), fasting insulin, HOMA-IR (a marker of insulin resistance), and assessing blood sugar markers can be useful in evaluating if this is the cause of their hormone struggles. From what we understand in newer research, visceral adiposity, or fat around the organs, is associated with a higher risk of inflammation, as opposed to having a bigger booty, thicker thighs, or curvaceous hips.[30] So what we're not gonna do is shame ourselves or anyone else when what I'm ultimately talking about here is some misbehaving cells poppin' off the inflammatory pathways. Working toward metabolic health means that the goal is optimal labs, hormones, and health.

To address inflammation, we need to figure out the cause. In most cases, you're going to do that best working with a naturopathic or functional-medicine physician, because digging deep is their MO. I will also be walking you through gut health practices, as well as providing you foods and lifestyle practices to help tame the flame in inflammation during the program. For some people, it will be as easy as making some dietary shifts, dropping stress, and getting better sleep. For others, it'll take treating infections, addressing autoimmunity, and figuring out where the source of their inflammation is.

More Stress. More Period Problems.

We did a lot of the stress talk in chapter 3, and at the risk of hitting the broken record vibe, it is a major reason for hormonal chaos, period problems, and extinguished sexual desire for some. Stress, whether the real thing (car accident, infection, boss yelling at you) or perceived (worrying about the what-ifs and psychologically working yourself up) causes shifts in your hormones that favor those that help you survive versus those that help you ovulate, have enjoyable sex, digest your food well, and relax. I think you get the picture.

But not all stress can be controlled, which is why we need to build a tool kit of resiliency to be able to handle the stress that does come our way. (I've got some tips for you on page 311 to help you do just that.) And for others, a life filled with the above-and-beyond stressors—like those that fall into the adverse childhood events (ACE) score category, microaggressions, racism, discrimination, caregiving, or living with a disability—takes more than a weekend yoga retreat, cup of tea, or a good-vibes-only shirt to strip away. (The only time I want to hear "good vibes only" is in a conversation about vibrators.) Allostatic load refers to the cumulative burden of life stressors and chronic events, and when it comes to your health, it's deadly.[31] It contributes to advanced aging, pregnancy complications like preeclampsia, diabetes, heart disease, hormone imbalances, cancer, and mood disorders like anxiety or depression.

So does this mean it's hopeless? Not at all. It means that if you've got the factors that lead to a higher allostatic load, you may need more support, boundaries, and self-care than others. And while I believe everyone does better with a mental health ally on their health care team, you definitely want to consider if you have access to these services. Mindfulness and meditation may feel like a fruitless endeavor in the face of such stressors, but research has shown us that we can change our brain, and how our body responds to stress, and thus shift our hormones to be less "start a riot" and more "I can handle it."[32]

To figure out if stress is causing your period problems, you'll need to evaluate your stress levels as honestly as you can. Don't fall into the trap of thinking *It could be worse* or *My life isn't as bad as it might be.* While perspective and gratitude are awesome, when it comes to cortisol, all that matters is how you perceive the stress in your life. On a scale of 1 to 10, with 10 being "I'm bananas-stressed out of my mind," and 1 "I'm as cool as a cucumber," ascertain your stress level at baseline. If you're teetering above 4, try to cut out as many stressful events, people, and tasks from life as possible, including stressful TV shows and social media accounts, which can also boost cortisol, even if you think you use them to "chill out." Make time to do gentle forms of exercise like yoga and walking, which will reduce cortisol, as will connecting with friends (the good ones, at least), getting at least seven hours of sleep, and doing the self-care practices that relax you, like meditating, taking long baths, reading a good book, or cooking a meal.

How Stress Affects Your Hormones

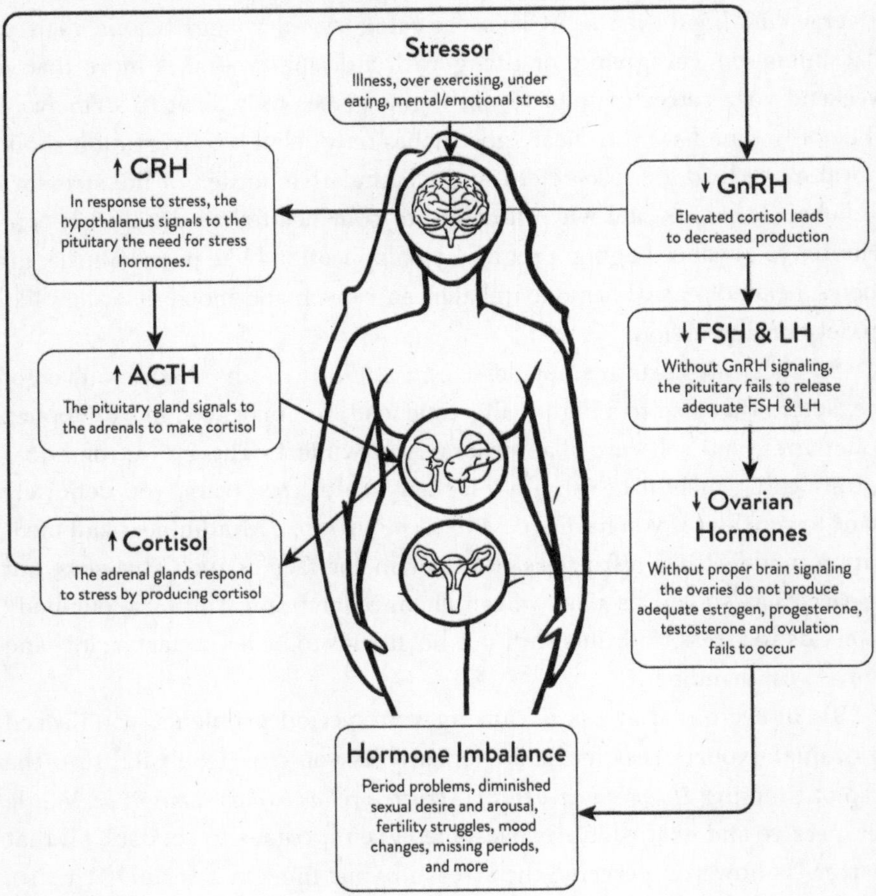

THE LOWDOWN ON LOW CORTISOL

Maybe you took the quiz on page 192 and found that your symptoms are pointing to low cortisol. Does that mean those adrenals are "fatigued"? Unless it is Addison's disease, a condition in which the adrenal glands are destroyed by the immune system, the adrenals aren't likely the issue. So what gives? Hypothalamic pituitary adrenal dysregulation or dysfunction (HPA-D), which is when the brain downregulates the signals or the receptors that receive the signals shift to prevent the adrenals from continuing to produce cortisol at a high rate, is often to blame.[33] High cortisol is bad news; you were never designed to pump it as hard as a frat boy's fist at a house party, or for as long as you do, so your body does what it can to keep you safe. In addition, the body also has other mechanisms, like binding cortisol via a protein called, aptly, cortisol binding protein, so that it isn't free to be used and instead converts it to cortisone, the inactive form. See the information in chapter 13 for more about low cortisol and what can help.

Circadian Rhythm: Your Ovaries and Other Glands Are on the Clock

The quality, timing, and duration of sleep means everything to your hormones, ovulation, period, sexual desire, and mood. That's because your body keeps tabs on its clock more than that white rabbit in *Alice in Wonderland.* And just like that rabbit is all flustered with fear that it'll lose its head, your body gets in a tizzy when there is chronodisruption, aka interference with the circadian rhythm. Your circadian rhythms, governed by the master timekeeper of the brain, the suprachiasmatic nuclei, are the physical, hormonal, behavioral, and mental changes that follow a twenty-four-hour cycle.[34] They are influenced by artificial light, temperature, illness, stress, noise, certain drugs, pain, sleep deprivation, and night-shift work.[35] Touchy little system, right? What you're probably most familiar with is the sleep-wake cycle, but just about every organ in your body is running on a clock. In fact, every cell of the ovary has its own molecular clock, which is why any disruption to your circadian rhythm can lead to missed or delayed ovulation, infertility, and period problems, and when it goes for too long, increased risk of cancer.[36] Timing is everything when it comes to the body's clock. The timing of hormone release daily and during your cycle is also why timing of hormone testing is so crucial. When our sleep is disrupted, it sets off a hormone cascade that can cause us to not ovulate and, so, lose our period, which, as you probably guessed, is a sign of major hormone imbalances. See the diagram on page 212 for how this is all connected.

When cortisol goes high, melatonin goes low (how it should be when you wake), which is why tending to your sleep habits to get cortisol in its place and encourage melatonin to do its thing is crucial to your hormone health. The natural rhythm is for cortisol to taper off in the evening and for melatonin to take center stage to lead you off into peaceful slumber. Bliss. Melatonin, heavily concentrated in the mitochondria, is one of the OG antioxidants, meaning it protects your ovaries and mitochondria. Making hormones produces free radicals, those little buggers that destroy cells and cause premature aging when in excess. Antioxidants tame them and protect the cells from damage. Yes, this is the same hormone you make when you sleep. It rises when the world gets dark, which corresponds with a decline in cortisol, which is why dodging artificial lights at night and sleeping in a completely dark room is a must. When melatonin is disrupted, our oxidative stress rises and cells age.

How Disrupted Sleep Affects Your Hormones

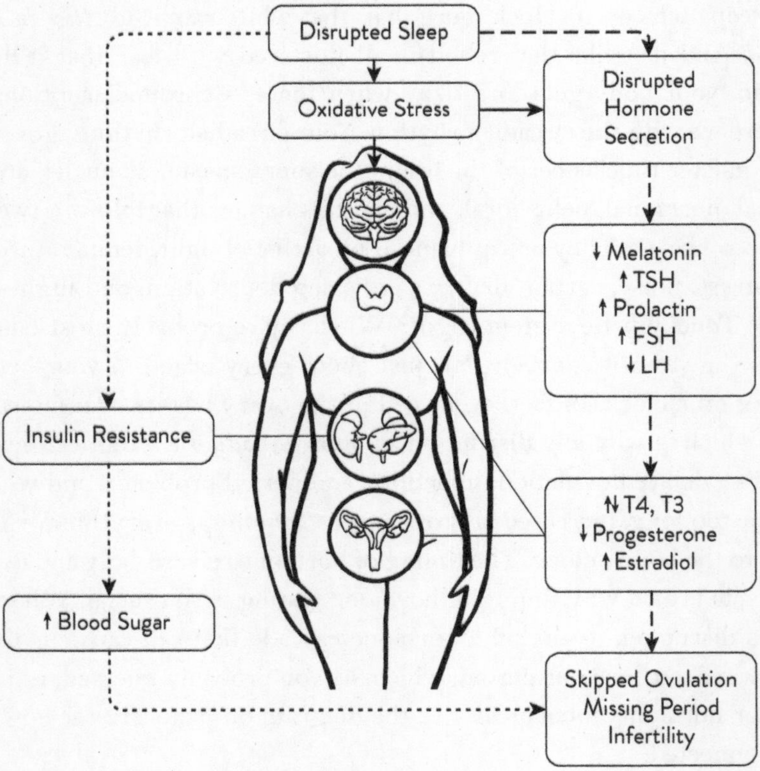

But sleep disruption doesn't stop there; our thyroid hormone is impacted, too. When we experience sleep deprivation or disrupted sleep it can lead to elevations in thyroid-stimulating hormone (TSH), the hormone that triggers thyroid hormone production from the gland. When TSH goes up, prolactin levels follow, as well as lack of ovulation, irregular periods, amenorrhea, anovulation, and recurrent miscarriages.[37] Got estrogen excess problems? In one small study, women with regular sleep patterns experienced 60 percent lower levels of estrogen compared to those with irregular sleep patterns, which may in part explain the correlation between sleep disruption and breast cancer.[38] Sleep is a pretty big deal, so we're gonna home in on getting the best, most restorative sleep in our 28-day program. And as promised in chapter 4, we'll be working on REM sleep, too, because again, sleepgasms!

TL;DR: ARE MY HORMONES NORMAL?

- Use the hormone quiz to help yourself identify which hormones are driving your symptoms. When you're ready to act, use the tools in chapter 13 to address your hormone needs.
- Hormone imbalance refers to when hormones are too high or too low and are causing symptoms. Hypothyroidism, low thyroid hormone, is an example of hormone imbalance.
- In most cases of hormone imbalance there are several factors that contribute to shifting hormones, and each must be addressed.
- When it comes to your sex life, endocrine-disrupting chemicals (EDCs) are the ultimate cockblock (an action that prevents someone from having sex). They can mimic hormones or block natural hormones from doing their job, leading to issues like estrogen excess symptoms, thyroid dysfunction, and inability to use testosterone.
- EDCs are linked to conditions such as endometriosis and PCOS.

- Your liver is responsible for processing EDCs and estrogen to be removed by the body.
- There are key nutrients your liver requires to effectively remove metabolic waste and environmental toxins. See the diagram on page 203.
- The estrobolome is the term for the microorganisms that interact with your estrogen and help maintain balanced hormones and a healthy vagina.
- Your gut microbes can reactivate estrogen via an enzyme known as beta-glucuronidase. Calcium D-glucarate is a nutrient that can prevent this enzyme from pushing too much estrogen back into its active state.
- Many people in the United States aren't getting optimal levels of the key nutrients needed to build hormones and keep them in balance. There's a chart for you on page 369 to guide you in how to eat to get the nutrients you need.
- Stress is one of the heaviest hitters when it comes to disrupting your hormonal harmony. To see exactly how stress impacts your period, see the image on page 210.
- Your ovaries have their own clock, as do other cells in your body. Your exposure to light and quality of sleep (or lack thereof) can seriously disrupt your hormones and cause your body to skip ovulation and miss periods.

CHAPTER 9

IS MY MENSTRUAL CYCLE NORMAL?

IS YOUR FLOW GOING WITH THE FLOW?

From your interest in sex, to lubrication, to you even wanting to be around your partner, the cyclical nature of your hormones has a lot of influence on not just your love life, but your life as a whole. While most of what we get by way of menstrual education is reduced to reproduction alone—aka here's how to avoid babies, and why periods suck—I'm here to tell you that your hormones give you legitimate superpowers. But it sure doesn't feel that way if you've got acne, bloating, irritability, anxiety, or any number of period problems. In my clinical experience, if you understand the hormone dance of your cycle and know what symptoms to track, you can solve a vast majority of sex hormone imbalances by making tweaks to your diet and lifestyle and, perhaps, building a supplement routine. So buckle in, because I'm going to give you the hormone talk that you should have gotten in sex ed, and the lowdown on how to troubleshoot the symptoms that arise when our hormones give us trouble.

Just how common are the hormone imbalances? Well, hormone-related symptoms affect upward of 90 percent of all cycling women,[1] but only 40 percent seek help from a provider, often because they don't know that what they're experiencing isn't normal. Instead, we're led to believe that we have to put up with bloating, PMS, cramps, and other hormonal symptoms simply because we have ovaries. What's more, many women feel too ashamed or embarrassed to bring up concerns with their medical provider about their sex life, menstrual cycle, or period—all of which can indicate hormone imbalances—because they've already had their concerns dismissed by a doctor in the past, been offered no help beyond a prescription for the pill, or been told to come back when they decide to have a baby.

As an integrative physician, I want to give you all the options, help you understand the cause of your symptoms, and equip you with the knowledge to advocate for yourself and have a more productive conversation with your doctor. Despite what you may have read online or heard from your doc, the pill isn't your only option for treating hormonal symptoms. So why is it all that many of us are ever offered? Well, in some cases, it can work really well to eliminate symptoms because it stops your own ovarian hormone production and replaces them with a steady dose of synthetic ones. Plus, there's the two-for-one of preventing pregnancy while clearing up acne or other symptoms, which makes it a good option for some people. If taking the pill is how you release the "don't make a baby" fear so that you can actually get in the mood, I respect that. But while great for symptom management, it doesn't address why you have them, and for a lot of women, taking the pill can make it more difficult to understand what's causing their hormone imbalances. Plus, as you'll soon learn, there's a lot of benefits your own hormones have to offer.

I'm board-certified in naturopathic endocrinology (meaning I'm a doctor who takes a holistic approach to hormonal health), so I treat hormonal irregularities on the daily by having my patients focus on nutrient density in their diet, optimizing activity levels, getting quality sleep, and dialing in a supplement routine, among other lifestyle habits, all of which can help them sustain hormonal health for their lifetime. I've included all these recommendations in my 28-day program to help you get in on all this goodness, too. In this chapter, I'm going to help you understand your menstrual cycle like you never have before, and give you the "why" behind common symptoms.

ASK DR. BRIGHTEN:

What are sex hormones and why do they matter?

Sex hormones are potent chemicals made by the body that influence how we develop, how we look, how we think and behave, how quickly we age, and if and when we're able to conceive. Contrary to popular belief, all bodies produce estrogen, progesterone, and testosterone, and everyone needs all three for healthy sexual function and development. Sex hormones belong to the class of steroid hormones because they're built from cholesterol (instead of proteins or amino acids) and are manufactured primarily by the ovaries or testes, but as we discussed in chapter 4, can also be made by the adrenal glands.

They are extremely powerful agents that shape how we view ourselves, our bodies, our partners, and our entire world. The health of our heart, brain, bones, skin, muscles, metabolism, immune system, and entire body all depend on our hormones. Your ability to move pain free, build memories, wake up energized for the day, maintain a sense of confidence, and handle stress without it wiping you out is all thanks to hormones that work for you. In other words, your hormones were designed to give you superpowers, not sabotage you on a monthly basis.

Estrogen, for example, turns your brain into a problem-solving machine, helping you learn, remember, stay sharp, and proceed with a clear mind.[2] Optimized levels of this hormone can make you feel like Beyoncé strutting across the stage, and increase sexual desire, vaginal lubrication, and your vulva and vagina's ability to be aroused. As estrogen rises at the beginning of your cycle and spikes just before ovulation, you may find your inclination is to suggest a night of Netflix and chill. Add in some testosterone, and it's a done deal.

Testosterone boosts libido in women, along with sexual fantasies and blood flow to the vagina and clitoris, which can increase arousal and makes sex more enjoyable and less painful.[3] It's no coincidence this hormone creeps up when you're most fertile, helping you see sex as much more appetizing. When your testosterone is just right, you'll wake up, kick ass, and set boundaries like a champ. This hormone is also crucial for body composition, allowing you to grow muscles and strengthen bones while burning fat.

While progesterone can put the kibosh on your sexual desire, without enough of this soothing hormone, you're more likely to experience PMS, anxiety, difficulty sleeping, and other symptoms that can indirectly sabotage your libido. When you get your progesterone dialed in, you'll be cool, calm, and collected, rarely stressing about the small stuff. But if you find yourself feeling that getting into a pair of sweatpants is much more appealing than getting into their pants the last week of your cycle, you're not alone. In some women, estrogen and testosterone stand no chance against progesterone's agenda, and their partner is going to need to bring their A game (helping release brakes and stimulate the gas pedal is discussed in chapter 3). Another cool feature of progesterone is that it helps solidify emotional memory and is neuroprotective, meaning it protects your brain.[4]

HORMONES OF THE MENSTRUAL CYCLE

- **Follicle-stimulating hormone (FSH)** is responsible for signaling to the ovaries to get an egg ready for ovulation and produce estrogen. FSH fluctuates over the course of your cycle and is highest in the follicular phase (period until ovulation). This hormone is secreted by the pituitary gland in the brain, which means your menstrual cycle actually starts in your head, not in your ovaries or uterus.
- **Luteinizing hormone (LH)** stimulates ovulation by telling your ovaries to release an egg, which is caught by tiny fingerlike projections called fimbriae that help usher it into the fallopian tubes. The hormone also tells your ovaries to produce estrogen and progesterone. Like FSH, LH is also produced by the pituitary gland.
- **Estrogen** is present in different amounts throughout your cycle, peaking right before you ovulate and rising again about a week before you get your period. On the first day of bleeding, your estrogen levels are lowest for the month. Estrogen helps thicken your uterine lining (endometrium) and encourages ovulation. Your ovaries are responsible for making most of the estrogen in your body—why the hormone is highest during your fertile years—although your adrenal glands, fat cells, and bones also contribute.

- **Progesterone** rises slightly before ovulation, then more sharply following ovulation, and peaks approximately one week before your period—the only time in your cycle when this hormone exceeds your estrogen levels. Like estrogen, progesterone also helps thicken your uterine lining. This hormone additionally prevents your uterus from cramping, protecting your body from prematurely shedding its endometrium. Progesterone is made by the ovaries by a temporary endocrine gland called the corpus luteum—more on this fascinating little hormone factory in a minute.
- **Testosterone** boosts your sexual desire before ovulation, when your testosterone levels are highest. If you have too much or too little testosterone, it can interfere with your period and affect your fertility, in addition to causing other troubling symptoms. About a quarter of your testosterone is produced in your ovaries, another quarter in your adrenals, and about half in the other tissues of the body.

Your Endocrine Glands (AKA Hormone Factories)

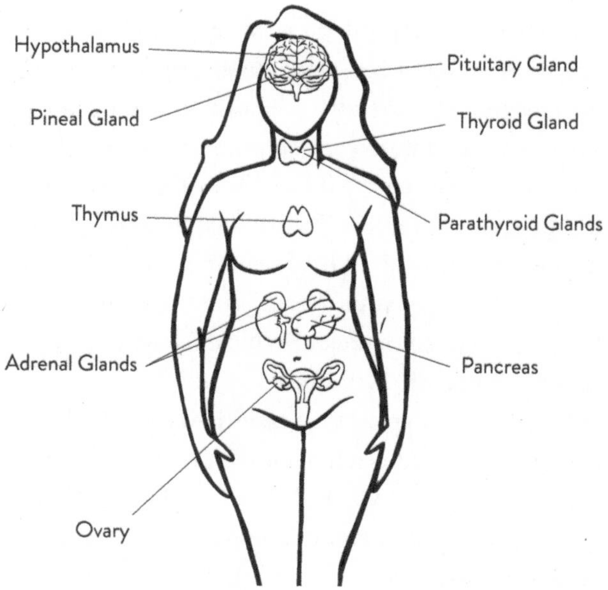

How the Menstrual Cycle Works

Your brain is boss in telling every endocrine gland (hormone-producing tissue) when to turn on and off production of their corresponding hormone. (See page 218 for a chart of glands and the hormones they make.) In chapter 4 we talked about the brain-adrenal connection. Now we're going to cover how your brain and ovaries communicate to produce an egg (ovulation) and a period. We are all taught that day 1 of our cycle is the first day we have a flow, and while this makes cycle tracking very easy, it places far too much emphasis on the period and does not give the main event of the cycle the play it deserves—ovulation. Nonetheless, I'm going to take it from the top with the period because it does lend itself to easier mastery of your menstrual cycle. Please note that all the days listed next to the cycle are more of an "ish" because each of our cycles are unique, and how many days we spend in each has variability. For example, you may have a period for only 3 days and ovulate on day 12 or day 18. All of that is normal.

PHASE 1: YOUR PERIOD (DAYS 1–7)

The entire point of the cycle is to get you knocked up. If you want a baby, there's some tips you'll find here to help you reach that goal. If you don't want a baby, these same tips can help you dodge the threat of semen in your womb. First off, let's get straight on what a period is. The period is the body's response to an unfertilized egg (when sperm and egg did not meet up). A fertilized egg that successfully implants in the uterine lining releases beta–human chorionic gonadotropin, commonly known as HCG (the hormone that pregnancy tests detect). The lack of HCG tells the body to drop it (estrogen and progesterone) like it's hot, faster than a Snoop Dogg song. In fact, this will be the lowest these hormones are for your entire cycle. When they drop, the lining of your uterus (endometrium) follows as prostaglandins (inflammatory hormonelike chemicals) take to causing your uterus to contract, otherwise known as cramps.

Bleeding ain't easy. You've taken a month-ish to build your uterine lining, and now your uterus is tasked with removing it all to start over. It's like putting up and tearing down wallpaper every month just to do it all over again. Sounds exhausting, right? And it can be, which is why a dip in energy is normal. But there are other things that aren't normal, which I'll be covering in detail in chapter 10. Although bleeding can hurt and add just another to-do (change tampon regularly, check) to your already busy schedule, there are some amazing things these hormones are doing within your body. Remember: estrogen is making your brain fire like a champ and never leaves you wondering where you put your keys, because it supports memory. See page 217 for a reminder of the superpowers these sex hormones provide.

PHASE 2: FOLLICULAR (DAYS 1–13)

The follicular phase is the name for the first half of your menstrual cycle and includes your period. I know, confusing AF, but I'll explain. Your uterus is doing one thing (a very important thing) at the beginning of the follicular phase—removing the endometrial lining. That deserves its own discussion, which is why I have a chapter for it. But even while your uterus is cleaning house, your brain and ovaries are working behind the scenes for another round of ovulation by maturing a follicle (ah, that's how this phase got its name). And since the entire point of this whole thing is ovulation, these names center around it (as they should).

Starting in the early days of your period, the brain (pituitary, to be exact) is pumping the follicle-stimulating hormone (FSH). FSH drops down to those ovaries and tells them to choose their champion; that is, get the winning egg ready to be released. Estrogen is on the rise and will be the main hormone of this phase, as it orchestrates the rebuilding of the endometrium at the end of your period. In the days leading up to ovulation, testosterone comes into play, and now you're feeling sexy, energized, and ready to mingle (wink, wink). When that egg is ready, estrogen levels spike like a flare signaling the brain that it's go time. The pituitary sends a surge of luteinizing hormone (LH) and tells the ovaries, "Release the egg." (Cue that "Release the Kraken!" voice from *Clash of the Titans.*) And *badaboom*, you just found yourself in the ovulatory phase.

PHASE 3: OVULATORY (DAYS 12–18)

It's a one-day event. The egg comes. The egg goes. Or the egg meets sperm and is transformed into a rapidly dividing ball of cells (how we all start out). And this, my friend, is the only time in your entire cycle you can get pregnant. I know—mind blown! (And if you knew that, congrats on being in the minority who've had a medically accurate sex ed.) That egg has a twenty-four-hour window to meet up with sperm, and your body provides you signs of when this event will take place. But wait! There's this thing called the fertile window. See page 224 for how to know when to time sex to get pregnant, or when to engage in any other kind of activity but vaginal sex if you don't. Of course, if you don't have sex with a penis, you may feel this information is unnecessary for you. Allow me to make a case why ovulation, and knowing that you're doing it, is a very good thing as we enter the luteal phase.

PHASE 4: LUTEAL (DAYS 15–28)

There's only one way to the magical world of progesterone, and you must go through ovulation to get there. Remember the corpus luteum from before? This little structure is responsible for progesterone production, which gives you a sense of calm, reduces bloating, alleviates cramping, and can make you feel a deeper connection to those you love. You may be asking yourself why life sucks so bad before your period, if all of this is true. To answer that, I invite you to explore the premenstrual syndrome (PMS) and premenstrual dysphoric disorder (PMDD) sections in this chapter.

So how about those sex desire–squashing effects? Well, as I told you in chapter 3, hormones are only part of the story. If you're someone (like most) who finds that feeling stressed, anxious, and having trouble sleeping kills your desire for sex, know that progesterone is your ally. It may help you ease the pressure on those brakes so you can get more of those gas pedal signals. You may need a little more stimulation to get in the mood, and this part of the cycle lends itself to a *Try to start something and see where it goes* kind of vibe.

If you get pregnant, meaning a fertilized egg has made your uterus its home, your corpus luteum will keep pumping out progesterone until the placenta takes over. If not, however, this little gland dissolves and the cycle starts over again, taking us back to your period. Feelings are mixed with that negative pregnancy result—celebratory or, as one patient told me, "Gutted to feel like I've failed again." If you're feeling the latter and have been trying for six months or more, use the steps on page 224 to time ovulation, leverage the information in the 28-day plan to optimize ovulation and progesterone, and schedule to meet with your provider.

Menstrual Cycle at a Glance

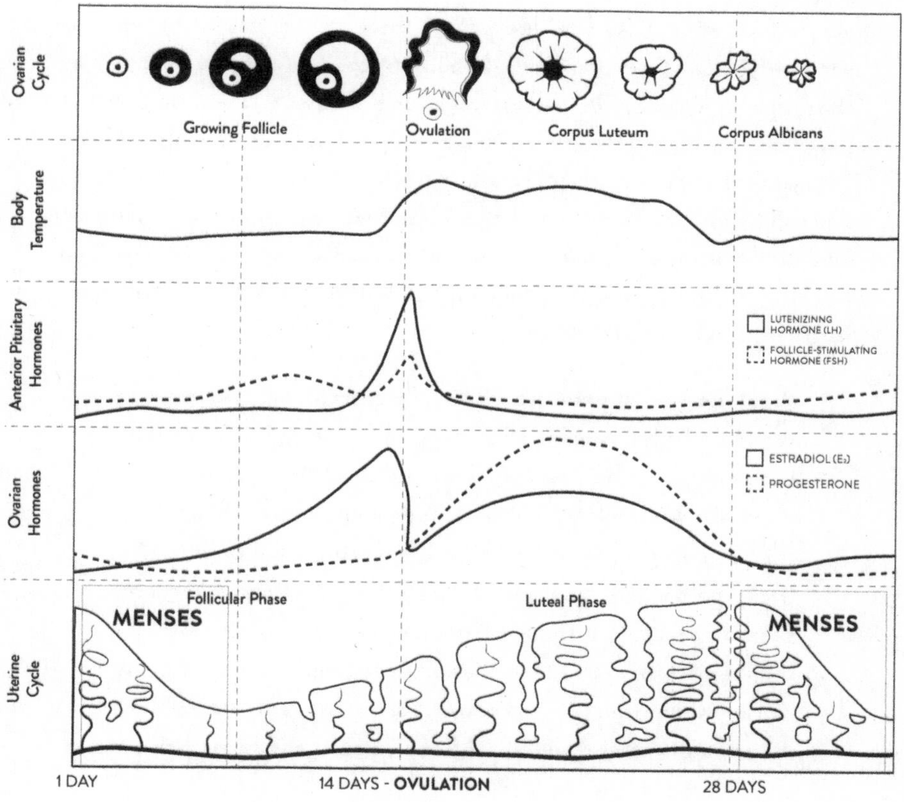

SIX OVULATION SIGNS FOR BABY-MAKING OR SPERM-DODGING (CHOOSE YOUR OWN ADVENTURE HERE)

The first thing you need to know: sperm be tricky little things! They will hang out (loitering, if you will) for the egg to be released 3 to 5 days before you ovulate. That means your fertile window (the days you can get pregnant) is about 6 days.[5] The math goes: Sperm lives up to 5 days + you're fertile for 1 day (the lifespan of the egg) = 6 days. Outside this window, you can't get pregnant. If you want to avoid pregnancy, don't let those sperm in 5 days before ovulation or the day of. If you want to get pregnant, trying 3 days before, and the day of predicted ovulation, can help you get the timing right. This data tracking can help you predict when you might ovulate, but I want to be clear that you cannot just count on ovulating the same day every month. Here are the signs to look for when tracking ovulation, part of a pregnancy pursuit or prevention called fertility awareness method (FAM):

1. **Basal Body Temperature (BBT) Increase.** The progesterone that follows the release of the egg causes a slight rise in body temperature, which remains elevated until the corpus luteum dissolves. To track BBT, take your temperature with a basal thermometer each morning before getting out of bed. The tricky part is that you need to take it at the exact same time every morning, first thing, before you do anything else. BBT is a tool helpful for confirming that ovulation occurred, versus predicting when ovulation will happen, since the temps usually rise immediately after ovulation. Alcohol, stress, and being sick can all influence this temp reading.
2. **Positive LH Test.** When you see the LH surge you can expect to ovulate in 1 to 2 days. LH surges to trigger the release of the egg.
3. **Fertile Cervical Mucus.** Your cervical fluid will shift to enable sperm to survive and successfully make their journey to the egg. This is the egg white consistency discussed in detail in chapter 7.

4. **Increased Sexual Desire.** If you find you're more receptive to sexual inputs (touch, thoughts, or visual stimulation) then it may be a sign you're about to ovulate. Estrogen and testosterone peak before ovulation, which gives you the nudge to have sex.
5. **Change in Cervix Position.** Your cervix will be higher than usual right before ovulation. It will also feel softer and slightly open.[6] When you aren't fertile, it closes up and feels lower, firmer, and drier. This is some next-level mastery in knowing your body, and can take time to learn.
6. **Ovulation Pain.** Mittelschmerz, what midcycle pain is called, can indicate ovulation. It feels like a sharp pain on one side of your lower abdomen. For most women, it's like a smaller version of a menstrual cramp that passes after a few hours, although some women describe a more severe pain, which is something that should be discussed with a provider. Otherwise, this discomfort is associated with the LH surge and linked to increasing prostaglandins.[7] Not everyone experiences this sensation, so if you don't, that's normal, too.

ASK DR. BRIGHTEN:

Do I ovulate every cycle?

Ovulation tends to occur around the same day in our cycle, however, it can shift and be affected by things like travel, stress, illness, light exposure, and other hormone conditions like thyroid disease. The best way to know when you ovulate is to use the signs in the box above. It is possible to skip ovulation every now and again and still have a period. This is what is referred to as an anovulatory cycle, which is doctor-speak for "no ovulation happened." If you're consistently not ovulating, as is the case with PCOS, you will not have consistent periods. If your periods are predictable, showing up at a regular interval, then you're more than likely to be ovulating. If you're on hormonal birth control that suppresses ovulation, then you are not ovulating (because otherwise you'd get pregnant) and that bleed is actually a medication withdrawal. More on this in chapter 10, along with why your period may be MIA.

Is it normal to not be in the mood every day of my cycle?

You may have noticed that at certain times of the month, you may look at your partner and think, *Yeah, you be lookin' good,* while other times it's, *Nah, I'm good, pass.* That's totally normal. Sometimes you'll be in the mood, sex will feel better, and your orgasms will come a lot easier (pun intended). Other times, though, you won't be super interested in sex, and being intimate with your partner may seem as fun as making a shopping list. That's all normal. A big reason for these wild pendulum swings is the hormones responsible for your menstrual cycle. As a cyclical creature, your mood, libido, lubrication levels, ability to orgasm, and ability to connect or even tolerate another human fluctuate according to your hormones (and life).

Unfortunately, we're not all aware of why it is we feel this way in the moment, and rarely are we told anything about our hormones outside of testosterone (let alone our cycle) in regard to sexual desire and arousal. In chapter 3, I explained responsive versus spontaneous desire, the latter being the *It's go time, all the time* kind of libido often depicted in the media. We talked about spontaneous desire being some people's default and, for others, it is something that is experienced only at the beginning of a relationship. But there's another layer here—some people tend to be much more in the mood during the days leading up to ovulation, when estrogen and testosterone are at their highest.[8] I have patients who totally identify with the responsive desire description most of the time, except for these few days out of the month where they report feeling that spontaneous vibe. Or, in other words, it may only take just the thought of something sexy to flip the switch on *all systems go* and take you full steam ahead into a super steamy session. In fact, some researchers have proposed that the 3 days prior to the LH surge, the day of, and 2 days following (doing the math for you—that's a 6-day window) be referred to as the *sexual phase* of the cycle due to the increase in sexual desire and fantasies some women experience during this time.[9] This all corresponds to ovulation, which is another reason why not only is ovulation a good thing, but your cycle is worth tracking.

In PCOS, a condition in which women may not ovulate or may do so infrequently, it has been found that there is impaired sexual function (arousal, lubrication, orgasm, and sexual satisfaction) that is independent of body mass index (BMI) and is heavily influenced by the lack of ovulation.[10] While BMI is bullshit (it was invented by a mathematician and basically places white male specimens as the standard by which we should all be measured), this is an important distinction in the research for three reasons: one, it is well documented that obesity and sexual dysfunction are associated;[11] two, women with PCOS often have their symptoms and concerns reduced to weight alone and are therefore told to just "eat right and exercise"; three, it underscores the importance of working toward creating healthy ovulatory cycles.

Physiologically, during our fertile window, we've got hormones doing what they do best, sending signals to our brain and other tissues, which lends itself to a clit that can swell on command and a vagina that says *No additional lube needed for me today, thank you very much.* But let me just remind you that needing lube and physical stimulation to get to a full state of arousal is also normal, no matter where you are in your cycle. During your fertile window you can experience a more spontaneous desire and feel more sexually charged. At other times in your cycle you may find you need more stimulation to even get your brain and body interested in sex, like we talked about in chapter 3. For example, if you're not interested sexually before your period, it could be that your progesterone levels are up. To add to the complexity, it could be you didn't ovulate, which lends itself to elevated estrogen issues coupled with low progesterone and all the PMS, anxiety, and *Could you just close your damn mouth* feelings you can imagine. (Psst: use the quiz on page 192 to determine what the heck is happening here.) But no matter what's up with your hormones, it's normal to need more foreplay if sexual intercourse is your goal. Use the journal prompts in the 28-day plan to track your sexual desire and how easy it is for you to become aroused throughout your cycle. You can use these to better understand yourself and communicate with your partner.

How Sexual Desire and Orgasms Change over the Menstrual Cycle

There's a lot that influences your sexual desire and ability to orgasm. Sure, there's hormones, but there is also stress, relationship dynamics, and whether or not you can get pregnant (to name a few factors). While hormones may say *Do it on this day* (hello, ovulation), your logical self may be more inclined to get it on when you know you're past that fertile window. What I'm outlining here are general guidelines of what you may experience, but it may not be exactly true of your experience. I encourage you to track your cycle, as we'll be doing in the 28-day program, and map out what is true for you over the course of your cycle. If you want to get to the next level in understanding your body's arousal and orgasm capacity, I recommend checking out the Lioness, which is a device that will record your arousal and orgasm each time you masturbate. It's a very sophisticated way to get in tune with your body while fine-tuning what gets you there.

Libido is complex. While your menstrual cycle influences your sexual desire, so do the many other factors we discussed in chapter 3. The bottom line: Get to know and trust your body. If you're down to get down, it doesn't matter where you are in your cycle. Either way, maintaining good communication with your partner and having plenty of lube nearby are excellent ideas for every day of the month.

YOUR PERIOD

- **Sexual Desire**
  With estrogen and progesterone down, testosterone is left to get you in the mood. Your desire may be greater, or period symptoms may have you wanting to put intimacy on pause. Masturbation may bring you relief from cramps and headaches. Also, the fact that you can't get pregnant may be releasing your brakes so more of the gas pedal signals get through.

- **Arousal**
  There's a lot going on in this area on your period and, for some, the increased sensations of menstruation also lend themselves to increased receptivity to pleasure.

- **Orgasm**
  If the goal is orgasm (and it is OK if it isn't), just know it may take a little longer to get there. Ugh! So frustrating! But when your body gives you the oxytocin and endorphin reward on the other side, it can feel

like just what the doctor ordered for relieving the common symptoms that accompany our period.

- **What to Know**

  While you might be in the clear for pregnancy risk (see chapter 10), period blood raises the pH of your vagina, and the presence of less estrogen during this time may mean less food for the lactobacilli. If you're the type of person who finds they experience BV after sex or periods, ejaculate is not your friend right now. Opt for a condom or ask them to aim outside the vagina when it's time.

  If you struggle with endometriosis or adenomyosis pain during your period, but your brain is still begging you to get some, opting for clitoral stimulation sans penetration may fit your body's needs best. Remember: there's lots of different kinds of sex, and while I'll preach the benefits of orgasms all day, they aren't totally necessary for a satisfying sesh.

  I had a patient share that she "loved getting railed," but wondered why it sometimes hurt. After a little tracking, we found that during her period, when the cervix is the lowest, she was more likely to feel pain when a penis collided with the lower end of her uterus. Yeah, that's a sensation that's not fun for a lot of us. If you find this is true for you, too, try different positions or an Ohnut (described in chapter 5), to accommodate your shifting cervix.

LATE FOLLICULAR

- **Sexual Desire**

  Estrogen and testosterone seriously have one-track minds, pushing your sexual desire up as you near ovulation. If you find yourself suddenly finding that TV star more attractive than ever before, or having a fantasy in the checkout line of the grocery, it's totally normal.

- **Arousal**

  If it is right after your period ends, you're going to need lube and probably more stimulation—both are normal. As you near ovulation, estrogen will make sure that self-lubrication comes easier, but know that more lube in the bedroom is rarely ever a bad thing.

- **Orgasm**
  Clitoral stimulation will always be the winner when it comes to going for the O, but you may also find that this is a good time to explore other areas of your body.

- **What to Know**
  If you want to try new positions, play with new toys, or experiment with a bit of kink, this is a phase where you'll likely be receptive and successful. Your breasts are less tender once your period begins, and your nipples become more sensitive once you enter the fertile window.[12] Once ovulation occurs, breast tenderness usually follows, so now is your window for trying a nipplegasm or just incorporating them into the mix.

OVULATION

- **Sexual Desire**
  If you're inclined to masturbate, know that most everyone else is, too, when ovulating (whether they do it or not) thanks to the surge of estrogen and testosterone. This is the time of the cycle when women report feeling most inclined to seek out sexual pleasure.

- **Arousal**
  If your sexual fantasies are increasing in frequency and they really get things moving down there, you're probably about to ovulate, and all of this is normal.[13] Your ability to self-lubricate is up and your genitals are more responsive to sexual stimuli. If you're in a heterosexual relationship, this is the phase when vaginal intercourse may bring increased genital arousal.[14]

- **Orgasm**
  If you find you get there quick, that's normal and seriously nothing to be concerned about or ashamed of. Heck, if you do, why not go back

for seconds? Orgasms are easier to achieve during this period, so it's a good time to try for multiples.

- **What to Know**
  Both deep penetration and doggy style are game on during this phase (if that is something you're into) because your cervix is at its highest position.

LUTEAL PHASE

- **Sexual Desire**
  Oxytocin is dropping, progesterone is rising, and you just may find that cuddles are where it's at as you get closer to your period. If you're struggling with progesterone, you may be irritated by your partner and find that every single thing slams on the brakes. If your progesterone is on point, you'll likely find yourself less critical of your partner and much more chill. While progesterone can decrease sexual desire, it does work for you by creating an inner calm that allows you to disengage brakes that would otherwise keep you from being interested.

- **Arousal**
  With progesterone up and keeping estrogen in check, you may find your genitals a little less responsive (give them time to get there) and that lubrication is lacking. It's all normal, and all a good reason to keep lube on hand, toys in the bedroom, and ask your partner for what you like.

- **Orgasm**
  While the clitoris may get larger around ovulation, it can also get a tad smaller as you approach your period.[15] I like to think of it more as an internal retreat, much like our energy and emotions do at this time of our cycle. If you're having partnered sex, oral sex may be your preferred way to orgasm. You can ask your partner to expose your clitoris further by retracting the tissue around it, or you can do it yourself.

- **What to Know**
  If you find you want to be alone during this time, that's normal. As we approach our period, energy can dip and we may not be that into partnered sex, or sex at all. If you have a partner, let them know that this is a normal time to see a drop-off in sexual desire. If you aren't into it, that's totally cool. But if you'd still like to be sexually active, this is a key time to communicate how to disengage brakes and what you specifically need in terms of pleasure.

Is it normal if I don't have a 28-day cycle?

It's actually way less common to have a 28-day cycle than what we've been told. In fact, according to recent research conducted by Swedish doctors, only 13 percent of all women cycle every four weeks to the day.[16] Depending on the source you're referencing, somewhere between 21 to 38 days is considered normal.[17] Anything shorter or longer than this range, however, is not normal. So a cycle less than 24 days or greater than 35 days may indicate a problem, which is why it is a good idea to bring your cycle length up with your doctor, especially if you have symptoms like what's listed in the chart on page 263.

In teens, whose brain and ovaries are just figuring out how to talk, their cycles may be irregular and anywhere from 21 to 45 days, which is normal.[18] And cycles may vary in length from month to month. This isn't necessarily a cause for concern. Although some doctors jump to prescribing the pill to "regulate" a new menstruator's cycle, not only is this not necessary in many cases but also uncharted territory, as we don't have studies that tell us what happens when we interrupt this necessary maturation process.

Why and How to Track Your Cycle

Tracking your menstrual cycle—not just your period—can help you identify any symptoms associated with hormone imbalances so that you can home in on where to focus your efforts. By tracking your cycle, you'll also be able to know what's normal for *you*, allowing you to notify your doctor when you experience any changes to your baseline health.

So how do you track your cycle? There are a few different options. You can invest in a journal where you can record your symptoms, download a cycle tracking app for your smartphone, or using a cycle tracking device like Natural Cycles, Clue, Flo, and Oura (be sure to check who shares your data). Start with the first day of your period, when you have real, legit blood flow, not just spotting. Make note of how heavy your flow is or how many tampons, pads, or menstrual cups you use and how regularly you change them (I'll explain why this is important in chapter 10). Pay attention to your skin's appearance and your mood, appetite, bloating, energy, and stress levels, and write down any changes. Also record how many days your period lasts, and whether it stops with spotting or just ceases altogether.

When your period ends, continue to make notes on your skin, mood, appetite, bloating, energy, and stress levels as your cycle progresses through the follicular phase. In a few days' time, start paying attention to your underwear, too. If it looks like someone blew their nose in it during allergy season, congrats: This snot-like substance is fertile cervical mucus and, unlike snot, it's awesome because it means your hormones are preparing you to ovulate. Unless you want to have a baby, don't have unprotected sex now. If you're trying to get pregnant, though, this is your window. If you want to know more about when you can get pregnant, I'd also suggest taking your basal body temperature—your temperature at rest—before you get out of bed every morning. When you see a little spike, or a bump by about 0.4 to 0.8 degrees Fahrenheit, you're ovulating. See the ovulation info on page 221.

After ovulation, as you enter the luteal phase, be on the lookout for any signs of PMS or other changes to your skin, mood, sleep, appetite, bowel habits, and vaginal discharge. Write down whether you experience any cramping, bloating, or headaches, and how severe the pain is on a scale from 1 to 10. When your period arrives, do the math to figure out how many days it's been since the first day of your last period: This is how long your cycle is. As you continue to track your cycle, keep this number in mind, noticing if your cycle is regular, meaning it occurs after the same number of days every month, or you're irregular, which happens when your cycle varies month to month by three or more days (more on this soon).

IMPORTANT CYCLE DATA TO TRACK

- When does your period start?
- How many days do you bleed?
- How many days do you spot? Beginning or end?
- How heavy is each day? How many tampons, pads, etc., do you use?
- Do you see clots? How big?
- How many days between the first day of your period and the next? (This is your cycle length.)
- How painful is it?
- Do you have to take time off from work or school?
- Do you have other symptoms like PMS, fatigue, diarrhea, acne?

ASK DR. BRIGHTEN:

Are my menstrual cycle problems normal?

While everything that can be off during your cycle often gets lumped in as a "period problem," some of these issues are a pre-period or an entire-menstrual-cycle problem. We'll talk period-specific issues in chapter 10, but for now, we're covering everything else.

Short cycles: Why is it I feel like I'm only getting a handful of weeks between periods?

OMG, is that my period again? When your period is showing up far too often it isn't just annoying, it's a problem. While the cycle length alone is a problem, we've gotta ask if you're ovulating, when you're ovulating, and how long your luteal phase is. For example, in some cases, a cycle less than 23 days can be a sign that you're not making enough progesterone to carry your uterus to the finish line, causing you to bleed sooner (depending on when you ovulate). This is what is known as a luteal phase defect (LPD), when the corpus luteum fails to produce progesterone for more than 9 to 11 days after ovulation.[19] So if you ovulated on day 14 and then bleed on day 22, this may be a case of LPD. As we enter our forties, we expect shorter cycles to arise due to our dwindling egg supply (although some can definitely get pregnant), which leads to the many symptoms of perimenopause.

If you're experiencing frequent periods or short cycles, it could also be due to primary ovarian insufficiency (POI), which looks a bit like perimenopause, but occurs before our forties. There can be many reasons for POI, and it doesn't always mean your periods are gone for good. POI is associated with a rare autoimmune adrenal condition called Addison's disease, which occurs when your immune system destroys your adrenal glands.[20] A third of women with Addison's will experience early menopause in their thirties. Other causes can be thyroid disease or the early signs that your period is about to bounce for good due to stress or poor nutrition, as can sometimes be the pattern with functional hypothalamic amenorrhea (FHA), although it is more common to see a missing period altogether. Other causes for bleeding showing up too early can be ectopic pregnancy, STI (see chapter 7), endometriosis or adenomyosis (see chapter 5), uterine growths, or some serious hormone issues—all of which warrant a check-in with a provider. If your cycles are frequent, having hormone testing (see https://DrBrighten.com/ITN-resources for the list of tests) to determine what is going on is an important step. Supporting your body's ability to ovulate and produce progesterone, and ensuring your other hormones are balanced, can do a lot for helping you have a healthy luteal phase. I'll be showing you how as part of the 28-day program.

Long cycles: What if I go a couple of months between periods? What does it mean to have an irregular cycle? What causes it?

If wearing white pants is the only predictable measure for when your period might show up (saboteur!), then it's time to start tracking. Just like a plane, there may be minor delays or early arrivals, but there should be some predictability to your period. If you're skipping a month three times out of the year or going beyond 35 days, it could be a sign of hypothyroidism, PCOS, FHA, or high prolactin, a hormone associated with milk production.

I'll be giving you tools to optimize ovulation and progesterone, but if you're finding your period is coming way too quick, staying gone for too

Perimenopause Symptom Check

As you approach menopause, your body's ovulatory cycles become less frequent. Basically, the ovaries are like, *This baby-making game was fun while it lasted, but it is now time to enter a new phase of life.* Our hormones can do wild things as we enter perimenopause, leading to a whole lot of symptoms that can span a decade before we finally do enter menopause. If you're over forty, these symptoms may be a sign of perimenopause, although these symptoms can start for some women as early as age thirty-five. If you're under forty, you shouldn't assume it's perimenopause, and your provider should be investigating what was discussed in the section above on short periods. Perimenopause doesn't have to be hell, and the sooner you create a hormone-loving lifestyle using the tips in this book, the easier you can make that future transition.

- ☐ Irregular, more frequent, or missing periods
- ☐ Hot flashes
- ☐ Night sweats
- ☐ Pain during sex
- ☐ Vaginal dryness
- ☐ Difficulty falling asleep, staying asleep, or insomnia
- ☐ Anxiety, panic attacks
- ☐ Depression, lack of motivation
- ☐ Mood swings
- ☐ Weight gain or difficulty losing weight
- ☐ Hair loss
- ☐ Headaches
- ☐ Changes in hair or skin texture or appearance
- ☐ Diminished sexual desire

long (does anyone ever miss their period?), or you haven't a clue if it'll ever show up, it's time for a trip to your medical provider to investigate the cause. Tracking your cycle can help you understand your normal and communicate more effectively with your doctor, which is why I have the deets on how to do that on page 234. We'll be diving into missing periods in chapter 10.

Polycystic Ovary Syndrome: More Than a Period That Rarely Shows Up

While it was once thought to be a rare condition, we now know that polycystic ovary syndrome (PCOS) affects as many as 20 percent of women worldwide.[21] Yet as common as the condition may be, many women struggle to get their doctor to listen to their concerns, never mind ordering any hormone testing. This is why nearly half of all women with PCOS see three or more health professionals before receiving the correct diagnosis, with one-third of all patients needing more than two years to reach the right diagnosis, according to research.[22] The same study found that only 16 percent of women with PCOS are satisfied with the information they receive from their doctor regarding the condition.

The truth is, we don't know what causes PCOS. It is a complex condition rooted in inflammation, gut dysbiosis (imbalanced gut flora), androgen excess, and insulin dysregulation that can lead to diabetes, infertility, heart disease, high cholesterol, and fatty liver disease if left untreated. While not true for everyone with PCOS, gaining weight and difficulty losing it can be a symptom. In some cases of PCOS, the body's ability to use insulin is impaired, which prevents the body from regulating blood sugar.[23] Because insulin is a nonnegotiable hormone, the body responds by increasing production when it's clear the cells are ignoring the signal. Unfortunately, the elevations in insulin stimulate the ovaries to produce testosterone, while also suppressing the production of sex hormone binding globulin (SHBG), a protein that binds testosterone (one of the androgen hormones), leading to symptoms of excess androgens—cystic acne, oily skin, hair loss on the head, and hair growth on the chin, chest, and abdomen. While your brain begs your ovaries to mature and release an egg, the excess androgens inhibit ovulation success. What is referred to as polycystic ovaries, which are sometimes seen on ultrasound, is actually a busy group of follicles trying so very hard to produce an egg. The ovulation issues are made worse by anything (stress, infections, inflammation, and other factors discussed in chapter 8) that causes the adrenals to increase cortisol, as this can interfere with ovulatory cycles. In addition, there is evidence that the adrenals may also be contributing to androgen excess in some cases of PCOS by way of DHEA, which is converted into testosterone.[24] (Props if you remembered that!) The inability to ovulate is why as many as 75 to 85 percent of women with PCOS will have irregular or long cycles, making anovulation a hallmark of this condition.[25] As discussed in this chapter, it may be the lack of ovulatory cycles that contributes to lower sexual satisfaction in women with PCOS.

Real talk for a second. Because body shaming and fat phobia are pervasive in medicine, I need to make this clear: *PCOS causes weight gain; weight gain does not cause PCOS.* Why is this so important? Blaming your symptoms on your weight is a classic move out of the sexist playbook, right up there with using "hysteria" to dismiss legitimate medical conditions. I've had patients tell me, through tears, how their doctor said that they caused their PCOS because they gained weight, or that if they could only lose weight, they'd cure the ailment. This is some major, dangerous misinformation. *You did not cause your PCOS and there is no cure—even if you lose weight.*

While there is currently no cure for PCOS, you can certainly effectively manage it and put symptoms into remission. Many of the symptoms of PCOS can be managed with nutrition, lifestyle strategies, and medications. And the concerns around heart disease and diabetes can be prevented.[26] Eating a nutrient-dense diet that is high in fiber and low in refined carbs can support healthy insulin levels while keeping inflammation in check. Including healthy fats (see the table on page 309) will also help support your blood sugar, as will building more muscle through exercise. And you can try supplements like inositol, omega-3 fatty acids, N-acetyl cysteine (NAC), vitamin D, zinc, and chromium, which research has shown can help mitigate PCOS symptoms. When it comes to hair loss on the head and unwanted hair growth on the face, saw palmetto, nettle root, EGCG, and reishi mushroom have been shown to decrease 5-alpha reductase activity, which is an enzyme that makes testosterone more potent by converting it into dihydrotestosterone (DHT).[27]

Other conditions like thyroid disease can mimic PCOS symptoms, which

PCOS Symptom Check

PCOS is a diagnosis of exclusion, meaning it can be confirmed only when other conditions that cause irregular periods and high androgens have been ruled out. If there is no other explanation for your symptoms, the diagnosis of PCOS is made when two out of the three symptoms are present, per the Rotterdam criteria.[28] If you have any of the following symptoms, please schedule with your provider to get worked up.

YOU MAY HAVE PCOS IF YOU HAVE TWO OF THESE THREE SYMPTOMS:

- ☐ Irregular or no ovulation (periods are more than 35 days apart)
- ☐ Signs of excess androgens: acne, hair loss on head, hirsutism (excess hair on chin, chest, abdomen)
- ☐ Polycystic ovaries on ultrasound

OTHER SYMPTOMS THAT ACCOMPANY PCOS:

- ☐ Anxiety, depression, mood swings
- ☐ Weight gain or difficulty losing weight, especially in midsection
- ☐ Infertility
- ☐ Skin tags (soft, skin-colored growths)
- ☐ Darker-than-usual, velvet skin in your armpits, groin, or neck
- ☐ Excess hunger
- ☐ Excess thirst or urination
- ☐ Sleep apnea
- ☐ Fatigue

is why it's critical to get the right tests if you have concerns. In addition, PCOS is associated with a higher risk of developing thyroid disease and autoimmune conditions, so there's nothing that says you can't have both. Ask your provider for the following tests to help identify PCOS:

- Free and total testosterone, which may be elevated
- DHEA-S, which may be elevated
- Sex hormone binding globulin (SHBG), which may be low
- Anti-Mullerian hormone (AMH), which may be elevated
- Fasting glucose and insulin, which may be normal or elevated
- Four-point urinary or salivary cortisol

Acne: Why Does My Skin Break Out Every Month?

Your hormones absolutely influence your skin, but in reality, there are several different mechanisms that drive acne, making it complicated in some cases. In acne, oil, skin cells, and dirt get trapped in pores. This is what people mean when they say "clogged pores." Some people's skin is more prone to oil production, which can be driven by testosterone and other androgens. There can also be issues with protein development within the skin cells that makes it more likely things like dirt and makeup will get trapped in a pore. Let's break it down:

Sebum (oil) production. Oil production by the skin is totally normal and necessary. But too much of it can fill pores and trap bacteria. Some people produce more oil, have a thicker consistency, or have an oil that supports bacterial growth.

Bacteria on the skin. Bacteria lives everywhere on and in our body. With acne, the most common offender is *Propionibacterium acnes*. An environment that is conducive to overgrowth of this organism or that doesn't support healthy flora can be problematic for acne.

Inflammation. If you've got bacteria trapped in your skin that does not belong there, you better believe your immune system is going to step in. With it comes inflammation. Inflammation leads to those red, painful, swollen acne lesions we all dread.

Keratin production. Keratin is a protein found in our skin. When there is an issue with how it is produced, we can experience more clogged pores. And within those pores we'll find oil and bacteria causing a ruckus. Your keratin production can also be totally normal, and dead skin cells alone can plug the pores and irritate the tissues.

Hormones. The sebaceous gland (oil gland) is very sensitive to hormones. In situations with excess testosterone (like we explored in earlier chapters), the gland can begin producing more oil. This is why women with PCOS often have acne as a symptom. During puberty, when our oil production is at one of its highest levels in our lifetime, testosterone can stimulate the glands to produce more. While the connection between estrogen and acne isn't well understood, it is thought that estrogen suppresses testosterone's effect on the sebaceous gland. When estrogen is low just before your period, it may be that androgens are allowed to ramp up oil production, leading to acne. This would explain acne just before and during your period. Use the solutions for high testosterone on page 340 to address this common hormonal cause of acne.

If you've already been struggling with acne and find yourself with scars, I've got tips for you as part of the 28-day program and on page 383. While we've all been told that acne scars are with us for life, there are things you can do daily to gradually banish them from taking up any more real estate on your face. Retinoids can help promote cell turnover, while vitamin C helps brighten skin and reduce dark spots. Both can be used topically daily to help you resolve your less favorable teenage memories. It's important to note that reducing and eliminating acne scars is something you'll have to be both patient and consistent with. Azelaic acid can also help fade dark marks on the skin and is another ingredient you should consider putting into your routine. In the morning after you wash your face, apply azelaic acid followed by sunscreen. When you get ready for bed, wash your face again and apply retinol followed by a moisturizer with niacinamide. Niacinamide is a vitamin B_3 derivative that can help even your skin tone and reduce hyperpigmentation. If you've got really stubborn or deep scars, make an appointment with your dermatologist to discuss laser treatments, chemical peels, and microneedling.

Supporting your skin from the inside is just as important as what you put on it, which is why I recommend following the nutrition guide in the 28-day program. Vitamin A is important for the health of your skin and regenerating new healthy tissue. Plus, it is involved in your immune health in a key way that can keep acne in check. Including egg yolks, liver, sweet potato, mango, and kale in your diet can help supply your skin with the vitamin A it needs. It's been found in the research that people who eat an abundance of plant-based carotenoids like those found in carrots, broccoli, butternut squash, and spinach are perceived as more attractive. Not too shabby a bonus.

Omega-3-rich animal sources like salmon, sardines, and mackerel provide your skin and body with anti-inflammatory support, which can reduce the redness of skin and new acne. These food sources also contain vitamin A and vitamin D, which has a bonus effect of helping your immune system keep acne in check. If you don't eat fish, aim for freshly ground flaxseeds, algae, and walnuts to be part of your daily routine.

Vitamin C is another key nutrient for supporting healthy skin and is crucial in maintaining your elasticity. You'll find vitamin C in more than just oranges. In the meal plan found at https://DrBrighten.com/ITN-resources you'll be incorporating vitamin C through bell peppers, strawberries, and leafy greens. Niacin and folate are two B vitamins that encourage increased blood flow and cell growth, and are beneficial for acne-prone skin. Including pumpkin, turkey, and lentils in your diet can help your body create renewed skin. See the table on page 369 for more food sources of these nutrients.

Premenstrual Syndrome (PMS)

Despite what you may have been told, all the significant mood issues, bloating, sleep problems, cramping, breast tenderness, out-of-control appetite, and other issues that millions of women experience every month known as PMS are *not* normal. Yes, PMS is extraordinarily common, with more than 90 percent of all women experiencing some PMS symptoms in their life, according to research.[29] But if you deal with the condition every month, month after month after month, and it is getting in the way of life—that's not normal, despite all the memes that would make it seem otherwise.

I address the common PMS symptoms individually here, as some people experience only singular or certain issues (FYI, breast tenderness is in chapter 11). But regardless of whether you get many or only a few symptoms, if you have PMS on a regular, consistent basis, meaning it's not just a one-off annoyance or annual fluke, then you likely have a hormone imbalance. While research isn't entirely clear on the exact cause of PMS, symptoms may stem from the interaction between sex and stress hormones and neurotransmitters with the brain. If you took the quiz on page 192, you'll likely identify the symptoms of PMS as being related to having too little progesterone, which leads to an excess of estrogen stimulating your tissues.[30] It's why it isn't uncommon to find that you have both symptoms of excess estrogen and low progesterone on the quiz—they go hand in hand.

While I detail how to identify and address these hormone imbalances in my 28-day plan, no matter whether your issue is estrogen- or progesterone-related, there's several things you can do to help. Eating more cruciferous vegetables like broccoli, cauliflower, kale, and Brussels sprouts will supply your body with diindolylmethane (DIM) and sulforaphane, which support healthy estrogen metabolism. You've likely heard this before, but you'll also want to focus on sleep: Going to bed and waking up at the same times as often as you can and getting a solid seven to eight hours per night can regulate a lot of hormonal problems. Stress management is also key since a high-stress state can suppress progesterone production. Making time to hang out with friends will also lower stress and boost progesterone, according to research.[31] Supplements like magnesium glycinate, vitamins C, B_6, and calcium, and the herb vitex agnus-castus, also known as chasteberry, can be helpful in getting symptom relief. You'll find dosages in chapter 13 but keep reading for more details on each of the symptoms that can arise before your period.

Premenstrual Dysphoric Disorder: Not Just "Bad PMS"

Despite what you might hear, premenstrual dysphoric disorder (PMDD) is not just "bad PMS." While the conditions share similar symptoms, PMDD is like PMS on steroids, with a greater intensity of emotions like anxiety, anger, irritability, and depression—some women with PMDD also experience suicidal thoughts. PMDD can last longer, too, with ten to fourteen days of symptoms, on average, while PMS typically occurs for five to seven days. PMDD affects 3 to 8 percent of all women who menstruate and, as one study estimated, women with the condition lose up to three years of their life due to the consistent misery this condition dishes their way.[33]

PMDD is not normal, and while it's 100 percent disruptive, it's also 100 percent treatable. This is one condition where oral contraceptives may help. We're not entirely sure of the cause of PMDD, but it appears there may be a genetic component that makes some brains far more sensitive to fluctuations of estrogen and progesterone during the cycle, making a medication that stops all fluctuations of hormones, like the pill, an effective treatment for some.[34] Other pharmaceuticals, like antidepressants and anti-anxiety drugs, can also be effective. There are also many supplements that can help complement pharmaceutical therapy and alleviate symptoms of PMDD. The first step, though, is getting a proper diagnosis.

To be diagnosed with PMDD, you need to experience five or more PMDD symptoms for at least six months out of the year.[35] Symptoms need to include at least one physical and one mental/emotional. Per the DSM-V criteria,[36] these include the following:

- Mood swings; sudden sadness; or tearful, increased sensitivity to rejection
- Marked anger, irritability, or major conflicts with others
- Significantly depressed mood, sense of hopelessness, self-critical thoughts
- Significant anxiety, tension, feeling on edge or "keyed up"
- Decreased interest in usual activities
- Difficulty concentrating
- Significant lack of energy, easily fatigued, lethargic
- Change of appetite, cravings, overeating
- Sleeping a lot or can't sleep at all
- Feeling overwhelmed or out of control
- Breast tenderness, bloating, weight gain, joint/muscle aches

PMS Symptom Check

There are differing opinions regarding the criteria for the diagnosing premenstrual disorders (PMDs); however, if you have one or more of the symptoms below for multiple months, and the symptoms arrive on the last week of your luteal phase and resolve within a few days of starting your period, and they inhibit your ability to function, it's likely PMS.[32] If you find you have more than five symptoms that are predominantly mood-related, they are present for most of your cycles, and they cause significant distress, it is time to be evaluated for premenstrual dysphoric disorder (PMDD), which we cover on page 243. If you don't have a period, but are still in your reproductive years with ovaries, look for cyclical symptoms. Using a calendar is a must for everyone who suspects they have PMS or PMDD.

PHYSICAL SYMPTOMS:

- ☐ Bloating
- ☐ Breast tenderness or swelling
- ☐ Headaches
- ☐ Joint or muscle aches
- ☐ Swelling of the hands or feet
- ☐ Weight gain

MENTAL/EMOTIONAL SYMPTOMS:

- ☐ Depression
- ☐ Anxiety
- ☐ Difficulty concentrating
- ☐ Prone to anger
- ☐ Irritability
- ☐ Socially withdrawn
- ☐ Tension
- ☐ Feeling on edge

If you suspect or are diagnosed with PMDD, testing hormones like thyroid, adrenal, or pancreatic (insulin) can help you understand if these hormones are behind your symptoms, allowing your doctor to give you more effective treatment options. It is also important to look at other markers of health like those that check for inflammation, iron deficiency, and vitamin D status. Many of the same therapies that have been shown to be helpful with PMS may also help ease symptoms of PMDD, like calcium, magnesium, vitamin B_6, and vitamin D. In my patients struggling with PMDD, I've seen great results with cognitive behavioral therapy (CBT), a form of psychological treatment shown by research to be highly effective in treating PMDD.[37] Since PMDD can have serious emotional consequences, a mental health specialist should be a key component of your treatment team.

Is It PMDD or Am I Neurodivergent?

Women are statistically less likely to be diagnosed with attention deficit/hyperactivity disorder (ADHD) and autism spectrum condition (ASC). And even when they are finally diagnosed, it tends to be later in life. I've had enough patients in my time come to me with a diagnosis of PMDD only to have their diagnosis of ADHD and ASC missed. This is, in part, because women are so damn good at compensating and masking their symptoms (that's called social adaptation, and is a literal survival tactic). But it is also because if you're a woman or assigned female at birth, you are expected to present with the same symptoms as men when you have these conditions. Let me be clear: we rarely have the same exact symptoms as a man when it comes to medical conditions (um, things be cyclical in these bodies), and this is no exception. The trouble with a diagnosis like PMDD is that once it's in your chart it can literally become all your doctor sees, blinding them to the fact that you're struggling in other ways, other times of the month. As much as women's hormone symptoms are ignored or largely passed off as normal, I feel these issues are amplified within the neurodivergent community. Does everyone with PMDD have ADHD or ASC? No. Can you have both PMDD and ADHD or ASC? Yes, and in fact, the few studies that have been done have shown a higher incidence of PMDD among those with ADHD[38] and ASC.[39] Can you not have PMDD, but have your ADHD or ASC symptoms dialed way up before your period? Absolutely! Cyclical hormones shift everyone's brain function. Neurotypical people's hormones can make them less tolerant to sensory input like sound, less able to focus, and more prone to emotional overwhelm, along with a whole host of body-wide symptoms. So if your brain is already dialed up on any of these, you better believe your hormones can amplify them. Your entire body is receptive to hormone stimulation. In my patients with ADHD, many of them find their medication just doesn't work as well in the luteal phase. Luckily, we've been able to mitigate it by supporting a balance of estrogen and progesterone during this phase with ample self-care. Clinically I have found that the same tactics we use for PMS can help improve the effectiveness of medication and mitigate the symptoms.

While getting a formal diagnosis of ADHD and ASC, along with the appropriate individualized treatment, is the ideal, not everyone has access to providers who can help with this. When it comes to women self-identifying with either of these conditions, women aren't often wrong about their symptoms, even when their doctors miss it.[40] But what we're not going to do is be flippant, like, "Everyone has a little ADHD," because no, they do not. And unless you actually have it, you haven't a clue how hurtful and harmful that sentiment is. If you do suspect you have ADHD or ASC, getting a formal diagnosis will allow you access to important resources.

ASK DR. BRIGHTEN:

Is it normal to be tired before my period?

Society was set up to favor a man's biological clock. If we lived in a matriarchy, a long time ago we'd have instituted work-from-home days for women whenever we have our period. That's because feeling tired when your body is getting ready to shed tissue it's built over an entire month is normal. Honor the need to slow down a bit by taking a rest day when you can, ignoring any inner or outer voice that tells you to step it up. Just like athletes need a recovery day to perform faster and stronger, when you take a rest day around your period, it can help you be more productive at work, home, or whatever you want to do.

What's not normal, though, is feeling so fatigued that you can't get out of bed, or sleeping twelve to fifteen hours just to be able to function.

This degree of constant fatigue can be a sign of hypothyroidism—when your body doesn't produce enough thyroid hormone—adrenal dysfunction, an autoimmune disorder, anemia, or another medical condition that merits attention from a doctor.

While you may find yourself wanting an IV of coffee running through your veins during this time of the month, I'd advise not to bump that daily caffeine intake, as it can lead to worse anxiety and, in some, may intensify menstrual cramps.[41] BTW, if you're sweating that I'm telling you to give up coffee altogether, I'm not. In fact, it supports more favorable estrogen metabolites (less-likely-to-cause-cancer kind), so a moderate intake may actually help your hormones this time of the month, so long as it doesn't contribute to anxiety. But it has to be caffeinated—the decaf version doesn't show the same benefit (she writes while sipping coffee).[42] Regular exercise has been shown to improve fatigue and bloating, plus, we know that exercise is also beneficial for a variety of mood symptoms.[43]

Are mood swings, uncontrollable crying, and *I hate everyone* vibes normal?

We're often made to feel ashamed, guilty, or like there's something wrong with us if we get emotional around our period. Some people accuse women of being moody, mopey, bitchy, irrational, or even unstable because of our period and, the worst, use it to validate why a woman should never be president. What these body-illiterate people don't know is that sex hormones actually make us smart and clear-headed by increasing gray matter (the area of the brain responsible for memory, decision-making skills, and a host of other critical functions),[44] by protecting our brains,[45] and by boosting our verbal skills.[46] Still, it's normal to feel a little emotional, irritable, anxious, ruminative, or weepy before your period, as progesterone levels decline at this time. Emphasis on "a little."

But if you feel like you can't go out in the world because you're so emotional, the sight of some people makes you want to go ballistic, you spend most of your time worrying or thinking the same thoughts, or you start sobbing during emotional movies, then that's a problem. See the symptom checklist for PMS, read up on premenstrual dysphoric disorder (PMDD), and definitely discuss with a medical provider.

If a mood issue keeps you from enjoying the things you want to do in life, your estrogen may be too high, your progesterone may be too low, and either may be causing unfavorable shifts in your neurotransmitters. Adopting my 28-day plan can help correct imbalances while offering tools to help you restore your emotional health. Lastly, there's never any shame in working with a therapist or mental health professional. Therapy is for everyone.

Is it normal if I look four months pregnant before my period?

A little bloat before and during your period is natural and normal as progesterone shifts, triggering your cells to retain more water and salt. You'll most likely notice this fluid retention in your face, hands, and feet, too. The first day you bleed can also be a bit of a doozy, since studies show this is when fluid retention peaks.[47] But while some bloat is normal, if your degree of distension or fluid retention is physically uncomfortable or causes you to amend your everyday activities, you may not be making enough progesterone. Progesterone is a diuretic, helping the body shed excess water weight, and while everyone's levels dip before their period, if yours never quite reached its ideal mark, you'll likely end up feeling beached-whale bloated. Having too much progesterone, on the other hand, can also cause bloating, since the hormone can slow digestion, triggering what some women call a "food baby" to form in their lower abdomen. (If period poops follow—as talked about in chapter 10—you may be asking, "How could I possibly have this much poop?" Progesterone, that's how.)

Increasing plants and proteins, while minimizing processed foods in the diet, can help with bloating. Fiber is your friend, which is why it's a staple in any hormonal-supportive meal. Drinking plenty of water and keeping active can also help relieve that bloated feeling. Including potassium-rich foods like potatoes, bananas, and avocados can help with some of the fluid retention as well. If you feel like your belly is giving you a six-months-pregnant vibe when you're not, ask your doc to evaluate your gut health. It may be a condition called small intestinal bacterial overgrowth (SIBO).

Is it normal if I find myself eating all the things? What about feeling like I gain weight before my period?

Retaining water can cause the number on the scale to go up. You may feel as though you've gained weight, but you really haven't: Water weight is not the same as fat or muscle and will clear when your hormones bring on your period. It's also normal to be hungrier or crave carbs at different times during your cycle, especially before your period. Your metabolic rate is also slightly higher during the luteal phase—studies vary, but experts estimate the increase to be between 8 percent and 16 percent[48]—as your body prepares for the possibility of carrying and nourishing another human.

When estrogen starts to fall toward the end of your luteal phase, your appetite can spike again for a few reasons. Estrogen acts as an appetite suppressant, so lower levels can leave you hungrier before your period.[49] When estrogen drops, it also reduces the body's production of serotonin,[50] which can lead to carb and sugar cravings as compensation, which give a temporary serotonin boost.[51] Some women also gravitate toward drinking more alcohol around the time of their period in an unconscious effort to try to combat lower progesterone and serotonin symptoms, along with consciously trying to alleviate possible PMS symptoms. While alcohol may seem like your ticket out of hormone hell, it's not it. Not unless you're looking to add some hot flashes, night sweats, swollen breasts, irritability, and irregular periods to your monthly mix.[52]

All these factors can lead to increased caloric intake, overconsuming, and, in some women, binge eating. If you consume too many calories, you can gain weight, especially if you do so every month while scaling back on physical activity at the same time. If you're routinely overeating, binge eating, or drinking too much at any time in your cycle, make an appointment to see a doctor, nutritionist, mental health practitioner, or other medical professional who can help you get to the bottom of what's going on. If you're not overconsuming but are still gaining weight, especially around your hips, butt, and thighs, you may have too much estrogen stimulating those fat cells to save up. You could also have a thyroid condition, which affects one in eight women in their lifetime (with some estimates reporting higher incidences), even though as many as 60 percent with thyroid disease don't know they have it.[53]

While most people associate food cravings with ice cream, chocolate, bread, and other fun stuff, some women feel the need to chew on dirt, clay, or ice. While relatively uncommon in nonpregnant populations, these kinds of cravings are not normal, and are a sign of an iron deficiency anemia. If you're experiencing this, ask your doctor for a complete blood count (CBC) and screen for anemia. I also order a ferritin test with my patients, as this screens for iron stores.

I can't sleep before my period; is that normal?

Tossing and turning every time you're about to get your period is not normal. It may take a few minutes longer to fall asleep before your period because of lower levels of progesterone, which acts like a natural sleep aid in the body.[54] But if you find you just can't fall or stay asleep, or you feel like you need to take sleep aids every time your period is about to roll up, your progesterone levels are likely low (see page 337 for progesterone support). Wake up at night feeling hot, sweaty, anxious, or hungry? It could be a blood sugar imbalance. Try adding a scoop of collagen and a bit of honey to your evening tea, or having a nutritious snack an hour before bed, to see if it helps. Just plain hot, sweaty, and not sleeping? Do the symptom check for perimenopause on page 236.

If you see a doctor for your sleep problems and are met with a prescription, I'd encourage you to ask them what your options are, what causes they've ruled out, and what are the risks with that prescription. It's important to know that some sleep aids form a dependency and come with a heavy warning about serious side effects.

TL;DR: IS MY MENSTRUAL CYCLE NORMAL?

- Your sex hormones, which regulate your cycle, greatly impact your sex life and almost everything else about you, including your physical health, emotional outlook, daily behaviors, and overall appearance.
- Knowing where you're at in your cycle can help you understand the times when you'll likely need more lube, foreplay, or TLC, as well as when you'll have an easier time climaxing. Remember: a lot of factors influence our arousal, desire, and sexual experiences, so honor what is true for you.
- When you tune in to your cycle, you're also able to tap into the power of your sex hormones, allowing you to optimize them to improve your sexual, physical, mental, and emotional health all at once.

- Not everyone has a 28-day cycle. Not everyone ovulates on day 14. All of that is normal. If you want to tune in to when you ovulate, see the list on page 224 of signs for ovulation.
- Thyroid disease is a common cause of short cycles, long cycles, irregular cycles, and period problems in general.
- Polycystic ovary syndrome is a common, yet often missed, condition that has symptoms of acne, hair loss on the head, unwanted hair growth elsewhere, and irregular periods.
- Shorter cycles (more frequent periods) can be a sign of perimenopause (there's a symptom checklist on page 236), but if this is showing up before age forty, you need to talk with a hormone expert.
- PMS is common but not normal. Use the symptom check to figure out if you have PMS or if you should be talking to your provider about PMDD.
- Mood swings, fatigue, bloating, and other symptoms that show up in your cycle do have a cause and aren't something you should just live with.

CHAPTER 10

IS MY PERIOD NORMAL?

RED, BROWN, SPOTTING, CLOTTING, AND MORE

I knew Danielle had something she wanted to ask. Fidgeting on the edge of the exam table, she stared past me with that look that patients get when they're considering whether they should ask me something they've never asked any doctor before. I tried to find her eyes, then gave her the same encouraging look that I give all my patients to let them know that whatever—and I mean, *whatever*—they want to say is not only acceptable, but also appreciated. I am their doctor, after all: If they are curious or concerned about anything that has to do with their bodies, physically, mentally, emotionally, or sexually, I want to hear about it.

A few seconds later she lowered her eyes to the floor and in an almost apologetic tone half whispered, "My period is really heavy the first couple of days and when it starts, I have to stay near a bathroom because I'm afraid I'll poop myself. It's just the first day. And sometimes I see brown stuff at the end of my period. My boyfriend and I almost always end up having sex while I'm still bleeding because I'm in the mood, but that's weird, right?"

Except it's not weird. The first day of your period is almost always the heaviest, and the same chemicals that cause your uterus to contract can also cause your intestines to contract. Brown blood at the end of your period is also normal—it means your blood was exposed to oxygen, which triggered a chemical reaction with the iron in blood cells that turned them brown. And feeling frisky during this time isn't weird at all, although some people would shame you into believing otherwise.

The period gets a lot of play in our minds, conversations, and medicine. Understandably, many of us count down the days to when we bleed every month, using our periods to plan our sex life, our outfits, our vacation time, even our weddings or major life events. We're anxious about getting our period when we're concerned about becoming pregnant or are trying to conceive, but the moment it arrives, we're just as restless to get rid of it again. Many of us worry about period problems like PMS, heavy bleeding, "period poops," and even so-called "butt lightning," some of which are normal and some not-so-normal, but treatable, even though most of us have been taught to either not talk about it or to just accept it.

If you're always stressing about your period, it can make having sex difficult, let alone enjoyable. Remember: These are the kind of worries that play out in the back of our minds and pump the brakes on any sexual desire. You may even stop having sex altogether in the days before or during your period, especially if you continually experience PMS, mood swings, bloating, cramping, or any other period problem that makes intimacy uncomfortable; if that sounds familiar, it may mean you're not having sex for at least one-fourth of your fertile years, depending on how long your symptoms last. That's a long time to go without getting it on!

We're taught to fear having sex on our period, but conversations often leave out the benefits: it can break tension both in your body and mind. But period sex isn't the only menstruation myth that needs to go away already. There's a ton of misinformation about the period on social media, the Internet, and even in your doctor's office. The biggest problem with all the myths and misinformation comes with buying into them and thus not getting the possible treatment you need. This can sabotage your physical, mental, and emotional health, not to mention your sex life. Even if you don't have period problems, knowing what's normal and not can relieve a lot of the anxiety and stress many feel every month. Here's the deal: You will menstruate for an average of thirty-nine years of your life, and not one of those years should suck because your period or hormones are acting up. While the conventional narrative is that periods and hormones do just suck, I want to assure you that symptoms are your body's way of signaling that something is wrong. You've already begun to problem solve in the previous chapters, so let's get into the specifics of what is and isn't normal about your period and what to do about it.

ASK DR. BRIGHTEN:

Are these period myths true?

Many myths are born from a place of wanting to control or manipulate an individual's decision; when it comes to sex, periods, and hormones, there are plenty of myths to go around. Some of them seem harmless—like menstrual blood attracting sharks—but at their core, they are stigmatizing and fear-inducing. So let me break down some of the big ones.

Is sex on my period safe?

When's the last time you saw a meme or heard a joke about how disgusting semen is during sex? Probably never. But when that "fluid" is female, suddenly we've got jokes for days about how disgusting it is. Funny how that works, eh? Most of us have been brought up to believe that period blood is somehow way more disgusting than any other liquid, and that we're unclean when we have our period. I'm not in the habit of debating people's beliefs, so if your religion says something different than the science and you want to go with that, no judgment. (Also, you'd be a good candidate for the outercourse we discussed in chapter 5.) But scientifically speaking, menstrual blood is just blood mixed with a bit of uterine tissue and vaginal secretions. It's certainly not going to harm, pollute, or tarnish you or your partner's penis, hand, or mouth if you do have sex, and when it comes to STIs, if you've got one, then you are at risk of passing it on whenever, but if you are bleeding there may be a slightly higher risk.[1] Regardless, if you have an STI, addressing that needs to happen before you have sex again.

Why do people even like to have sex during their period in the first place? There's actually a lot of ways it can support you through menstruation. Research shows that sex while menstruating can alleviate a lot of period problems, including cramps, stress, and headaches.[2] When you have sex, even if you don't orgasm, your body releases oxytocin, also known as the "love hormone," which helps lower cortisol and anxiety while promoting relaxation, sleep, and increased connection and trust with others.[3] While engaged in a sexual event, your brain also releases feel-good chemicals called endorphins—the same ones responsible for giving the "runner's high" after a hard workout—that can help fight pain from cramps.[4] And if you do have an orgasm, it can cause your body to shimmy out more menstrual blood, effectively shortening the length of your period.[5] Finally, if you like vaginal intercourse, having it can be akin to receiving an internal massage, which can help relax your pelvic floor and reduce cramping. Plus, some people are just into it, whether it be because all that attention their body is putting on down there is making them want to get down, or because there is a fetish involved; it's just some people's thing. And that's normal.

If you're thinking you're the only one, you'd be wrong. Eighty-two percent of women ages eighteen to fifty say they have sex on their period, according to a *Forbes* contributor who cites a poll conducted by the women's health brand Intimina.[6] Lots of women enjoy sex while menstruating for a number of reasons. Some of my patients, for example, say sex feels more sensitive, that they have a higher libido, or that they're aroused by the concept.[7] Remember that while libido-blocking progesterone dips at the start of your period, within days after, your estrogen is bumpin', which may leave you vibin' with your partner's offerings. For many, menstrual blood can act like a lubricant to get things going, but with estrogen low, it's a good idea to keep lube on hand. I advise that you don't rely on menstrual blood alone because while it is a fluid, it can dry out. I've also heard from men that they enjoy period sex.

If you want to try period sex, start by having an open conversation with your partner to make sure you're both on the same page. Using a menstrual cup, like a Ziggy Cup, Flex Disc, or Softdisc, can keep blood to a minimum and may make oral sex more enticing for you both. Still worried about the mess? Lay down a towel, or do it in the shower where cleanup is nonexistent. But please, do not have sex with a tampon in. It's bad news. And if you mistakenly do, see the guidance on how to retrieve it on page 270.

Can I get pregnant on my period?

It's a common scare tactic to tell women they can get pregnant any time in their cycle. But truth? The first day of your period is the least probable time you could get pregnant, for the simple fact that you're shedding the lining of the uterus where a fertilized egg would implant and there's no egg around to fertilize. But let's say you're seeing some spotting on day 7 of your period, and on day 10 you ovulate. Well, if you had unprotected sex on day 6 or 7 of your period, then you could potentially become pregnant due to the sperm's persistence, as discussed in chapter 9.

Does period blood attract sharks?

If this terrifying thought has ever crossed your mind and kept you out of the ocean, you're not alone: after watching an episode of Shark Week, I was once convinced that a single drop of blood would cause a feeding frenzy around me. But think about it: How many women are in the ocean at any given time? And is it possible that you're not the only one menstruating? But if you've seen the headline WOMAN WITH PERIOD ATTACKED BY GREAT WHITE, know that this is a myth, and an effective one at that.

Should you not work out on your period, or dial back your intensity?

Actually, some find they can go harder in their workout during their period, while others find they need to take more rests between sets or run a shorter distance. It really comes down to what is true for you. If your energy is lower, then honor that. If you feel a full-on beast mode rallying inside you, hit it. A great resource for training with your cycles is *Roar* by Dr. Stacy Sims.

What's a normal period?

The initiation to periods usually means: welcome to womanhood, here's a pad, and good luck. That about sums up what many people get when it comes to "the period talk." But as you learned in chapter 9, there is way more to the menstrual cycle than just a period, never mind all the stuff I'm about to explain about the period itself. Frankly, period stigma is so weird. It wasn't until my midthirties that I made the conscious decision to stop smuggling tampons up my sleeve as I went to the bathroom. Damned if the period stigma isn't so ingrained in us all. I share this because if you find you're still unable to ask the questions you need answers to, find yourself avoiding any talk that will bring up your period, and are sneaking off to the bathroom to change a pad, you are not alone. But knowing what isn't normal and when to seek help is necessary, which is why I'm so glad you're here.

How much pain is normal?

It seriously took a doctor saying that period pain is comparable to a heart attack for male doctors to take to the Internet letting us know that our pain is legit.[8] The kicker? This didn't happen until 2016, leaving about 50 to 90 percent of women (the estimate of those who deal with dysmenorrhea, or period pain) wondering why in hell it took so long for medicine to catch on.[9] But while the statement may have made men take period pain as seriously as a heart attack, the comparison doesn't make much sense, given that women are less likely to present with chest pain when having a heart attack.[10] Why did it take a statement like this to wake people up to a very real and debilitating problem impacting millions of women?

We've been conditioned to normalize period pain—to expect and accept it. I've lost count of the number of patients who have had their pain dismissed by medical providers, being told things like "Periods are supposed to hurt." Period pain isn't a badge of honor that we must wear month after month (although you're definitely incredible for all you do while dealing with cramps), and it isn't something you should just live with. And just so we're all on the same page, your period shouldn't leave you in tears, curled up in a ball, vomiting, unable to go about any of your normal activities, or missing work or school on the regular. If it does, that's not normal, and we need to understand if we've got endo, adenomyosis, fibroids, elevated estrogen, high inflammation, a magnesium or thiamine deficiency, or something else going on. Because it seriously shouldn't be like that.

Prostaglandins, hormonelike chemicals that cause the contraction of your uterus, are made from omega fatty acids.[11] Eat a diet rich in omega-6 fatty acids and these bad boys get potent, which can result in serious cramping.[12] Switch that diet to include more omega-3s and you can reduce their effect while still allowing them to do their job. Things that can help include thiamine, high-frequency transcutaneous electrical nerve stimulation (TENS) therapy, acupressure, acupuncture, topical heat, ibuprofen, birth control pills, and ginger. Magnesium can both relax muscle tissue and lower prostaglandins.[13] The Nutrient Food Sources table on page 369 can help you identify where you can get more magnesium in your diet, and the Cycle Symptom Relief chart on page 377 can offer guidance regarding supplementation.

If you're experiencing period-like cramps, but it is not time for your period, you'll want to meet with your provider to rule out endometriosis, pelvic inflammatory disease, pregnancy, and possibly gut issues like irritable bowel syndrome (IBS), inflammatory bowel disease (IBD), or appendicitis. Ovarian cysts are fluid-filled pouches that can range from very small to 10 cm or more. They produce symptoms like pain, especially around ovulation or with sex; irregular periods; spotting; a sense of heaviness in the pelvis; and difficulty or pain with bowel movements or urination. There can be significant pain when they rupture, sometimes with fever or chills. And in some cases, they can become so large they lead to the ovary twisting and cutting off blood supply, which is known as ovarian torsion. This is a go-to-the-ER-ASAP situation. Excess estrogen, endometriosis, pelvic infections, and even pregnancy can put you at risk of developing a cyst. While not common, the Mirena IUD is also associated with the development of ovarian cysts.[14] Many cysts will self-resolve, and you can help them along by increasing the number of plants you're eating and by following the recommendations in chapter 8 for supporting your body in processing estrogen. While the pill is typically prescribed to shrink ovarian cysts or to prevent you from ovulating, so you don't form one to begin with, this treatment hasn't been shown to be effective.[15]

How long should my period last?

It's normal to bleed for two to seven days when you have your period.[16] If your period lasts one day only, though, you should follow up with your doctor, as you could be pregnant and experiencing implantation bleeding, which occurs when a fertilized egg attaches to the endometrium. You could also be super stressed, exercising too much, eating too little, or have a medical condition like polycystic ovary syndrome (PCOS)—see page 239 for more. Being on the pill can also thin your uterine lining over time, resulting in shorter "periods."

If you're at the other end of the spectrum and bleeding for eight or more days on a regular basis, this is called menorrhagia, the medical term for prolonged or heavy periods. Menorrhagia affects one in five women, according to the CDC, so it's common, but not normal.[17] Unfortunately, many women don't seek help for the condition, either because they're too embarrassed to bring up their symptoms with their doctor, or they assume that bleeding as much or as long as they do is normal. But menorrhagia is treatable, and the tips in chapter 12 can help.

Could it be uterine fibroids?

It's estimated that by age fifty about 70 percent of white women and 80 percent of Black women may develop fibroids.[18] Fibroids are benign tumors that can develop in the uterus, along with polyps, which are smaller, benign tumors that form in the endometrium, can also cause menorrhagia. In addition to heavy periods, they are often longer in duration, and more painful. There can be other complications associated with fibroids like difficulty with urination, pain with sex, constipation, infertility, and miscarriage. Every uterus is at risk of developing fibroids, but the risk is higher among Black women, and their symptoms are often much more severe.[19] It's not that being Black is the cause of fibroids but, rather, differences in psychosocial stress, environmental exposures, perceived racism, diet, and lifestyle that account for the risk.[20] If you think you may have fibroids, use the Fibroid Symptom Check on page 262 and use those symptoms to communicate to your medical provider your concerns.

While surgery may be necessary to remove fibroids, there's quite a bit you can do through diet and lifestyle to lower your risk and improve your uterine health. Eating a diet rich in plants,[21] low in foods that disrupt blood sugar,[22] and reducing alcohol intake[23] have all been associated with a lower risk of developing fibroids. While higher red meat consumption has been shown to be associated with an increased risk, it is often less about the meat and more about the lack of plants in comparison to the meat.[24] In addition, vitamin A from animal sources lowers the risk. My advice: fill your plate with plants and, if you eat meat, vary the protein source (chicken, fish, beef, etc.); choose grass-fed, organic, or wild-caught whenever possible; and aim for a serving size of about the palm of your hand. Fibroids are estrogen dependent, so keeping your estrogen in check can go a long way in keeping fibroids in check.[25] We'll be covering how to do that in the 28-day plan, along with dodging endocrine disruptors, and how to make the dietary shifts I just mentioned.

How much blood is normal?

Losing anywhere from 5 milliliters (1 teaspoon) to up to 80 milliliters (16 teaspoons) of blood during your period is normal. Most women lose an average of six to eight teaspoons.[26] If you're using hormonal birth control, you likely have lighter bleeding, which is normal because these synthetic hormones lead to a thinner endometrial lining. See page 302 for details on this. But if you feel like the term "shark week" adequately describes your time of the month, you're probably losing too much blood. Having to change tampons, pads, or menstrual cups every two hours or less, doubling up with a tampon-pad combo or two pads, or waking up in the middle of the night to change one are all signs of menorrhagia.[27]

What color should my blood be?

If you peruse any of the period blogs written by supposed "hormone gurus," you might think that your period blood needs to be a bright, vibrant red—always. In reality, though, there are many different shades of red, and all of them are normal during menstruation. Have pinkish-reddish blood at the onset of your period? Totally normal because it means your blood just mixed with a little cervical fluid. Brownish-reddish blood at the end of your period is just blood that came into contact with oxygen. Anything outside the red spectrum, though, should be checked out. Greenish hues or a pearl-colored discharge can be early indicators of infection. See how to decode your discharge in chapter 7.

No matter the color, don't believe anyone who says you can diagnose a hormonal condition or any other ailment by the shade of your period blood alone. While various hues of menstrual blood can hint that something may be wrong, that's all it is: a hint, not a diagnostic tool. You can't identify hormonal imbalances with menstrual blood like you can use a Sherwin-Williams paint sample to match the color of your walls: hormone imbalances are more complicated than home decor.

Are clots on your period normal?

Seeing little clots on a pad or on a tampon is normal during your period. Anytime we bleed, platelets should be released to stop the bleeding by forming a clot, so some clots are normal. Typically, in the beginning, when the flow is faster, you will see bright red clots, and as the period progresses they will darken in color. If you experience clots larger than the size of a quarter, however, that could be a sign you have fibroids, polyps, a thyroid irregularity, or endometriosis.[28] If this is you, make an appointment to see your medical provider.

Fibroid Symptom Check

When a patient complains of lots of blood and pain every time their period comes, uterine fibroids are one of the first things we need to rule out. These symptoms can be similar to endometriosis, so if you find you're checking off boxes here, be sure to discuss all with your doctor.

- ☐ Heavy bleeding
- ☐ Long periods (more than 7 days)
- ☐ Pelvic pressure
- ☐ Pain with sex
- ☐ Significant period cramps
- ☐ History of miscarriage or infertility
- ☐ Lower abdomen pain
- ☐ Constipation
- ☐ Lower back pain
- ☐ Difficulty with urination, increased frequency, or pain
- ☐ Feeling of abdominal tightness

PERIOD POVERTY

Period poverty refers to the lack of access to menstrual products, hygiene facilities, waste management, and education. You can experience one or a combination of these, and while I often hear people argue that this is only a problem that developing nations face, it's not. Worldwide, 500 million people lack access to menstrual products and hygiene facilities.[29] The BBC reported 137,000 girls miss school every year due to lack of access to menstrual products.[30] In one study of women in college it was found that 68.1 percent of those experiencing period poverty had symptoms consistent with moderate to severe depression.[31] In reality, if we just eliminated the tax on menstrual products (some people pay up to 10 percent tax), we would be able to expand access to these necessary products.[32]

What if I'm spotting outside my period?

It's normal to experience light spotting in the days before or after your period. But if your spotting lasts longer than two days, it may be due to not making enough progesterone, which can be normal in perimenopause. You can also spot with ovulation, which is normal. But if you experience spotting outside of your period or ovulation, you're frequently spotting outside your period, it follows rough sex or trauma to the pelvis, lasts for more than a few days, you suspect you're pregnant, or it's accompanied by other symptoms like pain, easy bruising, or fever, see a doctor.

WHEN TO SEE YOUR DOCTOR ABOUT YOUR PERIOD

- Period consistently lasts beyond seven days
- Flow is so heavy you need to change a tampon or pad every one to two hours
- Require a tampon and pad in order to manage the flow
- You're waking at night to change your tampon or pad
- Cycles are longer than forty-five days or less than twenty-one
- No period by age fifteen
- No period three years after breast development
- No period and signs of eating disorder
- Pain that doesn't get better with over-the-counter meds
- Pain that keeps you from going to work or school
- Your period stops altogether after having it consistently

- Spotting between periods
- There is abnormal discharge or odor
- You have symptoms like fatigue, hair loss, acne, etc., that accompany changes in your period
- You're experiencing new or extreme symptoms like headaches, migraines, mood swings, pain, acne

Are period problems normal?

Between commercials, sitcoms, doctor's visits, social media memes, and sex ed classes, we are all given the message that periods are supposed to hurt, that the emotional roller coaster of PMS is to be expected, and that we should talk about none of this. *The truth, however, is that while period problems are common, period problems are not normal.* It's not normal to feel like you have to take fistfuls of Advil or Midol just to survive the pain, or cancel all your plans due to extreme fatigue. It's not normal to start crying out of nowhere, think you're going to poop yourself every time you bleed, or feel like your face needs copious amounts of strategically placed makeup just to be able to be seen in public. These period problems are all symptoms of hormone imbalances, not inevitable things you have to tolerate every month because you were born with ovaries.

Hormone imbalances related to your period are almost always treatable and, in most cases, can be resolved with lifestyle and nutrition modifications. But if you don't treat these irregularities, they can cause other complications, in addition to period-related problems. That's why it's so critical to identify what's going on in your own body and start addressing the issue as soon as you can. Not only can treating hormone imbalances resolve period problems, but it can improve your mental health, energy, and social life. Plus, it can lead to an increase in sexual desire, make you more lubricated during foreplay and sex, increase your ability to orgasm, and bolster your ability to connect with your partner.

Not all period problems are indicative of hormone imbalances, though. Some symptoms stem from other medical conditions while others are normal side effects of menstruation. That's why I want to give you the skinny on *all* the period problems, including a few most women are too embarrassed to bring up with their closest friends, let alone their doctors.

Why do I poop so much on my period?

Ever feel like you're going to poop your pants while cramping your brains out? It's not just you: Period poops are a common phenomenon for lots of women, and while extreme pooping is never normal, these poops don't mean your body has been storing up stool for a whole month. Instead, if your progesterone slows your digestion and you don't fully evacuate the bowels a few days before you bleed, and then the prostaglandins hit, it can feel like you just expelled everything you ever ate. But if you seriously do feel like you never stop pooping; or it hurts; or there's blood, mucus, or undigested food in the stool, then it's time to see a doctor. Otherwise, period diarrhea is usually caused by overproduction of potent prostaglandins, which are hormonelike molecules that trigger the body's bowels and uterus to contract—why period poops and bad cramps often go hand in hand. While prostaglandins are awesome at helping your uterus birth a small human and move out the endometrium you no longer need, they can also cause food to accelerate too quickly through your intestines.

I'm not saying you did it to yourself with your diet; what I am saying is that you can make some simple shifts to get the poop in check. Prostaglandins can be derived from omega-6, which is found in many foods, but most people in the US get it from cheap oils like soybean, corn, sunflower, and vegetable, which are the worst poop-inducing offenders. Instead include omega 3–rich seafood like salmon, mackerel, or sardines at least twice a week while taking 500 to 1,000 mg daily of an omega-3 supplement that's been third-party-tested for quality. Then the poops can become more manageable, plus less of those electrical shots in the butt (see below). I know that getting your hands on fresh, wild-caught fish can be difficult, but quality sardines that store well, well, those are an inexpensive way to bump the omega-3s. If you just made a *Imma vomit* face, please go to Pinterest and search the magical ways people have found to make these little guys more than palatable. Also try supplementing with 150 mg to 300 mg daily of magnesium glycinate, which research shows can decrease prostaglandins,[33] increasing your dose to 300 to 600 mg in the days before your period. Just be sure to choose magnesium glycinate and not another form like magnesium citrate: this less expensive variety can work like a laxative, increasing diarrhea rather than preventing it.[34]

Is it normal to get shooting pains in my butt on my period (aka butt lightning)?

Maybe you're walking down the street or getting up from the couch to grab a snack when suddenly you feel this stabbing pain right up your butt, like a bolt of lightning shot up from the ground and straight into your bootyhole. That, my friend, is what is referred to as "butt lightning," the slang term for the shocking rectum pain that many women experience during their period. In a TikTok video I did on the topic, almost 2 million people watched it in a matter of days, along with 2,500 comments expressing relief to learn that they're not the only ones. But what causes the pain-in-the-butt symptoms?

A handful of different conditions can cause butt lightning and its similar sister issue, crotch lightning—when that electric shock radiates up your front side instead of your butt. The nerves in your pelvis may be wired a certain way (normal), you may have a tilted uterus (normal), or you may be in your third trimester and your baby is putting a lot of pressure on your pelvis, stimulating the nerves down there to activate (also normal). But butt and crotch lightning can also be caused by abnormal conditions like high prostaglandins (see period poops, above), endometriosis, and some vaginal infections, in the instance of crotch lightning. If you recently participated in anal sex (for which your doctor should not shame you), or have any additional symptoms that indicate one of the ailments that we've covered in this book, make an appointment to see a doc.

Is it normal to feel like I'm getting sick before or with my period (aka period flu)?

If you're achy, your temperature is up, and you have joint pain, dizziness, headaches, and just want to go to bed due to low energy, like clockwork, then odds are you're experiencing the dreaded "period flu." When COVID-19 stepped onto the scene in 2020 we saw everyone become hyperaware of any flu-like symptoms they were experiencing. What resulted was my practice and social media being inundated with concerns about cyclical flu symptoms showing up just before or at the onset of menstruation. While no one is sure what causes period flu, one hypothesis is that excess estrogen interfacing with histamine may be the culprit. Estrogen can bind to mast cells, the cells responsible for releasing histamine, and make them release more of this chemical, which can give you itchy eyes, brain fog, runny nose, headaches, and even hives. And histamine can lead to more estrogen production. In animal studies it has been shown that estrogen also slows down diamine oxidase (DAO) production (the enzyme that breaks down histamine) in the gut.[35] Progesterone, which opposes estrogen, inhibits histamine and is also anti-inflammatory, so when it drops, it may open the doors for inflammation.[36] And then there are prostaglandins (again, I know, right?), which are inflammatory themselves and may lead to the achy, icky, and I-need-to-go-to-bed symptoms.

If you suspect you suffer from period flu more than a one-off (because you could legitimately be sick), track your cycle to be sure your symptoms line up consistently with the days just before your period or day 1 or 2 of your cycle. If it looks like period flu for you, leveraging the estrogen- and progesterone-optimizing strategies as part of the 28-day plan can help you begin to rein in symptoms. Additionally, vitamin B_6 and vitamin C, which also support progesterone levels, help increase the DAO enzyme so you can clear histamine more efficiently. Eliminating foods high in histamine like wine, avocados, hard cheeses, fermented foods, and vinegar may help you feel better. Some foods, like cocoa, citrus, and tomatoes, which aren't necessarily high in histamines but can stimulate histamine release, are worth reevaluating as well. If you're considering eliminating high-histamine foods to see if it helps, work with a registered dietician or certified nutrition specialist to ensure your success.

PANDEMIC PERIODS

In the late spring of 2020, after several months of national lockdown due to the COVID-19 outbreak, I started seeing an increasingly common phenomenon among my patients: Their periods were freaking out as much as the country was. Some were getting much longer periods, or bleeding was getting heavier, or their PMS symptoms were way worse, or they had lost their period altogether. I wasn't the only practitioner who was seeing this happen, either: According to the *Guardian*, London-based gynecologist Dr. Anita Mitra conducted an informal survey that found that 65 percent of more than 5,600 women experienced a change in their cycle during the pandemic.[37] Which is a lot. In one study, 25 percent of women who had COVID reported a change in their period.[38]

The phenomenon, now known as "pandemic periods," is something we've seen before—hormones go off the rails due to stress, and it's normal to experience that temporarily. Whenever you're stressed, whether you lose a job, move, go through a breakup, contract a serious virus like coronavirus, or live through the worst global health crisis of our lifetime, your body produces more cortisol and other stress hormones that, in excess, will tell your ovaries and other endocrine organs to stop any hormone talk of babies and to even skip ovulation sometimes. In addition, the endometrium is responsive to immune changes, so when the body decides it is time to crank out the immune defense, it can lead to changes in endometrial function. There were many women who contracted coronavirus and found their period changed—that's normal. And there were others who got the vaccine and discovered they, too, experienced changes in their period, which rightly freaked everyone out because no one bothered to track menstruation or even talk about it in the vaccine research.[39] But what we've seen is that once the body has time to recover from the stressor, normal menstruation resumes. I know this may sound bad, but it's actually what your body should be doing: if you're under a lot of stress, your body knows that now is not the best time to become pregnant. Pretty smart, right?

Are period headaches and migraines normal?

Having to deal with headaches or migraines every month around your period is not normal. A one-off headache that comes right before you bleed? Nothing to be concerned about, as it may not have anything to do with your cycle. But if your searing headache accompanies your period or shows up in the days just before, every month, that's a sign your estrogen may be too high and dropping too quickly, which can trigger brain pain. The information in chapter 12 can help rebalance high estrogen levels while also stabilizing hormonal dips and spikes. Either way, if you suffer from migraines with an aura, be sure to avoid taking the pill, as the drug can increase your risk of stroke. Many of my patients respond well to 600 mg magnesium glycinate at the onset of a headache or migraine. If you suffer from cyclical migraines, try taking 300 mg of magnesium glycinate daily. Ensuring you're well hydrated, rested, and stretching regularly is another way to stave off headaches. Another trick: if you do get headaches or migraines, consider having sex. Research shows that orgasms can alleviate head pain for some women, working more quickly and effectively in some instances than pain medications.[40] Rx: take two orgasms and call me in the morning. I must caution, however, that for some people, an orgasm can be the cause of their head pain (coital cephalgia) and can be due to a serious issue, so it is best to discuss with your provider.

There is also evidence to suggest that those who suffer from migraines may be at the mercy of mitochondrial dysfunction. Remember those little powerhouse cells I told you in chapter 8 were rich in your ovaries? They're also rich in your brain and any tissue that requires serious energy production. If your mitochondria are being impacted by oxidative stress (when free radicals produced in the body, or that come in through the environment, pummel cells), are not receiving adequate nutrients to do their job, or are dealing with serious toxins like heavy metals, they will struggle, and headaches can follow. Nutrients like thiamine (B_1), CoQ_{10}, magnesium, niacin, carnitine, alpha-lipoic acid, vitamins B_2 and B_5, folate, and vitamin B_{12} can help your mitochondria function, and have been shown to help migraines.[41] Melatonin is also beneficial to mitochondrial health because on top of being a sleep hormone, it is a really kick-ass antioxidant, which may also reduce migraines.

CAN I LOSE A TAMPON UP THERE?

Lots of women forget to change their tampons: They're too tired or busy, they get sick, or something else happens that throws them out of their regular routine, and they don't realize the mistake until they notice a foul odor or feel discomfort during sex or after inserting another tampon. We've all been there. I once found my own little treasure waiting for me after a twenty-three-hour flight delay which left me exhausted and muttering "WTF" when I finally reached my bathroom at home. But contrary to urban myth, a tampon will never get "lost" in your body. There's no physical way a tampon can wander out of your vagina and make its way into your stomach—those body parts don't have a secret passageway connecting them. Toxic shock syndrome (TSS), a potentially life-threatening condition caused by a bacterial infection, is still a concern with forgotten tampons. But since tampon manufacturers started labeling absorbency levels and we began educating women on changing them every four to six hours, TSS annual cases dropped from 890 in 1980 to only 61 by 1989, not all of which were even menstrual-related.[42] But since all tampon users are still at risk, I recommend the following to prevent TSS:

- Change your tampons every four to six hours, and aim to never go beyond eight
- Use the lowest absorbency necessary
- Wash your hands whenever inserting or removing tampons
- Use a pad or clean menstrual cup instead of a tampon if you're concerned you might forget the latter

HOW TO REMOVE A "LOST TAMPON" (OR CONDOM)

- Wash your hands and make sure your nails are filed down (no sharp edges).
- If you're doing this solo, squatting down may be the easiest position. If you have a partner, they can assist with you lying on your back, like for a Pap smear.
- Insert your index and middle fingers into your vagina and perform a sweeping motion to feel for the object. Your cervix will feel a bit like the tip of your nose; if you feel that, try to do a sweep behind it (toward the tailbone side), as things sometimes like to hide there.
- Once you've located the object, pinch it between your two fingers and gently pull so that it eases out without you losing your grip.

- While this whole thing is stressful, try to breathe and relax, as this will help your vaginal muscles relax, too.

If you do forget about a tampon and can't pull it out using clean hands for any reason, you will need to have it removed by a medical professional. Doing so is no reason to feel embarrassed or ashamed: I see plenty of women who just need a little help with a tampon for whatever reason, and I'm more than happy to administer care. If your doctor shames you, find a new doctor. You can also contact your local Planned Parenthood or community clinic, which may be able to offer you a low-cost or free visit to remove a "missing" tampon for free.

Is it normal to get itchy down there on my period?

Feeling a little scratchy down there during or right after your period is normal, as menstrual blood can disrupt your vagina's incredible balance of flora by causing a slight uptick in yeast, which can trigger mild itching. Changing pads and panty liners regularly, washing the vulva daily, and even using a baby wipe or other non-fragrance-filled product to gently clean the area during the day can cut down on the itch that period blood can cause. But if your scratching is anything more than mild, there's something up: you could have a sensitivity to your menstrual products, a yeast infection, vaginitis (a form of inflammation), or another infection. See chapter 7 for more on these conditions and what to do about it.

Where's my period? Is it ever coming back?

We often dream of the days where we never have to deal with our period again, but when it happens, or, er, doesn't happen, the red alert goes off in your mind. Am I pregnant? Definitely first question if you've had a recent encounter with sperm. Am I sick? Also a very good question, as a significant illness can throw your cycle off. Don't sweat your period ghosting you one time, but if it's staying gone for three months or more, then we definitely want to know why.

Amenorrhea is the medical term for when your period stops before you reach menopause (the average age of which is fifty-one for women in the

US[43]) and stays gone for an extended period of time. If your cycles have been coming at a predictable pace (plus or minus a few days is still regular), but now have been gone for at least three months (six months if your cycles are irregular), that's amenorrhea. For my patients, we don't wait around for a three- or six-month mark; come month 2, I want to know what's up.

What I just described is secondary amenorrhea—you had a period once and now you don't. But there's another type called primary amenorrhea, when that period never comes. If you don't reach menarche (fancy medical term for the first time you get your period) by age sixteen, it's time to investigate conditions like anatomical issues, hypothyroidism, genetic variations, elevated levels of follicle-stimulating hormone (FSH), and PCOS.[44] If you've had no signs of puberty at all by age fourteen, your doctor will likely want to investigate the cause. While less than 1 percent of women experience primary amenorrhea,[45] the incidence of secondary amenorrhea is higher.[46]

So what things can cause our period to stop for several months, as is the case with secondary amenorrhea? PCOS (see symptom check in chapter 9), hyperprolactinemia (when you produce excess prolactin, the hormone responsible for milk production), thyroid disease, and primary ovarian insufficiency, which happens when your ovaries stop producing hormones before age forty.[47] If you're breastfeeding, it's normal to not have a period, and some women do not resume menstruating until they wean. All that bleeding postpartum was part of after-birth healing, not a period. Menopause is diagnosed once you have had twelve consecutive months of no periods. If you're in your late forties or fifties, this missing period may be the sign of a transition into menopause.

Certain lifestyle habits can cause your period to stop, especially those that the body perceives as a high-stress situation like overexercising, undereating, and/or losing a lot of weight. These three stressful habits can be seen in athletes who overtrain and underfuel, or in disordered eating, or in having an eating disorder. Functional hypothalamic amenorrhea (FHA) is the diagnosis that is given when there is no other discernible cause and there are high-stress factors at play. FHA occurs when the brain (hypothalamus, to be exact) stops making gonadotropin-releasing hormone (GnRH), which is what sets off the FSH and LH hormones discussed in chapter 9 that are responsible for ovulation and menstruation. Without brain hormones there can be no sex hormones and, thus, no ovulation or period. If you have painful, heavy, or what you feel are dreadful periods, then you may be thinking *Sign me up*. But there's a hell of a lot more than just a period that goes missing here. With FHA your estrogen plummets. Remember this hormone is giving you the ability to self-lubricate, and influences your desire for sex. It's also keeping your bones strong, brain healthy, and cardiovascular system in tip-top shape. Without your ovaries cycling hormones you can find yourself anxious, experiencing hot flashes, noticing your skin is thinning, confused, and exhausted. No one wants to be signed up for that.

We need to know why the period is MIA to treat appropriately. While most doctors jump to "Just take the pill to fix your period," that's actually not the best move. First, the pill doesn't fix your period, it just makes you bleed (see page 302 for details), and it doesn't protect bones quite as well as we previously thought.[48] But the biggest issue—and why the Endocrine Society warns against using the pill as treatment for women with FHA—is that you'll never know if the lifestyle and nutritional treatments you're employing actually work, because the pill's primary mechanism is to stop ovulation.[49] To recover your period, it takes addressing the stressors—like easing up on exercise or changing the routine, increasing caloric intake, stress management practices, and eating a nutrient-dense diet—to reclaim ovulation. If you're diagnosed with FHA and suffer from an eating disorder (ED), you need to work with someone who is an ED specialist to ensure the best and safest recovery.[50] While I'm providing you nutrition tips throughout this book, it's important that you work with a professional to guide you in the best dietary approach for your needs.

LAB TESTS TO CONSIDER FOR A MISSING PERIOD

- Pregnancy test
- Follicle-stimulating hormone (FSH)
- Luteinizing hormone (LH)
- Estradiol (sometimes docs won't test estrogen, but if they don't, then they're missing info on how the ovaries respond to the brain signals)

- Prolactin
- Thyroid panel
- Free testosterone
- Androstenedione
- Dehydroepiandrosterone-sulfate (DHEA-S)
- 17-OH progesterone
- Cortisol
- Fasting insulin
- Glycated hemoglobin (HbA1c), fasting glucose, or glucose challenge

Will you need all of these? Maybe. Maybe not. This is where an experienced clinician can help.

IS IT ← PCOS OR FHA? →

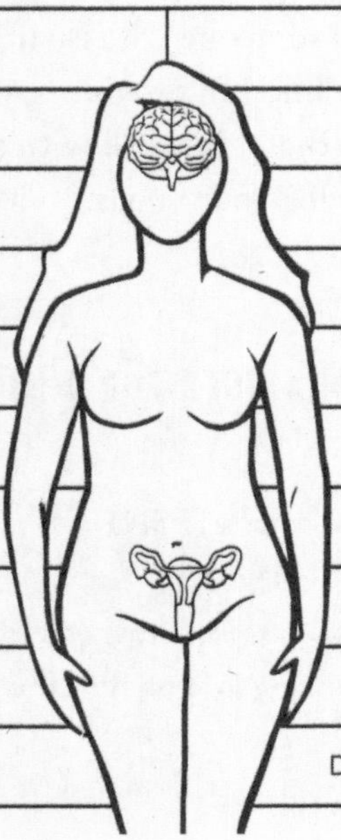

PCOS	FHA
Irregular Period	Missing Period
Elevated Androgens	May Have Slightly Elevated Androgens
Polycystic Ovaries	Polycystic Ovaries
Any Body Weight	Low or Normal Body Weight
Low SHBG	Normal SHBG
Normal or Elevated Fasting Insulin	Normal or Low Fasting Insulin
Normal or Elevated Fasting Glucose	Normal or Low Fasting Glucose
Elevated AMH	Normal or Slightly Elevated AMH
Elevated Cortisol	Elevated Cortisol
Increased Endometrial Thickness	Decreased Endometrial Thickness

If I don't need a period on the pill, why do I need a period at all?

I commonly hear: "My doctor told me it was bad I wasn't getting my period and prescribed me the pill. But then they told me I don't need a period while on the pill." Confusing, right? If you've been wondering what gives, you're not the only one lost by the nonspecific use of the word "period."

As you learned in chapter 9, HCG (the pregnancy hormone) stimulates the corpus luteum (what produces progesterone in the ovary after ovulation) to continue pumping out progesterone when a fertilized egg has implanted. If no pregnancy occurs, the lack of HCG leads to the corpus luteum stopping progesterone production, which causes your period. The drop in hormones triggers the brain to begin FSH production as the body sets out to ovulate once again. Meanwhile, your uterine lining sheds (period) and then rebuilds through the month due to the stimulation of estrogen. It's complex.

In contrast, on the pill, you take synthetic estrogen and progestin (not progesterone) every day until you don't, and then you bleed. With the pill, there's no corpus luteum, progesterone, brain hormones stimulating your ovaries, significant building of the uterine lining, and no cyclical symphony of hormones playing through your month. There are hormones and then there's not, which is why this is called a medication-induced withdrawal bleed and not a period. This is all because the pill prevents pregnancy by providing exogenous (outside) hormones that suppress the brain from secreting hormones that tell your ovaries to ovulate. Because the pill's hormones don't build the uterine lining like your own hormones, there's no real need to bleed. With your actual menstrual cycle, hormones stimulate the growth of the endometrium, and it must be shed (period) to avoid endometrial hyperplasia (when it gets too thick) and the risk of endometrial cancer. Not having a period can also be a sign of something serious (see the section on amenorrhea) and can have consequences like bone loss, vaginal atrophy (shrinking vaginal tissues), vaginal dryness, pain with sex, declining brain health, and increased risk of cardiovascular disease due to the hormone imbalances at play.

So just to recap, legit periods are necessary. Pill periods or, more accurately, withdrawal bleeds, are not necessary. You can skip your period on the pill, just don't skip your period if you're not on it. For more specifics on birth control and its effects on hormones, please read my book *Beyond the Pill.*

TL;DR: IS MY PERIOD NORMAL?

- Period sex is safe (and even fun). Using menstrual cups, a towel, or taking to the shower can make cleanup easier.
- In general, you can't get pregnant at the start of your period, but if you ovulate within five days of unprotected sex, then you could get pregnant.
- Normal periods aren't excruciatingly painful, don't significantly interfere with your life, and don't go beyond seven days or require you to double up on menstrual products, and shouldn't produce clots that could play a slot machine.
- Periods are necessary. Pill bleeds are not necessary (see page 275 for why).
- Period poop, butt lightning, and period flu may all be related to hormonelike chemicals called prostaglandins. But there's some other causes too that I discussed that are worth mentioning to your doctor.
- Migraines and headaches are not normal parts of having a cycle, and can point to estrogen issues and in some cases low magnesium.
- I taught you how to fish out a tampon, a condom, or other object. It's a good idea to bookmark that page, just in case.
- There are several reasons why your period may disappear for a while, and none are normal.

CHAPTER 11

ARE MY BREASTS NORMAL?

BIG, SMALL, POINTY, ROUND, AND EVERYTHING IN BETWEEN

Fun fact: Humans are the only mammals in the animal kingdom who develop breasts that stay with them for life. Every other species only sports a set when it's time to mate or feed their offspring.[1] What gives for humans? Well, we don't know why we rock the pair our whole life, but scientists think that when we took to standing, our bodies made the switch from an enlarged anus to breasts to signal that we're potentially fertile.[2] Personally, I'll take the breasts.

When it comes to breasts, there's an endless number of combinations in terms of shapes, sizes, colors, areola colors, and nipple shapes. They're all normal, but what we often see in the media are sets that represent only a small percentage of the population. If, like me, you grew up in the nineties, then you're all too familiar with the gravity-defying, *Baywatch* bounce of Pamela Anderson's boobs, which sparked a trend of bigger is better, making women (and girls) everywhere think that D and beyond were the breasts to aspire to.

Plus, until recently there had been a diversity desert of breasts in billboards, magazines, and the bras of Victoria's Secret, leaving many questioning if that is what we're "supposed" to look like and if that is normal. All those natural breasts are normal, as are every single one (or two) of the breasts that fill women's cups across the globe. While augmented breasts are a deviation from the original normal of the body they are on, we're not going to call those abnormal because everyone has the right to alterations in their appearance (although there are some things you should be aware of that I discuss on page 293).

And moving on to nipples, which feel like the ultimate taboo of the upper body with platforms like Instagram keeping a strict ban on any images depicting breastfeeding until 2020. With so little exposure to what nipples look like, let alone breastfeeding, and breasts themselves, it's no wonder I get so many questions about what's normal when it comes to how breasts look, and that women feel so isolated in their breastfeeding journey. So, running with the theme of this book, let's normalize normal bodies and normalize conversations that should have never been made taboo in the first place.

ASK DR. BRIGHTEN:

Is my breast size normal?

We are conditioned by marketing to want what we don't have. Got itty bitties? *Men like them bigger, so you should want them bigger* is a message that plays out time and time again, which may account for why 47 percent of women surveyed in over forty nations said they wanted bigger breasts (23 percent wanted smaller).[3] BTW, in a separate survey, almost 70 percent of men said they were happy with their partner's breast size.[4] Small breasts are normal. In fact, all breast sizes are normal. But there are breasts so big that bra straps leave a permanent imprint in shoulders and cause backaches all the time. Big breasts are normal, but that doesn't mean they can't cause you serious problems, which are rarely talked about. In fact, when women complain about their large breasts they are often met with "You should be so grateful." When your breasts interfere with your ability to live comfortably, studies show that breast-reduction surgery may improve quality of life in patients for ten to thirty years afterward.[5] If your breasts are a real pain in the back, then surgery may be helpful. Outside of medical concerns, there is no reason to have breast surgery unless it is something you truly desire.

Breast Anatomy

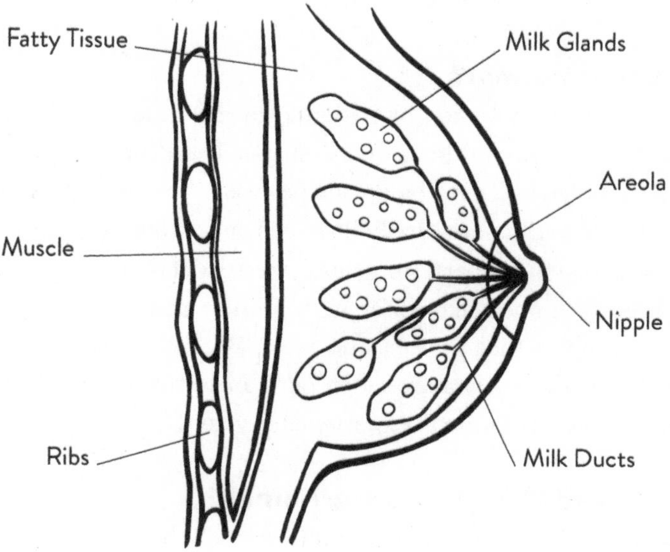

When do breasts stop growing?

Typically, breasts stop growing a year or two after your first period. But for some, they'll continue to grow into your late teens or early twenties. And just because they've stopped growing doesn't mean this dynamic tissue can't change, as is the case with pregnancy, weight gain, and entering menopause. Fat is what gives your breasts volume, which is why your breasts can increase in size if you gain weight. And I want to note that gaining weight is normal after your early twenties, so your breast size may change.

Many experts believe that breasts have not undergone full maturation until after lactation. That's because while your breasts may have stopped growing after puberty, they undergo major changes after breastfeeding. I want to assure you, however, that you do not need to ever be pregnant to have healthy, normal breasts. During pregnancy, hormones cause milk-producing tissues to grow—estrogen stimulates breast duct cells, and progesterone stimulates the milk glands. In the last stages of pregnancy and following birth, prolactin stimulates milk to be produced. BTW, those bumps on the areola (Montgomery tubercles) are going to pop up, and you may notice your chest is covered in a highway of veins, which is due to increased blood flow that is part of a normal pregnancy. Your nipples will also darken as you approach your due date, and may or may not return to your original normal when you're done breastfeeding (normal).

Are tube boobs normal?

I have been asked this question by patients several times. What's meant by "tube boob" is a narrow and long breast shape. Teardrop and round, sometimes called "bubbles," seem to be the shapes we're sold most by augmented breasts in the media. But some are bell shaped, and others are close together while others are farther apart, and there are sets that are more muscular. There are breasts shaped like cones with nipples pointing straight ahead, and there are nipples that go east and west. Breasts come in all different shapes and those shapes change as we age, breastfeed, lose weight, gain weight, and just live as humans experiencing gravity.

Can I breastfeed if my breasts are small?

Yes. Breast size isn't an indicator of whether you'll be successful in breastfeeding. I encourage any mom with concerns about this to schedule with a lactation consultant soon after your baby is born. No matter how many babies you've had, an objective eye outside your body can always give pointers to help. While we're on size, it also doesn't matter when it comes to sexual pleasure, either, since most of the breast's nerve endings are concentrated in the nipple.

Is it normal for one of my breasts to be bigger than the other?

Your body isn't symmetrical. Divide it down the center and you'll find your breasts to be no exception. Asymmetrical breasts (uneven) are incredibly common, with estimates that over half of women do not have a matching pair.[6] So, normal. Not only is it normal for one to be bigger than the other, but your breasts can also differ from each other in shape, volume, positioning, and density. If you notice one is suddenly bigger than the other, or feeling more full or heavy, speak with your provider.

Why are my breasts itchy?

There's a lot of answers here. Detergent, dry skin, irritating fabric, new lotion, and a poorly fitting bra can all explain why you may feel the urge to scratch. But if that itching won't stop and you have a rash, you need to get it checked out. It could be a few things, but a condition called Paget's disease, which is associated with breast cancer, is one we definitely want to rule out.

Breast Changes to See Your Medical Provider About

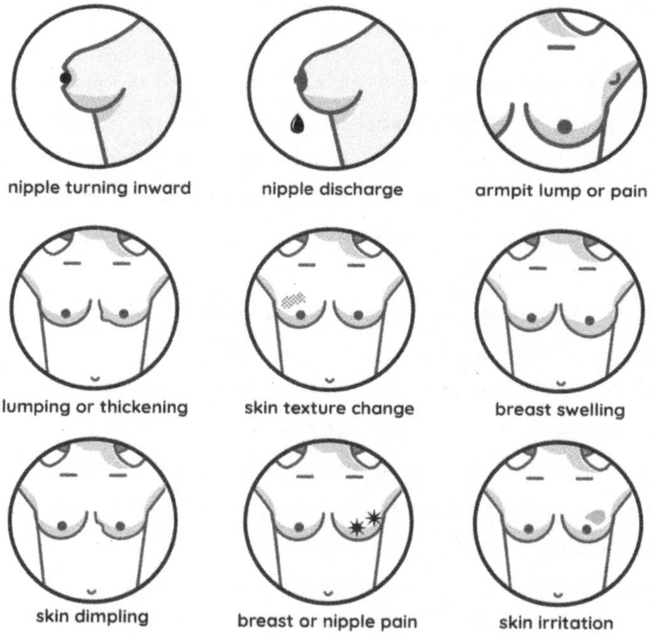

We expect breasts to change throughout our lifetime; however, abrupt changes should be examined by a provider. These nine changes are ones you should definitely get checked out.

Is it normal if I have stretch marks on my boobs?

Stretch marks are normal on your breast, butt, thighs, abdomen, or anywhere else tissue has seen a rapid growth spurt. While every breast development book shows this slow and gradual growth, sometimes those buds become full-on Bs seemingly overnight due to the hormonal agenda outside our control. The same can happen in early pregnancy, or when your milk comes in during early breastfeeding. If it happened to you, you're not alone, as up to 70 percent of women develop stretch marks before delivery.[7] If any body part expands quickly, the skin has got to stretch to accommodate. You're more likely to get stretch marks if you're dehydrated, so drink plenty of fluids and apply moisturizer. Protein, zinc, and vitamins C, E, and D may all help your skin in adapting to the growth. See the nutrient chart on page 369 for foods that contain these. Topical vitamin A, glycolic acid, or laser therapy are a few of the treatments to discuss with your doctor.

Is boob sweat normal?

This is like asking if armpit sweat or groin sweat or (gasp!) butt sweat is normal. It all is. Any tissues that come together can get hot and, in response, your body will release sweat to cool you down. If you've got boob sweat but don't want it, try these tips:

- Choose cotton fabrics, as opposed to synthetic ones that don't breathe and can trigger your body to sweat.
- Padding is like insulation to your breasts. So if you're trying to avoid sweat, you're going to want to avoid padding.
- Try a sports bra, which is generally made from breathable, moisture-wicking material, meaning it will pull sweat away from your breasts.
- Wear loose-fitting tops that allow for ample airflow.
- Use cotton pads (yeah, like the kind for breastfeeding) to absorb some moisture, and change them during the day.
- Do a quick bird bath with a baby wipe in the bathroom to remove sweat and irritation-inducing moisture.
- There is special "for the breast" deodorant available and some antichafing options, which can be helpful if irritation becomes an issue.

Is boob acne normal?

Oh, breast-ne, why you gotta suck like that? Yes, boob acne is a normal (and lame, since you have to deal with it) occurrence. It can show up where your bra rubs, because you put sunscreen on (as you should), or because your breasts come together in such a way that they rub or sweat. The occasional pimple here or there isn't anything to be too concerned about. But chest-ne that makes it so you feel you can't ever wear a bathing suit (you still can) is something to bring up with your doctor. There can be situations where acne isn't just a bacterial issue, but fungal in origin. Your doctor can help you troubleshoot and resolve it. In the meantime, use the solutions on page 381.

Is it normal for my breasts to droop or sag?

Unfortunately, collagen and estrogen don't have our backs for life. As we get older, our levels of estrogen and collagen decline, which can cause breasts to fall as connective tissue known as Cooper's ligaments stretches, and any gravity-evading tactics fail. If your breasts are larger, you have lower estrogen levels, you're in menopause, or you smoke, your breasts can drop or droop more quickly. Fallen breasts due to low estrogen can also start to wrinkle, lose volume, and gather at the bottom, which some describe as having "rocks in their socks." If you have these symptoms that suggest low estrogen, speak to your provider about it.

What color should my nipples and areolae be? Is it normal if they change color?

Nipples and areolae (the plural of "areola") can be any shade from pink to dark brown. The color of your areola (remember: that's the disc that surrounds your nipple) may also be darker than the nipple itself, which is normal and common. Your areolae may also have an outer ring that is darker than everything else surrounding it. Totally normal. But if you notice they are changing color for no reason, suddenly have red, purple, or dark purple making an appearance, or you have scaling over the areola, or there's any change to how the nipple looks, that's not normal. Ask your provider if there's something going on.

Hormones have powerful and varying effects on our breasts. If your hormones just changed—like when you're pregnant, breastfeeding, going through menopause, or begin to take oral contraceptives—then your nipple color may, too. The shade of your nipple and areola can also darken at certain times during your cycle. And there can be a mismatch of color, where one side is darker than the other. A patient I saw with this concern called it her "David Bowie boobies" because they were mismatched, like the rock star's eyes. Pretty cool spin to put on it. And still entirely normal. However, some people get areola tattooing to correct the color. I don't recommend it, though, since changes in your hormones later in life may result in there being inconsistencies showing up once again. While most of the time these changes that accompany hormonal shifts are totally benign, I always encourage my patients to have any and all breast changes examined. See the image on page 281 for changes to see your provider about.

Could my nipples be too big?

Nipples and the saucer they sit on, the areola, can vary in size. Sometimes it's based on breast size and other times it's based on genes. I've had many patients concerned about nipples that are too big but, when I examine them, I find they are normal.

Is it normal for my nipples to get hard when I am cold?

Everyone's nipples get hard when they're cold, thanks to smooth muscles around the areola. It's the same mechanism that causes you to get goose bumps.

Does having an innie nipple mean there's something wrong with my breasts? Does that mean I can't breastfeed?

Up to 20 percent of all people are born with one or both nipples inverted, meaning they don't protrude.[8] It's also normal if your nipples are flat. And inverted or flat nipples shouldn't inhibit your ability to breastfeed, but whenever you struggle to breastfeed, get that lactation consultant on speed dial.

If I have a nipple piercing, can I still breastfeed?

Yes, you can, as long as the piercing was done properly and impacts only the nipple (not the ducts or glands).

What if I have a third nipple?

Milk lines—not like you're queued up to get some milk, but the actual embryonic lines that breast development follows in utero—extend from your armpits to your groin. Before your body exited the first trimester, these lines were isolated to where we typically think of breasts being (although your breast tissues extend into your armpit and are referred to as the tail of Spence). Sometimes there's a little hiccup in development, and you end up with breast tissues or a little nipple somewhere on that line. This is where some people can have a third nipple, also called a supernumerary nipple. It is normal and common. About 1 percent of people get a nipple complete with its own breast tissue, while about 2.5 percent have just a solitary nipple.[9] Many people with supernumerary nipples mistake them for a mole, although it can become noticeable if they swell, get sore, or start producing milk, which can happen with nursing. Actor Mark Wahlberg revealed he has a third nipple, just in case you're looking for celeb cred.[10]

Is it normal to have bumps around my nipples?

Yes! Those bumps are called Montgomery glands or tubercles, and not only are they normal on your nipples and areolae, but they also serve an important function by producing oil to keep your breasts moisturized and soft during breastfeeding. While these tubercules may look like clear pimples, don't treat them like pimples and squeeze them, which can cause irritation and infection.

I have hair on my nipple. Is that normal, and what should I do about it?

A hair or two is normal and common. A lot of hair, however, especially if it is thick or coarse, can be a sign of a hormone imbalance or polycystic ovary syndrome (PCOS), which can be caused by excess androgens, a group of sex hormones that includes testosterone. See chapter 9 for more about PCOS. Please do not shave here. Ingrown hairs on your breasts can get real nasty real quick. If you must, pluck.

Why are my nipples leaking if I'm not pregnant or haven't had a baby?

This isn't normal. It's a go-to-the-doctor-ASAP situation. One test they will likely order is prolactin, which is the lactation hormone. As we discussed in chapter 8, prolactin can increase in cases of hypothyroidism, so it's best practice to take a thyroid-stimulating hormone (TSH) test to see where the elevated prolactin is coming from. If it's not your thyroid, we look for other causes. Certain medications like antidepressants, birth control, blood pressure meds, and certain painkillers can lead to the drip of galactorrhea (milk production). A benign brain tumor known as a prolactinoma can also cause milk production. I know that sounds bad, but it isn't a dangerous cancer lesion. It can impact vision, however, due to structural changes, so if you're making milk and having trouble seeing, it's a doctor's visit for you. In rare instances, a lot of nipple play can trigger the body to make milk.

How can I incorporate nipple play and my breasts into sex?

As I shared in chapter 4, some people can have a nipple orgasm, just like they can when their clitoris is stimulated. That's because like the clitoris, your nipples increase in size, become erect, and light up the same areas of the brain (the sensory cortex) that correspond to sexual pleasure when aroused.[11] If your clitoris and nipples are erect, does that make it a triple lady boner?

A study in the *Journal of Sexual Medicine* reported that 81.5 percent of women experienced increased arousal when their partner stimulated their breast or nipples.[12] Of course, not everyone is into this, and if you're not, you're among about 7 percent of others in the study who found this a turnoff. Timing can be everything, as we discussed in chapter 9, when you set out to explore nipple play. Play with those breasts the week before your period and it might be a *Hell no* from below. But come at them in midcycle, or just after your period, and you may get the *Green light, go.* That's because hormones can change the way our breasts feel.

How to Incorporate Breasts into Sex

These multitasking mavens become erect, enlarge, and produce an odor that gets both you and your partner turned on. Breast tissue is full of sensitive nerves, which is why they can act as an erogenous zone in both women and men. Nipple stimulation also activates the same area of the brain as the genitals do, providing a similar sense of sexual pleasure.[13] Your breasts will likely be less tender while on your period, and your nipples will increase in sensitivity during your fertile window, which makes the follicular through ovulatory phase the perfect time to try out some breast and nipple play. Following ovulation, breasts can get tender. But don't worry, I have solutions for breast tenderness coming your way. Here are some tips for partnered sex to help you incorporate this highly erotic tissue. (Note: you'll probably want to share this with your partner before things begin to heat up.)

Get Into You. If you're among the 71 percent of women unhappy with your cup size, you may feel inclined to keep your shirt on during sex or completely disconnect from that area of your body.[14] While society will tell you all day, every day, the girls *should* look a certain way, that's just some arbitrary standard that someone else (read: men) invented that keeps us disconnected from this incredibly sensual part of our body. Getting comfortable with yourself is essential in the quest for more pleasure. I'd encourage you to spend some time with your breasts and getting acquainted on a more intimate level. Try this: Next time you get out of the shower, stand in front of the mirror and apply lotion or oil to your breasts. Take your time applying it and explore not just how your breasts look, but also how they feel. What pressure do you like best? Is there a direction that feels best? How sensitive are your nipples, and does that feel good?

Titty Talk (But Make It Dirty). This is a major turn-on for so many and your partner can leverage it to help put you at ease during sex. Communicate with your partner about how you'd like to incorporate your breasts into sex. Having them tell you "Your tits are so hot" or "Oh my God, I love your boobs" can go a long way in helping you get into it. When that *bow-chicka-wowwow* vibe hits, your partner will know exactly what to whisper to help disengage the spectator brake (that self-critical observation that kills desire). Well, maybe. It could take some practice, like anything new and worth doing.

No Honking, Please. Whether it's to break awkward tension or because your partner genuinely thinks it's funny, honking, jiggling, or slapping without consent isn't the right foot forward.

It's Not Target Practice. There's a whole lot more than a nipple, and while it does resemble a bullseye, heading straight for the center can be a straight turnoff for some. Start from the outside and work toward the nipple. Try different pressures to find what feels best. Using a hand with fingers spread wide and grasping the breast with a slow and gradual squeezing toward the nipple, is one example of how to do this.

Mouth, Tongue, Teeth. Kissing, licking, or caresses with the lips are sometimes a preference over hands for some. And while some enjoy rough breast play, not everyone does, so tugging, biting, and teeth in general need permission before you proceed. Just because you gotta ask doesn't mean it's gotta disrupt the vibe. "Do you like that?" "Would you like more pressure?" or "I want to nibble it, is that OK?" are all ways to get consent without feeling like you're stopping to have a dialogue.

Make the Temp Drop. Ice cubes will make the nipples erect and may increase the sensations. Just be sure not to leave the ice on one area too long (yes, some people are really into that), as it can cause tissue damage.

Pinch, Clamp, Suck. You can buy nipple clamps, suckers, and other devices that stimulate the nipples. But some people prefer a pinch between two fingers. Just like biting, though, you want to make sure your partner is into this first.

Bring the Clit Along. Stimulating the clit while engaging in other activities will almost always make it more pleasurable. You may find that nipple and breast play are much more pleasurable combined with other types of sex.

ASK DR. BRIGHTEN:

How common is breast tenderness?

Nearly three-quarters of all women experience sore or painful breasts at some point in their lives.[15] Cyclical breast pain (aka mastalgia), the kind that shows up around ovulation or before your period every month, isn't generally anything to worry about. While it is a real pain in the boob, it is often due to cycling hormones. Sure, these are normal times for breast tenderness to show up, but if you can't jog, let alone walk, that's not normal.

Noncyclical breast tenderness, the kind that comes out of nowhere, generally isn't hormone-related and is more concerning, depending on the cause. Noncyclical breast pain should never be considered normal or ignored.

Is it normal for my boobs to ache before my period?

Mild cyclical breast pain is normal and the most common cause of mastalgia.[16] Your breasts may feel sore, tender, dull, achy, or heavy around ovulation or right before your period. The pain can affect one or both breasts, range from mild to moderate, and radiate into your armpit and even down your arm. Anything more than moderate discomfort should get checked out.

When estrogen goes up, as is the case around ovulation, it can lead to breast tenderness. Similarly, if there is a higher amount of estrogen before your period or if you're making more of the 16OH-E1 metabolite we discussed in chapter 8, you may also experience sore breasts. Abnormal levels of prolactin, the hormone that causes milk production, can also cause breast pain and is elevated in some non-milk-producing people.[17] There are several steps you can take to banish boob pain that is due to hormones. In addition to the suggestions in the 28-day plan, the suggestions in the Cyclical Symptom Relief Chart can also help you get relief.

What are fibrocystic breasts and can they become cancerous?

Super common and, yet, not commonly discussed, fibrocystic breast change is found in 80 percent of patients during their reproductive years.[18] This condition can cause your breasts to feel lumpy or ropy due to the formation of fibrous tissue and fluid-filled sacs beneath your skin. They can also feel increasingly heavy as you near your period. Fibrocystic breasts can cause pain and tenderness, especially right before your period, but not everyone feels sore.[19] Fibrocystic breasts are a normal development, affecting half of all premenopausal women—doctors call the condition "fibrocystic breast change" rather than "fibrocystic breast disease," since it's not a disease or disorder.[20] If you ever feel a new or different mass in your breast, however, make an appointment to see a doctor. Sure, fibrocystic breasts aren't thought to increase your risk of cancer, but you do want to be sure that is what you're dealing with.

While we aren't totally sure what causes fibrocystic breast changes, the predominant theory is hormones—estrogen, progesterone, prolactin, and testosterone may all play a role. Because hormones soar in pregnancy, that's also a common time to see fibrocystic breast issues crop up or get worse. Both vitamin E and flaxseeds have been shown to reduce lumpiness and breast pain.[21] Iodine, which is concentrated in breast tissue, impacts both structure and function of breast tissue, which is why it is important to include iodine in your diet.[22] With hormones as the likely culprit, you'll find lots of tips in the 28-day program to help you optimize hormones and reduce breast tenderness.

Symptom Check:
Is it pregnancy or PMS breast tenderness?

PMS is a tricky one, as it can mimic early pregnancy. But there are some major signs that it's time to stop by the drugstore for a pregnancy test.

- [ ] **Ouch! My breasts are killing me**
- [ ] **My period is late**
- [ ] **My mood swings haven't come to visit**
- [ ] **The thought, smell, or sight of food makes me want to vomit**
- [ ] **I've seen brown or irregular spotting**
- [ ] **My nipples are darker**
- [ ] **I am noticing little bumps on my areolae**
- [ ] **I'm bloated and constipated**
- [ ] **I recently had unprotected sex, a condom broke, or I was otherwise exposed to semen**

If semen was permitted any passage into your vagina and you're waiting on an expected period to show up, grab a pregnancy test or schedule a visit with your doctor, because all of these symptoms can be a sign of pregnancy. If, however, your period's due date hasn't yet arrived or you don't have sex with penises, you may be in the clear.

What if I just started having breast pain out of nowhere?

This isn't normal and can be due to totally benign reasons, like your bra isn't fitting right, or might be more serious. See page 288 for signs you should see your doctor. Noncyclical breast pain can affect one or both breasts and be sporadic or continuous.[23] Breast pain caused by factors not related to your cycle is rarely due to cancer.[24]

Here are some of the leading causes of noncyclical breast pain:

Pendulous breasts: That's doc-talk for really large breasts. Sometimes sheer size can cause breast pain, in addition to headaches and neck, back, and shoulder pain. If you're experiencing pain due to the size of your breasts, speak with your provider about treatment options, including breast-reduction surgery, which may be covered by insurance if you get a medical diagnosis.

Trauma: If you feel pain in one breast, it could be due to an injury, like an accidental elbow to the breast, a fall, or a poor-fitting bra. Breast trauma can also cause a benign lump to form. Depending on the degree of trauma, or if the pain gets worse over time, it is best to meet with a provider.

Birth control pills, hormone replacement therapy, fertility drugs: Starting any of these medications can cause you to feel breast pain, but they may also help relieve the condition, according to studies.[25] If you've begun a new hormone medication and are experiencing breast pain, speak with your provider.

Nonhormonal medications: Some medications like antidepressants, antibiotics, and heart medications can lead to breast pain. If you're taking one of these medications, speak with your provider about alternatives that may not leave you with sore boobs.

Pregnancy and breastfeeding: That first-trimester breast expansion is no joke and, plus, later comes the milk production, which can make things sore. Higher levels of hormones like estrogen and progesterone can make your breasts feel sore when you're pregnant. While estrogen drops after you give birth, you produce more prolactin, which can cause breast pain. Your breasts can also become engorged when breastfeeding, which can make them feel tight and painful. If being postpartum is where you need support, my book *Healing Your Body Naturally After Childbirth* can help.

Ductal ectasia: Your breasts have ducts, also called milk ducts, that bring milk to your nipple. Regardless of whether you're breastfeeding, these ducts can become inflamed and even blocked or clogged, which is more common as we approach menopause. (This is different than a plugged milk duct that can lead to bacterial mastitis in breastfeeding women.) You may also experience discharge, skin thickening, and redness around the nipple. And while you may have a fever, the inflammation and pain aren't due to an infection, like we see in mastitis (see below). An ultrasound can help your doctor understand if ductal ectasia is the source of your pain.

Mastitis: Before you glaze over this one, thinking it's for breastfeeding moms only, it's not. Mastitis is an infection that develops in the breast, and while it's more common when women are breastfeeding, you can develop it when you're not lactating, too. Classic signs of mastitis include a red, painful, or swollen breast that may be accompanied by fever and chills. Smoking cigarettes increases the risk of mastitis. If you suspect mastitis, see a provider immediately.

Inflammatory breast cancer: I used the C-word here, and that usually causes a panic. First, know that this is a rare form of breast cancer, accounting for only 1 to 5 percent of all breast cancers diagnosed.[26] It is aggressive, and the symptoms are not subtle, which means you won't miss them and should see a provider immediately. With inflammatory breast cancer, the tissue becomes red and swollen, and the skin looks like an orange peel (think texture, not color). There may also be a rapidly growing lump. It can sometimes be mistaken for mastitis, so if you're treated with antibiotics and symptoms don't improve, call your provider.

Cysts and other lumps: If you feel a smooth lump in your breast, it could be a benign cyst, which may or may not cause tenderness. You may also have fibroadenoma, a solid, smooth lump that is usually tender, but is the most common cause of benign lumps.[27] That lump may also be a fat necrosis, which occurs when benign, damaged fatty tissues form into a mass.[28] Whenever you feel something new in your breast, schedule a visit with your provider and pay attention to whether the area changes with your cycle. The only way to distinguish a benign mass from a more problematic mass is to have imaging done, most often an ultrasound.

Smoking: Some studies show that smoking may contribute to breast pain.[29] If you do smoke, there's a whole lot of reasons to consider stopping, including that it might alleviate your breast pain.

Caffeine: The evidence is mixed for whether eliminating caffeine will eliminate breast pain. Clinically, I've absolutely seen patients' breast pain and fibrocystic breast symptoms resolve with cutting out caffeine completely. But I've also seen patients who employed the same therapies I'll share in chapter 13 and then brought caffeine back in without the return of symptoms. Should you cut it? It couldn't hurt. (Did you just decide we're not friends?) But it will take about four to six months to know for sure if caffeine is your issue.

IS BREAST IMPLANT ILLNESS REAL?

Breast implant illness (BII) is a term used to describe a range of symptoms some women experience after having implants placed. Symptoms of BII can include chronic fatigue, joint pain, breathing problems, hair loss, rashes, brain fog, headaches, depression, and anxiety.[30] While women have been gaslit (about this and loads of other BS) for years, BII is real and can manifest in different ways in different people. But since the data is lacking, we don't actually know how many women have BII.[31]

I want to be clear that I'm not for or against breast implants. Instead, I want to give you all the information you need to make the best medical choices for you. If you're considering implants, choose a board-certified plastic surgeon with whom you can discuss your full medical history and health concerns. If you already have implants and suspect BII, there's no test to diagnose the condition, but you can speak with a provider and undergo testing to rule out other, similar medical issues and autoimmune disorders. You should also speak with a board-certified surgeon who has experience with BII about treatment options, including explant surgery, or the removal of breast implants.[32] Explant surgery doesn't always resolve symptoms, but small studies show the procedure can be effective.[33]

TL;DR: ARE MY BREASTS NORMAL?

- Humans are the only mammals who have permanently enlarged breasts. So ask a llama if your breasts are normal and it's a "Hell no." But who really cares what a llama thinks anyway?
- There's no perfect size of breasts, and size does not correlate to pleasure. While a significant number of women report being unhappy with their breasts, a significant number of men report being happy with their partner's breasts. Houston, we have a disconnect.
- Big breasts can be a big pain in the back. If your breasts are interfering with your quality of life, chat with a provider about it.
- There are some serious signs that signal it's time for a medical exam. Check out the table on page 281 to get familiar with them.
- Everyone is capable of orgasm from nipple stimulation alone, but it certainly takes mastery, and with the clit being a sure bet, you might not be into this pursuit. Want some tips on nipple and breast play (because why not pull in this highly erotic area)? They are on page 286.
- Brain imaging shows that nipples stimulate the same pleasure-related area of the brain as our genitals.
- Having dark nipples and areolae, a third nipple, inverted or flat nipples, or some hair around your areolae is totally normal. Most breasts don't look like what we see in the movies.
- Breast tenderness caused by your menstrual cycle is normal, unless it's impacting your ability to just live. Seriously, annoying. Head to chapter 13 for tips on how to eliminate breast pain.
- Breast implant illness is real, and there are options to help mitigate it.

Part 3

THE 28-DAY PROGRAM

CHAPTER 12

WELCOME TO THE 28-DAY PROGRAM

LET'S GET DOWN TO BUSINESS (NOT *THAT* KIND, BUT HELPFUL FOR THAT KIND, TOO!)

This is the moment where we're going to take everything you've been learning and incorporate it into a focused 28-day strategy. We're building a lifestyle that will ultimately lead to balanced hormones and more pleasure. I'll be taking you through the core of the program that everyone will follow, and have provided you with resources to customize it to your needs. You'll find the Hormone Symptom Check results to help you target the hormones that need your help, plus advanced protocols (Cycle Symptom Relief on page 377) to target cycle-specific symptoms and hormone-related conditions.

How to Follow the Program

We're going to kick off this plan on day 1 of your cycle, starting with getting some serious period symptom relief. But you don't have to start on day 1 if you're eager to go now, as I'll explain. Remember: day 1 is the first day you have your period. I've outlined a plan for you to follow with check-ins and instructions each week of your cycle to keep you on track to creating easier periods, less PMS, better moods, and more pleasurable sex by the start of your next cycle.

I am providing guidance on nutrition, which you'll begin incorporating at the start of your cycle. If you're someone who does well with more guidance, I have a full 28-day meal plan to support you at https://DrBrighten.com/ITN-resources so you can print it out and take it with you to the grocery, or put it on the fridge. If you have a medical condition, a history of an eating disorder, feel your relationship with food isn't what you want it to be, or are following a specialty diet, then here's a few things I want you to know. First, this food talk is a guide focused on nutrient density, supporting your hormones, and feeling good throughout your cycle. We don't do "good" or "bad" foods or dietary dogma in my clinic, and you won't find that here. If you have specific medical needs, please run this by your health care provider to make sure this plan is in your best interest. But if you've been burned by the "this food is bad so you're bad if you eat it" kind of approach that runs through the wellness industry, I want you to know that isn't what I'm about.

You will find tools in this chapter on how to reduce stress, get better sleep, exercise, and set your body on a course of healing. I'll be prompting you during each week of the program with suggestions of what might be most helpful based on what your hormones are doing. But while I'll be offering guidance, I truly want you to be the one making the call on what is best for your body, because no one knows it better than you. But it can feel confusing to understand what is causing what. This is where tracking your cycle, symptoms, sexual desire, and the other areas I'll be asking you to check in on can make a huge difference. I've already taught you how to identify key signs during your cycle and what symptoms tend to crop up when, but now we're going to pull it all together. At the end of this program, you should have a deeper understanding of your hormones; have identified the nutrition, lifestyle, and supplements that are most effective in helping you feel your best; and know how to tend to your sexual needs. If you're someone who just wants to get your hormones in check and could give AF about your sex life right now, I encourage you to focus on what you feel you need. I'm confident that somewhere on your journey you'll find this sex talk helpful, so when you're ready, it's here for you.

My goal in this program is to provide you with the information I wish every patient had before coming to me and, in truth, a lot less of them would need to see me. That's because the things that keep you out of the doctor's office consist of the intentional steps you take every day toward your health. Your doctor dedicated their life to medicine, but they haven't lived your life and they can't give you all you need to optimize your health and hormones in a single visit. What I am providing you is a way to improve your hormones, eliminate the symptoms that can be managed with diet and lifestyle, remove the obstacles to your sexual desire and pleasure (close that pleasure gap), gain a deeper understanding of your body, and, ultimately, learn practices to set you up for a lifetime of health. And I want to caution you against falling into the trap of "I already know this" or "This is nothing new." Instead, ask yourself, If I already know this, how well am I doing this? Because what I often find is that my patients do already know some of this stuff and yet, for whatever reason, they're not doing it.

Listen, it ain't a quick fix and I'm not going to be one of those doctors who tells you, "Do this and you'll reverse everything in a matter of weeks." Healing takes time; in fact, healing cyclical symptoms usually takes two to three cycles to see significant results. Things will get better sooner, but to really move the needle, you gotta be in it. And for these changes to stick, the strategies you're implementing will need to go with you for the long run, which is why you're going to track. This way you can identify what's most beneficial for you. If we want to keep acne in check, periods regular, and moods stable, then there's going to be some nonnegotiables in your routine, which you will define for yourself using this program.

So why 28 days? Because it is the framework in which we are taught about our cycle, which I've found makes it easy for my patients to wrap their head around the program. It's a small commitment, relatively speaking, to invest in creating habits that will give you the results you're looking for. Now, if you're like me, impatient as all hell and ready to jump into the program, you may find yourself frustrated that I'm asking you to begin with day 1 of your cycle when you're just now on, for example, day 8. Here's the thing: You can jump in right now if you'd like, but I ask (or rather, beg of you) to please, please start it all again on day 1 of your cycle so you can get the full 28-day experience. This will enable you to put it all together and make the most sense of this beautiful body you live in.

Here's what's in the plan:

Eat foods that support your hormones. Use the table on page 369 to see the foods that have the nutrients you're after. I've provided you several food lists and tips that you are welcome to implement on your own. If you're looking for more guidance and like meal plans, I've made one for you to download. For the next 28 days, commit to leverage the nutrition guidance here. I find my patients are most successful when they give themselves a week to prepare, so if that's what you need, take it. I recommend marking on the calendar when you'll start so that you're committed.

Begin to master stress management. Be gentle with yourself because this takes practice and consistent implementation. And just when you've got it, life throws a new stressor at you to test those skills. Notice when stress gets the best of you in your cycle and be sure to track the tools that help you most. You can set an alarm in your phone on those cycle days to remind you to breathe deeply or take an extra walk that day.

Take steps to improve sleep. If you focused only on sleep and stress management you'd see a lot of improvement, so please do not skip this part. It's a crucial step in creating exceptional hormones. Be sure to track where sleep is more difficult, and use the tips on page 313 to help.

Employ hormone-specific solutions from the Hormone Symptom Check. Customize the plan for your needs by using the nutrition, lifestyle, and supplement suggestions on page 317.

Clitoral commitment. OK, it's not all about the clit, but if you aim to close the pleasure gap in your life, it kind of is. You'll get guidance on when your sexual desire might change, how your ability to self-lubricate may shift in your cycle, pleasure practices to experiment with, and be tracking it all. If you want to see shifts in this area of your life, I highly recommend that you commit to doing the work here. If this part of the program isn't for you right now, that's totally fine. It'll be here when you're ready for it.

Track your symptoms, cycle, and sexual desire. Keep a record of where you started, what you've implemented, and what you experience. I encourage you to retake the Hormone Symptom Check on page 192 after a full cycle of the program to see what improvements you've made.

Level up with advanced protocols. I've provided you a list of advanced protocols (Cycle Symptom Relief) to troubleshoot cycle-specific symptoms and hormone-related conditions. If you need to level up the program to match your needs, you can pull in some of these specific tools.

WHAT IF I HAVE NO PERIOD?

There's this handy cosmic event that happens to be about 28 days—the moon cycle. From the new moon until the next there are technically 29.5 days, but it's close enough and easy enough to follow if you don't have a period. Your day 1 will be the day of the new moon. Go google it and write it down. It's OK, I'll wait.

WHAT IF MY CYCLE ISN'T 28 DAYS?

Welcome to the Totally Normal Club. Most cycles aren't 28 days. Remember: 28 days is just a framework for teaching, learning, and exploring your cycle. If your cycle is shorter than 28 days, you can read ahead and incorporate some of the additional tips that fit your needs. If your cycle is longer than 28 days, then you can continue the luteal phase practices until your period. As I take you through the program, I'll explain how you can modify this for your own cycle so you can make the program your own and continue to use it even after your first round. In addition, there will be journal entries I'll ask you to make. This will help you identify what helped you most so you can go back to that solution in the future and understand what may have made symptoms worse, which will be handy should they come back. You're basically your own lab experiment, and this will help you build your user manual. You can use anything you like, but buying a cute journal may be in order.

What will you be journaling? I'm so glad you asked. I have a section for you on page 314 on setting up your journal. This is the exact data I ask my patients to track, and the only way that, as a physician, I can get a complete insight into the health of their hormones. Nope, labs aren't everything. How you live and what you experience in your body is crucial data, too.

WHAT IF I'M ON HORMONAL BIRTH CONTROL?

Not all hormonal birth control works by stopping ovulation like the pill, the patch, and the ring. The progestin-only versions, like the mini-pill or hormonal IUDs, don't always stop you from ovulating. If you're on a form of birth control that stops you from ovulating or has stopped your period, follow your pill pack or the moon cycle for the program (see "What If I Have No Period?" on the previous page). If you're still having a period with your IUD, you can follow your cycle. Know that everything I talk about won't apply since your natural hormones cycle in a way that these don't. In addition, contraceptives like the pill can squash testosterone and your libido, which can leave you asking *What's wrong with me?* It's not you, it's the birth control, and you can talk to your prescriber about other options. Remember: the fear of unintended pregnancy is a big brake for a lot of people, which is why I recommend finding reliable birth control that works for you so you can release this worry.

Eat a Nutrient-Dense Diet

As a physician who has studied nutrition extensively, here is something essential I want you to understand: your diet and lifestyle absolutely influence your hormones, and every day is a new opportunity to create balance. We don't do any good food/bad food talk around here. What we are going to do is start building a way of eating that focuses on nourishing your body so it can make the hormones you need and discard the ones you're done with. We'll also tackle blood sugar balance, lowering inflammation, supporting gut health, and fueling our mitochondria. The bonus is that all of this supports sexual desire, our ability to respond to sexy cues and self-lubricate, as well as maintain our vaginal health so we can dodge those BV and yeast infections that can follow a really good time (if you know what I mean). Yes, it is essentially a sex meal strategy that will whet your appetite in more ways than one. To ensure your success, I've provided you with a downloadable four-week meal plan and recipes to accompany the program in this book, at https://DrBrighten.com/ITN-resources. They are gluten free and dairy free to accommodate those who need it and, I promise, you will not miss those foods with how delicious they are, but you're welcome to substitute as you like. You'll also find helpful charts here on foods that might help your sexual desire, the best fats to choose, and how to support hormone detoxification and elimination with food.

WHAT SHOULD I EAT? HOW TO SET UP YOUR PLATE.

I'm always asked about portion size, and the answer I always give is: It depends. Did you work out today, and how strenuous was it? Are you in your luteal phase approaching your period? That's a time when caloric needs go up. Are you sick and have no appetite? Honestly, there's no way to provide a portion size to someone I don't know (although I feel we're really well acquainted at this point), and even if you were my patient, I wouldn't rob you of your own food independence and ability to self-regulate by giving you strict portion control guidelines. It's not how I roll because it doesn't respect that you ultimately know your body best.

What I can provide you is a guide on how to fill your plate. This is a general template to help you get the most nutrients, provide your body with variety that keeps blood sugar stable, and ensure you're getting the fiber you need daily. Cut your plate in half and fill one side with plants, including starchy vegetables and fruits. Take the other half and split it in half again; one quarter will be for protein and the other quarter is for the carbohydrates of choice. Then add two tablespoons (or more, depending on your needs) of fat to the meal. You might be thinking, *Does this mean we're eating low-carb?* Nope, because while we've mostly been taught by the food pyramid that "carbs" means grains, plants are an excellent source of nutrient-dense carbohydrates and full of fiber, too. Got a missing period? You may need more carbs and fat, in addition to the protein. Have insulin resistance, as we sometimes see with PCOS? You may need less starchy or root vegetables and more leafy greens and zero grains. It's really about working with your body. And always, variety is key to getting you the nutrients you need and signaling to your gut that all is well.

Carbohydrates. Plants are an excellent source of carbohydrates and offer vitamins, minerals, antioxidants, and fiber that your gut will love. Choose leafy greens, estrogen-detoxing cruciferous, and root vegetables like sweet potatoes, yuca, beets, turnips, and carrots. Fruits like berries, kiwi, pineapple, and citrus have anti-inflammatory compounds and provide an array of nutrients that support your endocrine glands. Plants are rich in antioxidants that drop inflammation (your adrenals love this), fight free radicals, and support mitochondria health (hello, healthy sex hormone production), so we want plants–lots of them.[1] They can also help with insulin sensitivity, which is part of the foundation of hormones that work for you.[2] Beans are fiber-filled friends of your microbiome. If you eat whole grains, avoid letting them dominate your plate, as they aren't as nutrient dense as the plants you could be eating. When it comes to grains, opt for the types that don't typically spike blood sugar, like quinoa and brown rice, and couple it with plants, fat, and protein.[3] New to eating so many plants? Start with one serving a day until you build a plate that has them well represented at every meal.

Fat. Polyunsaturated omega-3 fatty acids, monounsaturated fats, and saturated fats are what we want to be the core of the fat on our plate. Grass-fed butter on my broccoli? Don't mind if I do. Guac on my burrito bowl? Yes, please. A handful of nuts on your salad, seeds tossed in a smoothie, and coconut oil on your roasted vegetables are all ways to incorporate fat. Avoid trans fats, which have zero health benefits and a hell of a lot of health consequences like increased cardiovascular disease and diabetes.[4]

Protein. In every meal we're going to include protein so we can build hormones and keep ourselves full. Aim for the size of the palm of your hand and the thickness of a deck of cards as a serving size. Can't finish it? OK, put it in a storage container. Hungry within an hour of eating? Probably needed more protein. If you can access organic, grass-fed, and growth hormone–free meats, excellent. If not, I encourage you to do the best you can. Select wild-caught fish whenever possible, and don't forget that those economical sardines are also rich in omega-3 fatty acids, selenium, and iodine, which your breasts, groin, and hormones need.

WHAT ABOUT ALCOHOL AND CAFFEINE?

Can you give yourself 28 days alcohol free? You may just learn a lot about how it is affecting your body, your relationships, your sexual desire, and how much you enjoy sex. If you do find yourself at a special occasion and wanting to have one drink, have the drink and make note of how it makes you feel through the next day.

Caffeine could be behind your anxiety, night waking, hot flashes, and tender breasts. Or it may just be a cup of comfort each morning. There are some people who do not process caffeine efficiently (this is you if you drink coffee after noon and find yourself up all night) and there are people (and cultures) who enjoy espresso in the evening without any difficulty falling asleep.

HOW OFTEN SHOULD I EAT?

Fasting is primarily studied in men, but ubiquitously applied to women as if we're just the version of a man that comes with baby-making accessories. Does fasting have benefits? Absolutely. Is it for everyone? Absolutely not.

In general, most of us are going to feel better with a twelve-hour fast—that is not eating after dinner and then eating breakfast about twelve hours from when dinner was. You're probably already doing this. Allowing your body a break while you sleep allows your migrating motor complex (the fancy little street sweeper of your intestines) to do its job, and promotes deep sleep. But if you're someone who wakes up feeling hungry, hot, and anxious at night, you may benefit from a snack an hour before bed to keep your blood sugar from dropping. What about longer fasts? They can also have benefits, but for this program, we're not focusing there. The reason is, if your hormones aren't right, fasting is rarely the place to start and can be more problematic for your adrenals, thyroid, and blood sugar. If you already fast, know that for women, fasting in the follicular phase is generally better because caloric needs go up and insulin sensitivity goes down slightly (normal) in the luteal phase.

How often should you eat? Well, eat when you're hungry. If you eat a meal and you're hungry an hour later, you need to tweak your meals to have more protein, fiber, and fat. If you find that you need more calories because you're in your luteal phase, you worked out more, or your body says *More,* then choose protein, fat, and fiber snacks over refined carbs or high-sugar snacks, which will ultimately make your blood sugar unstable and cause your body to compensate with shifting hormones. We live in a society that tells us that our appetite can't be trusted, our calories must be counted, and that feeling hungry all the time is some sign of moral superiority. That's all bullshit. Yes, there are cases in which fat cells produce excess leptin, a hormone that tells us we're full, which our brain may not interpret, known as leptin resistance.[5] We're not sure what causes this, but we do know that decreasing inflammation, getting restful sleep, exercise, and eating foods high in fiber and protein while avoiding large amounts of refined carbohydrates can help.[6] That's literally everything I'm providing you in this program. In the case of leptin resistance, you may need additional support from a provider, but to say in general that you can never trust your appetite just because you've got ovaries—that's wrong.

PLEASURABLE PLATE: APHRODISIACS

Everyone is always looking for that one aphrodisiac to get them or their partner in the mood. I'm often asked about oysters and spicy food, and if there is any truth to any of this food-for-your-mood business. Yes, there are foods associated with increased arousal, sexual satisfaction, desire, and helping you get in the mood. But remember how context matters? Is it that the oysters alone make you want to skip the restaurant dessert for another kind of dessert, or is it that you're having a relaxing meal, enjoying your partner's company, and setting aside time for something special? It could be the latter. It could be both. So why not employ all of the above? Here's a list of foods that, when combined with everything else we've talked about in this book, might give you the assistance you need in the bedroom. But remember: there's no magic pill or potion that will change your sex life.

- **Saffron.** Remember when we talked in chapter 3 about the sex-sabotaging effects of (sometimes very necessary) SSRIs? Well, in one study, saffron was able to help mitigate that side effect.[7] Saffron can help you get aroused, get wet, and in some cases, reduce pain. Other studies have been mixed, some showing increased sexual satisfaction only, while others showing it supports arousal and lubrication.[8] Bonus: saffron has shown some benefits for PMS, cramps, and irregular periods.[9]

- **Watermelon rinds.** Rich in citrulline—Mama Nature's Viagra—watermelon rinds help the blood get to where you want it to go—the erectile tissue of the clitoris.[10] Not sure how the heck you'd eat that? Try a pickled watermelon rind.
- **Oysters.** A great source of zinc for testosterone production and the amino acid tyrosine, which is needed to make dopamine, oysters (in a high enough quantity) might give you the nutritional edge to support your sex life.
- **Other zinc-rich foods.** Other than oysters, pumpkin seeds, beef, chickpeas, and lentils are other ways to get more of this testosterone-supporting ally.
- **Magnesium-rich foods.** What doesn't this mineral do? When it comes to magnesium, it may help your testosterone stick around a little longer to stimulate the tissues that need it most.[11] See the table on page 369 for magnesium-rich foods you can eat.
- **Antioxidant-rich foods.** Figs, strawberries, pomegranates, cherries, and dark chocolate are often depicted as sexy food and I have to agree, antioxidants are sexy. They protect your body from free radical damage, are excellent at supporting ovarian health, and support testosterone production. They're also good at supporting the blood vessels that cause your tissue to become engorged, wet, and ready for sex. Some studies have even found that they are great at preventing erectile dysfunction.[12]
- **Spicy foods.** Well, in male rats, at least, there is evidence that it decreases the refractory period, the time between ejaculation and your ability to cum again, but it also made it so they came a lot quicker. Not sure if that's really what we're looking for here.[13] But beyond that, it is true that spicy food or, rather, the capsaicin that's in it, can get the blood flowing and release endorphins.
- **Maca.** A popular addition to smoothies, maca, a Peruvian medicinal plant, has been shown to have a positive effect on sexual desire and may also help with the sexual dysfunction that accompanies SSRI use.[14] In postmenopausal women, maca has been shown to decrease anxiety, depression, and symptoms of sexual dysfunction.[15]

5 WAYS TO IMPROVE DIGESTION

Use these simple tips to improve your digestion so you can absorb the nutrients you're consuming.

1. **Chewing.** When you think you've chewed enough, chew some more. It seems simple, but when you mechanically break down your food and mix it with the enzymes in your saliva, it can improve absorption. In addition, this gets the entire digestive tract, which your mouth is the beginning of, primed for digestion.
2. **Calm.** Eat in a calm environment. Try to avoid eating at your desk, on the run, or in the car.
3. **Hydration.** Dehydration leads to constipation (and sometimes hemorrhoids from straining). Aim to drink at least 60 ounces of fluid daily, more if you work out, breastfeed, or live in a hot climate. Most experts agree to aim for half your body weight in ounces of noncaffeinated, nonsugary fluids daily. So if you weigh 150 pounds, then this would be 75 ounces of water.
4. **Mindfulness.** Be present with your food. How does it smell, taste, look, and feel in your mouth? This is a simple act of mindfulness that can translate to other areas of your life.
5. **Probiotics.** Foods like kimchi, sauerkraut, miso, and pickles can help reseed your gut while providing you with prebiotic fiber to feed them. You can also take a probiotic supplement. See page 206 for more on probiotics.

FOODS THAT SUPPORT THE LIVER–GUT ESTROGEN PATHWAY

These foods supply your body with the nutrients it needs to create the best estrogen metabolites and then remove them from the body via the gut. Try to incorporate these foods into your diet daily, and rotate what you eat throughout the week. These foods are also rich in fiber, which means they will help you poop regularly and feed the good bacteria in the gut. Remember: those bacteria help your vagina get the sugars it needs to feed the lactobacilli that keep the yeast and BV at bay.

- Beets
- Broccoli
- Brussels sprouts
- Burdock root
- Cauliflower
- Celery
- Garlic
- Grapefruit
- Jerusalem artichokes
- Kale
- Legumes
- Onions
- Turmeric

FATS TO MINIMIZE, FATS TO MAXIMIZE

There are definitely fats that are going to support your hormones, bring in anti-inflammatory benefits, and reduce symptoms like acne. And then there's those other fats—the cheap ones that get used in almost all processed foods because, well, they're cheap. But they're oh so expensive when it comes to the trouble you'll deal with down the line if they are a main staple in your diet. Artificial trans fats, like partially hydrogenated vegetable oil, shouldn't even be in food. They are so ridiculously bad that the FDA banned them, but alas, they persist, although in smaller amounts, in fast food and fried foods (especially those where the oil is reheated multiple times) due to the processing methods. This is another reason why whole foods, as often as you can, are the best choice.

FATS TO MAXIMIZE

- Cold pressed olive oil
- Coconut oil
- Avocado oil
- Ghee
- Whole avocado
- Egg yolk
- Nuts and seeds (not their oils)
- Cold-water fish
- Whole olives

FATS TO MINIMIZE

- Sunflower
- Corn
- Soybean
- Flaxseed
- Canola
- Peanut oil

How can I manage my stress?

Mental and emotional stress increase cortisol, DHEA, and testosterone, but drop estrogen, progesterone, melatonin, thyroid hormones, and growth hormone. So I'd say it's a pretty big deal when it comes to optimizing hormones. Chronic elevations in stress lead to alteration in adrenal output of stress hormones, reduced insulin sensitivity, and elevated blood sugar.[16] I'd love to tell you to just have an orgasm to relieve the stress and make a rapid hormone shift, but when stress is up or we're stressed about having sex, that can keep cortisol up and sexual desire down.[17] As explained in chapter 8, stress can be behind the hormone symptoms you struggle with. It can also lead to anxiety, often worst before our period, and is definitely behind sabotaging some people's sexual desire. If you find you need more stress support, head to page 360 for additional resources.

MEDITATION

Meditation can have profound impacts on our mood by reducing anxiety and balancing our hormones.[18] It has been shown to help modulate the HPA axis, which means less stress hormones and more feel-good hormones.[19] And meditation can help you improve the quality of your sleep.[20] Plus a meditative practice may lead to higher levels of dopamine.[21] Studies have shown that women who meditate score higher in sexual desire and function.[22] And you don't have to be doing it perfectly, for hours on end, or be a meditation master. How can you get into meditation, especially when your mind feels like a circus? These steps tend to work well for most of my patients:

1. **Get comfortable.** You do not have to sit with a straight spine in a full lotus pose. Just be comfortable. Try this at your desk, lying on the floor, sitting in your car, or any way where you won't find yourself fidgeting.

2. **Close your eyes and focus on your breath.** Just breathe and notice. Did your breath change because you decided to focus on it? Normal. Did you stop breathing for a second? Normal. But try to stay with that breath.

3. **Let the lion go free.** In that circus, if you notice the lion is getting riled up, acknowledge it–it's interesting–and then let it go. Trying to control thoughts will cause thoughts to control you. Just let that shit go. You do not need to tame every lion. Perfection isn't the goal. You're not a "bad meditator" because you get distracted. You're a badass meditator if you notice the distractions and learn to just let them go.

MINDFULNESS

Your ability to stay present during any intimate endeavor can amplify the sensations you're experiencing. Mindfulness during the early stages of arousal, or when you start to engage in sexual activity, may not only enhance the feelings of sexual arousal, but may also create concordance between what your mind and your genitals are into.[23] Remember when we talked about arousal nonconcordance back in chapter 3, where the brain says, *Yes, let's do it* and the genitals are like, *Huh, I didn't quite get that*? Well, mindfulness during sexual activity (not talking just intercourse) can help your clitoris get engorged and your vagina self-lubricate in some cases. So mindfulness can increase your desire for sex, your ability to get turned on, increase your enjoyment of sex, and can even boost your self-esteem. Need I say more?

Now, here's the deal: One does not just enter into sex a mindfulness expert, and frustration is the only guarantee of what you will experience if you try your first act of mindfulness with zero idea of what that will bring you. It takes practice. And like a lot of things, solo practice is a better way to train the skills. Sure, you could have a solo sex session, but with my patients, I like to start much more simply by removing the sexpectations and, instead, using mindfulness in the day-to-day stuff like experiencing the senses, being present while you eat, going for a walk, and just focusing on your thoughts.

If you can practice mindfulness in one area of your life, you can do it anywhere with practice. Think about how you could apply this in the bedroom. If you're neurodivergent, as is the case with ADHD, or you just get easily distracted and your mind carries you away with the stress of the day, try mixing up the senses. Put in earplugs, strap on a blindfold, and focus on touch. You can also bring feathers, ice, leather, lace, and other items with varying textures and sensations to pull your mind into focus. The bottom line on all of this: You're not going to do it wrong. You're going to practice, make it your own, and find what works for you. And then, when it doesn't work, you're going to change it again for your needs.

BUILD STRESS RESILIENCY

There's no one stress management practice that works for everyone or works in every situation. Find what brings you joy, helps you shake off the stress, and allows you to focus on what is most important in life. Stress will always be there, but that doesn't mean it needs to always get the best of you. You may need additional mental/emotional support from a mental health professional and that is always encouraged. Don't hesitate to leverage the amazing professionals who are available.

In addition, start to employ daily practices like box breathing, dancing, gratitude journaling, and self-care routines that help you cultivate calm. And don't forget: taking social media breaks, blocking hurtful people online, and building boundaries are all forms of self-care.

EXERCISE

Exercise always wins in the research regarding anxiety, depression, and other mood symptoms. It helps modulate the HPA axis stress response and improves brain-derived neurotrophic factor (BDNF). In stress-related mood disorders, it is often found that BDNF is lower.[24] Movement also helps keep our bowels regular, improves insulin sensitization, and helps our body activate our thyroid hormone. Not to mention it will help us lower the effects of stress and sleep better.

Everyone has an opinion on what exercise is best, especially for women. In reality, a variety of exercises that builds muscles, reinforces a healthy core and pelvic floor, challenges your cardiovascular system, and enables you to remain flexible and able to move without pain is what's best. And maybe most important, it should be something you enjoy. While exercising every day may not be possible, movement, like getting up from your desk, stretching in the morning, and engaging in the activities that modern life has otherwise simplified for you (hello, elevators) can make an impact on your overall health. With that said, aim to exercise at least thirty minutes a day, most days a week. Doesn't have to happen all at once; instead, your movement throughout the day can be added up to total thirty minutes. While exercise is great for your health, more isn't always better. Sometimes it's just more and that turns into a stressor itself, which can result in hormone imbalances and missing periods. It's not uncommon to feel stronger and like you can exercise hard in the follicular phase, and then feel like you need to dial back in the late luteal. If that's true for you, honor it.

Sleep Is Sexy

No, I'm not talking sexsomnia, a sleep disorder where people engage in sexual activity while asleep.[25] Instead, I'm talking about how sleep can improve your sex hormones, stress hormones, skin, mood, and sex life. Yeah, that kind of sexy. Quality sleep is a must for all our hormones to function at their best and, with insulin, studies have shown that sleep deprivation can lead to reduced insulin sensitivity.[26] That means inflammation, cortisol chaos, and difficulty balancing any other hormones. If you find you need additional sleep support, especially before your period, head to page 386 for more. I also promised you sleep tips for sleepgasms, so here we go:

- **Establish a routine.** Go to bed around the same time most nights and have a routine to help you wind down at the end of the day.
- **Dark and cool.** The room needs to be pitch black or close to it. Melatonin needs it dark. Cortisol likes the light. So give melatonin what it needs. Sleeping in a cool room—60 to 67 degrees Fahrenheit is optimal—helps your body get more restorative sleep.[27]
- **Eliminate screen time.** At least thirty minutes, if not two hours, before bed, get off the melatonin-disrupting light devices.

- **Exercise daily.** It only takes twenty to thirty minutes to improve your sleep, so get moving.
- **No to the nightcap.** While alcohol might make you sleepy, it actually doesn't help sleep. In fact, it disrupts REM sleep and will definitely block your chances of a sleepgasm.
- **Time the caffeine.** Not that you can't use it, but for a lot of people, once the clock strikes twelve—p.m., that is—any use of stimulants can sabotage your sleep. BTW, we all know cigarettes are bad and they can make sleep, cramps, and PMS worse.
- **Rotate pillows.** Replacing your pillow annually can help keep you comfy, but so can rotating your pillows out nightly.
- **Consider blue-light-blocking glasses.** If you need the screen (late-night deadlines, I've been there) then wear glasses that block the blue light and protect your melatonin.
- **Expose yourself.** Not like that. Expose yourself to sunlight in the morning to encourage a healthy circadian rhythm. And if you do want to expose your body to the light, too, it'll help your vitamin D production. Just don't flash your neighbors.

How to Set Up Your Journal and Customize Your 28-Day Plan

OK, so the truth is that adopting the nutrition strategy I've given you is going to help, but it is unrealistic to expect that you'll be 100 percent on your game. Not every day will be perfect, and some days the best you can do is make sure your vegetable intake is on point. I've heard so many times from patients how previous endeavors failed because they had an *all-or-nothing attitude.* Can we adopt an *all-or-something attitude*? I recommend picking the key things you will focus on in your nutrition at each phase (write it in that pretty journal) and giving yourself a big high five (I'm old like that) for doing something from that list. Use the Hormone Symptom Check guide to help you fill in what you'll be focusing on based on what you found. If you need additional symptom support, you can also pull in the information from the advanced hormone protocols (Cycle Symptom Relief). You'll find there's some overlap in what will help, which will keep the program from becoming overwhelming.

The Nutrients/Foods I Will Focus On During My __________ Phase:

____

____

____

____

There are many lifestyle strategies that can help you achieve optimal hormone health. What my patients have found most success with is focusing on incorporating a handful at a time. Choose three to five strategies that feel right for your body to incorporate over the next 28 days, and divide what feels best into the phases. You can always add more in the future once you've got a good schedule going. I'll be giving you prompts during the program to help remind you of these.

The Lifestyle Strategies I Will Focus on During My __________ Phase:

____

____

____

____

____

While supplements are not required to follow this plan, they certainly can be helpful in achieving your goals quicker. You may be someone who needs extra nutrient support because of your health, your lifestyle, or because it makes you feel better. There is no shame in leaning on a supplement to support you in your journey—a lot of people need this kind of support. I find with my patients that supplements that are part of a healthy foundation of nutrition and lifestyle can be a total game changer in helping them have more energy, better moods, and easier periods. If you're planning on using this plan to get pregnant, definitely start your prenatal now. Use the protocols that match your Hormone Symptom Check results and add in any advanced protocols (Cycle Symptom Relief) you may need. This is another reason it is wise to give yourself a week to plan your start date for the program.

WHAT SHOULD I LOOK FOR IN SUPPLEMENTS?

It's no secret that the supplement industry isn't well regulated, meaning what is on the supplement label might not actually be what's in the capsule you're taking. Here's what I share with my patients: First, if you're purchasing supplements in bulk at a big box store and feeling like you just scored the biggest deal of your life—you are in fact getting exactly what you paid for (or maybe less). That's because to make a super cheap supplement you need to use super cheap ingredients, like the kind your body doesn't readily use. And supplements break down over time, meaning they become less potent, which means the bigger the bottle, the higher the probability this is happening. Second, you want to look for a company that does third-party testing. Not a lot do because it's expensive. But third-party testing is how companies ensure that what they say is in the bottle is in fact true. After over two decades in the field of nutrition and working as a physician with thousands of women, I formulated the Dr. Brighten line of superior supplements in order to offer women a trusted source with the highest-quality ingredients and third-party testing. It's one option you can trust should you choose to use supplements during this program.

WHAT IF I HAVE A HARD TIME TAKING SUPPLEMENTS?

This is me. I am this person. So I feel you and have a few hacks. One, take them with something fizzy. Sparkling water is my go-to because something about it helps me get my throat open and those supplements down. You can also try changing up beverages. I will sometimes take mine with some sparkling water, then add some lemon and keep going. Other times I switch from water to kombucha to sparkling water with a splash of juice. Whatever keeps my brain distracted. Another trick is to put them in the fridge if you are someone who is sensitive to taste or smell (every woman who has ever been pregnant knows this). Keeping them cool will make it harder to smell and taste. Lastly, you can take them throughout your meal. Take a few bites, then take a capsule or two. I know people say not to drink with your meals, but seriously, sometimes you gotta do what you gotta do.

DAILY DATA TO TRACK DURING THE PROGRAM

Flow: none, light, medium, heavy, spotting
Cervical fluids: none, tacky, creamy, stringy, stretchy, fluid, chunky, dry
Mood: happy, calm, peaceful, anxious, depressed, sad, excited
Energy: energized, wired, tired, fatigued
Stress: low, medium, high
Sleep: fair, good, excellent
Appetite: normal, absent, increased
Sexual desire: none, low, medium, high
Skin: clear, glowing, oily, dry, acne
Cramps: scale of 0 to 5, with 0 being no cramps and 5 being *I am in so much pain I cannot move*
Basal body temperature (optional): _______ F/C

Now to make this plan your own! If you haven't yet, do the Hormone Symptom Check on page 192 and use those results, and the corresponding guidance on what to do about it, to fill out the tables provided in order to individualize this plan to your hormones' needs. I'll be giving cycle-specific suggestions for diet, lifestyle, and supplements throughout the program. Try them out and write down what works best for you. For the entirety of the 28 days you'll want to focus on the core nutrition, lifestyle, and supplement strategy based on your results.

CHAPTER 13

THE 28-DAY PROGRAM

ONE CYCLE TO CHANGE THEM ALL

Welcome to your first 28 days and congrats on getting here! To start, we'll go through your Hormone Symptom Check results so you can make notes of where to customize this program to fit your needs. After that the program starts with Phase 1: Your Period. (Remember: you can skip to the phase you're actually at to start; just be sure to keep going so you complete an entire cycle of the program.) The days next to each phase are an estimated period of time you might be in that phase, or when it might take place in your cycle. They're there for guidance and aren't rigid time frames your body must follow. Use a journal and the guidance provided in chapter 9 to figure out how long each phase lasts for you.

When it comes to journaling, I recommend you make it a daily practice. I know that sounds like a lot, but it's important. You'll be writing down the cycle data tracking information from page 234, and I'll be providing you additional prompts to work on during each phase of your cycle. To get the most out of this program, do the assignments to the extent that you're comfortable. You'll find additional resources for the program in the appendixes, like the supplement table and Nutrient Food Sources table, as well as the Cycle Symptom Relief table with solutions and advanced protocols. If I reference a chapter you skipped, take that as an invitation to read up on it, as it will be even more pertinent to where you are in your cycle.

So You've Got a Hormone Imbalance. Now What?

My approach to eliminating unwanted hormone symptoms is to address the root of the issue, while also getting symptom relief. It's all about feeling better fast and seeing the healing through. In the 28-day program you'll be building a hormone-healing lifestyle that will enable you to rein in the symptoms and set yourself up for a lifetime of happy, balanced hormones. You'll begin by focusing on the base of the hormone pyramid to ensure your efforts stick. That means stress management, restorative sleep tips, and nutrient-dense foods for everyone! See page 320 for guidance on creating a hormone-balancing lifestyle. Use this chart to identify the areas where you need to focus, and use the Nutrient Food Source table on page 369 to help you dial in the plan that is best tailored to fit your needs.

High Cortisol

Common Causes:	Associated Risks:
High stress	High blood pressure
Autoimmune disease	Low sexual desire
Inflammation	Osteoporosis
	Insulin resistance
	Metabolic syndrome
	Anxiety
	Hypothyroidism
	Headaches
	Thinning skin
	Ovulatory issues and infertility

WHAT CAN HELP:

LIFESTYLE

Use stress-reducing tools. Leverage stress-reduction practices (see page 310).

Bedtime routine. Support your body in getting restorative sleep by following the guidance on page 313.

Reevaluate relationships. Do they fill you up? Do you leave the interactions feeling happy, confident, or peaceful? Or do you find yourself replaying the conversation with a ball of stress in your stomach, dreading their text messages, or making excuses why you can't meet up? Our relationships are crucial to our health, and if they are bringing you nothing but stress, it's time to reevaluate them.

Gentle exercise. When stress is high, sometimes we want to run, lift, or push ourselves even harder. Working with your body to move into the rest-and-digest aspect of your nervous system (parasympathetic nervous system) can help you keep your cortisol in check. If you're going to increase the intensity of your workout, do it in the morning, when cortisol should be high, and keep it gentle in the evening. Try out tai chi, restorative yoga or Yin Yoga, Pilates, and walking.

Addressing the autoimmunity. If that is what is behind your symptoms, this is key in getting your cortisol levels balanced. Work with an experienced naturopathic or functional medicine provider to address the common triggers of autoimmunity.

Make box breathing your bestie anytime you feel stressors taking hold. This will help calm your system and retrain the stress response. See https://DrBrighten.com/ITN-resources for how to do this.

Unapologetically prioritize the hell out of your needs and the things that make you feel good and bring joy. High cortisol is a signal that there's not enough of the good stuff filling up your day.

Embrace boundaries. Make your boundaries and stick to them. Your follicular phase is a perfect time to set some boundaries, so do it. When you feel tempted to take on too much or put up with too much, keep those boundaries and hold them down.

Get out into nature. Being among plants drops our stress levels and even our blood pressure, so consider adding more plants to your work space.

NUTRITION

Foods for your gut. Eating fiber and antioxidant-rich plants will support your gut health, which is where hidden inflammation can lie and cause cortisol to go high. Use the guidelines in the program to bring these foods into your meals.

Anti-inflammatory foods like cold-water fish, turmeric, berries, ginger, avocados, mushrooms, and green tea can help lower the inflammation that the high cortisol is trying to control.

Magnesium. Bring in the magnesium-rich foods that support the HPA axis and help with keeping the nervous system calm.

Zinc is an important nutrient in the aspect of the brain that tells the HPA axis *Yo, chill* when it's misfiring the stress response.

Eat your Bs. Vitamin B_5 is especially important for adrenal health, but all the B vitamins are at play for nervous system function, hormonal health, and keeping your mood and emotions even.

SUPPLEMENTS

Phosphatidyl serine, 50–200 mg nightly, can protect against the effects of high cortisol. By lowering cortisol, it can improve mood, memory, and metabolism.[1]

Magnesium glycinate, 300 mg on its own or combined with **30 mg of vitamin B_6**, can help reduce feelings of stress.[2]

Rhodiola, 100-400 mg daily, can help improve your stress response.[3]

Ashwagandha, 100 mg daily, works on the HPA axis to help modulate the stress response.[4]

L-theanine, 200-400 mg daily, can help reduce stress and anxiety.[5]

WHEN TO SEE A DOCTOR:
Cushing's disease and syndrome are serious conditions that manifest with high cortisol, rapid weight gain, purple-colored stretch marks, and a very round face. While rare, these require medical intervention.

Low Cortisol

Remember back on page 210 when I told you low cortisol is a result of chronically elevated cortisol? That means many of the strategies for high cortisol are going to apply here, too. There's no adrenal fatigue, but there's adrenal insufficiency (see When to See a Doctor below).

Common Causes:	Associated Risks:
Chronic stress	Post-traumatic stress disorder (PTSD)
Inflammation	Burnout
Blood sugar imbalances	Brain fog
Disruption in circadian rhythm	Chronic infection
	Chronic fatigue syndrome[6]
	Fibromyalgia
	Depression

WHAT CAN HELP:

LIFESTYLE

Charge up your stress battery pack. Resiliency in the face of stress takes having a fully charged system because, let's face it, that ish is depleting. If you put the self-care in up front, that can help you have more in the battery stores to pull from when stress hits. Your system is already in need of recalibration, so doing whatever self-care looks like for you is nonnegotiable. This strategy is going to be your go-to for life. Yes, I just told you to prioritize what makes you feel good in life.

Lower social media stress. Get that phone right out of your hands in the evenings. I'm as guilty as the next person for scrolling TikTok leading up to bed. Because if your FYP isn't filled with nothing but humor, puppytok, or other feel-good stuff, then you're gonna be messin' around with your cortisol and sleep.

Permission to block. Hit that block button online and in real life. If you're experiencing fatigue, then you have no extra energy to be giving to people who just consume, rather than fill you up.

Light/dark rhythm. Tend to your circadian rhythm (dark and light cycles for sleep) like you're the CEO of sleep excellence. See the tips on page 313.

Exercise right. Exercise in a way that doesn't leave you depleted, sore, or exhausted three days after the activity. It's normal to feel sore after a heavy lift for a day or two. But if you feel like you just can't recover, you've gone too far. You gotta Goldilocks that workout to be just right, not too much or too little. This is highly individualized, and you're the expert on your body here.

Manage PMS. Working on your PMS, if you have it, it also a must. PMS goes together with HPA-D and it's a cycle of one feeding into the other. You'll find a PMS protocol in Appendix 2 beginning on page 384.

Gratitude. Be grateful for what's good. This doesn't make the sucky stuff go away, but it does give you an opportunity to calm the system, down-regulate the inflammatory response of emotions (the literal biochemical response), and it just makes you feel good. So why not give it a go?

Oxytocin boost. Laugh, hug, pet an animal, or have sex to get oxytocin up. It mitigates the effects of cortisol, which will help your body shift into a state where it makes it so you can use the cortisol you're making.

Handle hidden infections. Yeast, parasites, bacteria, and viruses aren't always as apparent as we might think. Working with a licensed health care practitioner to address any of these that might be present is a wise move in healing your hormones.

NUTRITION

No hangry here. Maintaining regular meals is a must in getting these adrenal glands to chill and stop pumping out the cortisol.

Bye, alcohol, bye. It may feel like it takes the edge off (true, but not without consequences) and helps you sleep (false), but it ultimately hits all your hormones hard. Drinking alcohol to feel better is like making some kind of deal with a wicked fairy-tale character, and you just know they're going to come back around demanding more than you were ever willing to give.

Stay hydrated. Dehydration is a stressor, and your adrenal glands must respond with hormones to keep your blood pressure in check in the absence of adequate fluids. Add a pinch of salt to your water to give yourself electrolytes.

Focus on anti-inflammatory foods. Bring in the turmeric, cold-water fish, walnuts, olive oil, spinach, and kale.[7]

Ditch dieting. I'm talking here about the extreme caloric restrictions that weight loss programs promise are all women need to lose weight. Nah, that ain't it, and in fact, it's gonna mess with your cortisol and other hormones in ways that will sabotage weight. If you want to lose weight, nourishing yourself, exercising appropriately, and working with a registered dietician or certified nutrition specialist is a better route to go. If you're just wanting to shrink yourself because the predominant message is that smaller is better, please know that the people behind those messages don't know you or have your best interest at heart. If you're struggling with adrenal symptoms, take care of your hormones before trying to lose weight rapidly.

SUPPLEMENTS

Vitamin C, 1,000–4,000 mg daily, can help support your adrenal function. The adrenal tissues contain among the highest concentrations in the body of vitamin C because they seriously need this nutrient.

Magnesium glycinate, 300 mg daily, can help support adrenal gland health and promote restful sleep.

B-complex. Vitamin B_5 is the one for the adrenals, but you need all those Bs for the nervous system, sex hormones, and more. So be sure to get the full spectrum of Bs.

Holy basil, 100 mg daily, is an adaptogenic herb that helps promote energy and mood, while reducing fatigue.

Rhodiola, 100–400 mg daily, can help improve your stress response.

Ashwagandha, 100 mg daily, works on the HPA axis to help modulate the stress response.

L-theanine, 200–400 mg daily, can help reduce stress and anxiety.

WHEN TO SEE A DOCTOR:
Addison's disease, an autoimmune disease that causes insufficient adrenal hormones, will show symptoms of low cortisol. If you have severe fatigue, weight loss, and your skin color is darkening, seeing a doctor for evaluation is a must.

Insulin/Blood Sugar Dysregulation

Common Causes:	Associated Risks:
Skipping meals	Nonalcoholic fatty liver disease (NAFLD)
Eating a high-carbohydrate or refined-sugar diet	Heart disease
Inflammation	Elevated cholesterol
Chronic stress	Type 2 diabetes
Low thyroid hormone	Obesity
	Neurological symptoms, dementia

WHAT CAN HELP:

LIFESTYLE

Build muscle. Strength training helps insulin sensitivity so your body can effectively use it and get your blood sugar to the cells that need it.

Sleep. Get quality sleep to improve your insulin sensitivity. Use the list of recommendations on page 313 to help. If you need more support, see the protocols in Appendix 2, page 386.

Stress check. Tend to your stress, which will help your adrenals stop poppin' off those "release the sugars" hormones. Make a list of major stressors and if you can cut them, do that. If you can't, use the list of ways to manage stress on page 310.

Target visceral fat. Work on losing the visceral fat, not just weight or body fat. It's the fat that hangs out around our organs that is problematic in releasing hormones that make us insulin resistant. Limiting added sugar to no more than 25 grams daily, aerobic exercise for thirty minutes daily, and quality sleep can help you achieve this. Not smoking also goes a long way here.

NUTRITION

Nutrient-dense diet. Fiber, protein, fats up, and refined carbs down is one of the best dietary approaches to help your body regulate your blood sugar and not feel the need to pump out so much insulin.

Anti-inflammatory foods like cold-water fish, olive oil, berries, turmeric, and ginger will help the cells use insulin more easily.

Blood sugar-supporting spices. Add garlic, fenugreek seeds, turmeric, and ginger to your meals.[8]

Eat cinnamon with your foods, 1/2 to 3 teaspoons daily. Cinnamon may mimic insulin or enhance the ability of cells to utilize insulin.[9]

Drink green tea, which can help improve blood sugar levels.[10]

Limit fructose, not from fruit, the added-to-your-food kind like high fructose corn syrup.[11]

SUPPLEMENTS

Chromium picolinate, 200–1,000 mcg, has been shown to improve insulin's ability to usher sugar into the cells.[12]

Omega-3 fatty acids, 2,000 mg daily, can help with lowering inflammation and insulin sensitization.[13]

Inositol, 2 g with 50 mg of D-chiro inositol daily, can help with insulin sensitization in women with PCOS.[14] When combined with 400 micrograms of folic acid, 4 grams of myo-inositol daily has been shown to improve insulin in gestational diabetes.[15] Some people need to pump the inositol up to 2 grams twice daily.

Magnesium glycinate, 150–300 mg, on its own or coupled with chromium, can help with insulin sensitivity and has been shown to result in lower blood sugar averages.[16] Most studies use magnesium chloride, which often requires higher doses due to low bioavailability.

Berberine, 500 mg three times a day, has been shown to be beneficial for insulin sensitization in those with type 2 diabetes and has shown benefits in those with PCOS.[17]

WHEN TO SEE A DOCTOR:

If you're constantly thirsty, peeing all the time, noticing skin tags, have darker-than-usual, velvety skin on your neck or groin, or are ravenously hungry, it's time to see your provider. Catching diabetes early can make all the difference in your health and in managing it.

High Thyroid

Common Causes:	Associated Risks:
Graves' disease (autoimmunity)	Insomnia
Thyroid nodule	Tachycardia
Thyroiditis	Heart failure
Too-high thyroid medication	Anxiety and depression

Common Causes:	Associated Risks:
Too-high iodine intake	Eye disease
	Osteoporosis
	Thyroiditis (inflammation of thyroid)

WHAT CAN HELP:

LIFESTYLE

Address the autoimmunity. This is a condition where working with a licensed medical provider is a must. You'll likely need medications to control the symptoms of excess thyroid. You can also take steps to reverse the autoimmune condition.

Tend to trauma. Trauma chips away at everyone's health, and having survived trauma can be a trigger for autoimmunity, including the kind that leads to hyperthyroidism. Work with a mental health practitioner who specializes in trauma.

Exercise to protect bone health. The bones take a major hit with this condition, so be sure to do weighted exercise, jump rope, trampoline–all the things to build and maintain strong bones.

Prepregnancy care. Getting established with a practitioner who can manage Graves' disease in pregnancy is a must if you have a personal history of it. Pregnancy is a common time to see Graves' disease come on, and things get a whole lot worse, so get the support you need. If you have a family history of Graves', discuss this with your provider.

NUTRITION

Eat iron-rich foods. It is more common to be low in iron when you have hyperthyroidism, so use the nutrient chart in Appendix 2, page 369, to bring those foods in.[18]

Low iodine. Your doctor may recommend a low-iodine diet before treatment. Please discuss with your provider first. You can use the nutrient chart in Appendix 2, page 369, to identify these foods. I also recommend seeing the American Thyroid Association's sample meal plan at https://thyroid.org/low-iodine-diet/.

Cut caffeine. If you've got the jitters and anxiety, don't add to it with caffeine. Now is the time to bring all the chill you can to your nervous system.

Pre- and probiotics. Eat your fiber and fermented foods, and consider a probiotic. The immune system is primarily living in your gut. So we need to tend to home base to help the immune system find its balance.

SUPPLEMENTS

Selenium, 200 mcg daily, may help restore normal thyroid levels as an adjunct therapy.[19]

L-carnitine, 2–4 grams daily, helps manage some of the symptoms associated with hyperthyroidism and aids in bone remineralization.[20]

Omega-3 fatty acids, 1,000–2,000 mg daily, to help lower inflammation.

WHEN TO SEE A DOCTOR:

Graves' disease is an autoimmune disease in which the thyroid antibodies stimulate the thyroid gland to make excess thyroid hormone. If you have a tremor, are losing weight rapidly, feel like your heart is pounding out of your chest, are sweating all the time, or feel extremely hot, you need to meet with your provider. Hyperthyroidism is beyond of the scope of this book and absolutely requires medical attention. While I've provided some tips on what can help, I'm not giving you a pass on skipping a doctor's visit. You will likely need a medication to manage this condition. I included this in the symptom check so you can identify the issue and have a list of symptoms to discuss with your provider.

Low Thyroid

Common Causes:	Associated Risks:
Hashimoto's thyroiditis (autoimmunity)	Depression
Certain medications (e.g., seizure meds, lithium)	Goiter
Surgical removal	Infertility
Radiation	Miscarriage
Insufficient nutrients	Pregnancy complications
Infections	Weight gain, obesity
Environmental toxins	Heart disease
Hormone resistance	High cholesterol
	Hair loss
	Postpartum depression
	Digestive issues, gallbladder disease

WHAT CAN HELP:

LIFESTYLE

Move daily. Even on the days you don't feel amazing, some movement will definitely help your body activate thyroid hormone.

Get outside. Sunlight on our skin helps us generate vitamin D, which is important for thyroid, hormone, and immune health.

Stress management. This is so vital to thyroid function and immune health. Use the tips on page 310.

Handle hidden infections. Yeast, parasites, bacteria, and viruses aren't always as apparent as we might think. Working with a licensed health care practitioner to address any of these that might be present is a wise move in healing your hormones.

NUTRITION

Eat foods that contain iron, zinc, B vitamins, vitamin A, vitamin C, selenium, and iodine to support thyroid health, hormone production, and help your body use your hormones or the ones you may need to take.

Consider an elimination diet. Removing gluten and dairy, among other common food sensitivities, can be helpful as part of healing. I recommend working with a nutrition expert before trying this.

Watch your blood sugar. The thyroid depends on your adrenal health and insulin (remember: they are the base of our hormone pyramid) to function optimally. Be sure to eat regular meals and use the tips under the adrenal section as well.

Pre- and probiotics. Eat your fiber and fermented foods and consider a probiotic. The immune system is primarily living in your gut. So we need to tend to home base to help the immune system find its balance.

SUPPLEMENTS

Inositol (also known as myo-inositol), **2 grams** daily can help reduce thyroid antibodies and improve thyroid function and hormones. The research shows it works synergistically with selenium.[21]

Ashwagandha, 100–600 mg daily, can help normalize thyroid hormones.[22]

Vitamin D, 1,000–5,000 IU daily, can help support thyroid and immune health. Your dosage should be based on your lab results.

Selenium, 200 mcg daily, supports the production of the antioxidant glutathione and has been shown to help thyroid antibodies.

Omega-3 fatty acids, 1,000-2,000 mg daily, can help lower inflammation, allowing your body to utilize the thyroid hormone you're making and supporting balanced immune health.

WHEN TO SEE A DOCTOR:

Because the most common cause of hypothyroidism is autoimmune destruction of the thyroid gland, it is possible you may require medication to replace the hormones your body is unable to produce. Thyroid hormone, like insulin, is a nonnegotiable in life, which means if you can't make it, you must replace it. Untreated hypothyroidism can be a cause of infertility, hair loss, and lead to nerve damage and heart complications. Low thyroid can also present as depression; if you're ever experiencing mood symptoms that interfere with your day-to-day living, seek help.

High Estrogen

Common Causes:	Associated Risks:
Endocrine-disrupting chemicals (EDC)	Weight gain
Estrogen replacement therapy	Cancer: breasts, ovaries, endometrial
Inadequate fiber intake	Autoimmune disease
Estrogen-containing birth control	Hypothyroidism
Gut dysbiosis (microbial imbalance)	Gallbladder disease
Poor liver detoxification	Endometrial hyperplasia
Inflammation	Fibroids
	Fibrocystic breasts

WHAT CAN HELP:

LIFESTYLE

Avoid xenoestrogens. Download the free guide at https://DrBrighten.com/ITN-resources.

Exercise for at least thirty minutes most days of the week.

NUTRITION

Eat cruciferous vegetables, aka sulfur-containing foods, which provide your body with what is needed to process estrogen through the liver.

Add broccoli sprouts two to three times per week. It's a very economical and easy way to increase sulforaphane.

Consume prebiotics and other fiber-containing foods to support estrogen elimination through the gut.

Eliminate alcohol. If high estrogen is your issue, then alcohol has got to go until you can get it in check. Don't freak out–this isn't forever–but reducing or eliminating can go a long way in improving your symptoms.

SUPPLEMENTS

DIM (diindolylmethane), 50-100 mg daily, supports phase 1 estrogen metabolism, so you make less cancer-causing estrogen metabolites. More is not better; in fact, it could lead to hot flashes and persistent headaches. Why supplement if you can get it from broccoli? You have to eat, like, 2 to 3 cups per day to get the same benefit. If you can do that, more power to you. Otherwise, there's a supplement that can help.

Sulforaphane, 100 mg, especially when coupled with both myrosinase and vitamin C to make it more bioavailable, supports phase 2 liver detox, as well as an enzyme that makes your 4OH-E1 less of a pro-cancer molecule. It's also an anti-inflammatory antioxidant that has shown promise in cancer research.[23]

Calcium D-glucarate, 500 mg daily, helps keep the estrogen moving out by mitigating the effect of beta-glucuronidase.

B-complex taken daily will provide you with nutrients your liver needs to process estrogen, plus what your body needs to build hormones.

Magnesium glycinate, 100-300 mg daily, supports estrogen metabolism to make less dangerous forms.

WHEN TO SEE A DOCTOR:
Elevated estrogen is associated with the development of certain cancers, which is why regular screening exams are important. If you find that you have very heavy periods and/or large clots, it's important to meet with a provider, as it may be a sign of endometrial hyperplasia or fibroids (see chapter 10 for details).

Low Estrogen

Common Causes:	Associated Risks:
Menopause	Heart disease
Primary ovarian insufficiency	Vaginal atrophy
Poor energy intake (extreme dieting, disordered eating, or eating disorder)	Pain with sex
Overexercising	Increased UTIs
Low body fat	Osteoporosis, osteopenia
Chronic stress	Compromised brain health, Alzheimer's, dementia

Common Causes:	Associated Risks:
Postpartum (temporary)	Infertility
	Depression

WHAT CAN HELP:

LIFESTYLE

Assess your exercise. If you're training hard and lost your period as a result, you may need to increase your caloric intake or dial back the intensity.

Aim to orgasm regularly, which can support hormones, reduce inflammation, and improve immune function.

Is it menopause? If you're entering menopause, you can speak with your provider about hormone replacement therapy (HRT).

NUTRITION

Eat fat. Increase your daily fat intake. You may want to increase your fats to fill a quarter of your plate.

Caloric increase. You may need to increase your calories if you're struggling with a missing period and low-estrogen symptoms due to overtraining or undereating. Working with a nutrition expert can help.

Eat phytoestrogens like flaxseeds, beans, and broccoli. Phytoestrogens were once thought to contribute to cancer; however, research has shown that they are actually protective against certain cancers like breast cancer.[24] If you've lost your period or are postmenopausal, you may benefit from organic soy in the form of edamame, tempeh, natto, or miso. Be aware that soy is a top allergen.

SUPPLEMENTS

Vitamin D, 1,000-5,000 IU or based on your lab results, to support estrogen production and bone health.

Vitamin E, 400 mg daily, can help support estrogen production.

Black cohosh, red clover, dong quai, and vitex have been shown to have estrogenic effects. It is best to work with a provider to find the right dose for you.

WHEN TO SEE A DOCTOR:
We expect low estrogen after menopause and no time before it. Using the tools in this book can help, but I would still advise meeting with a doctor because low estrogen can lead to bone loss and a decline in brain and heart health. While a missing period might feel like a blessing, it's a major flare-level warning from your body that danger is ahead.

Low Progesterone

Common Causes:	Associated Risks:
Chronic stress	Fibroids
PCOS	Fibrocystic breasts
Primary ovarian insufficiency	Infertility
Anovulation	Miscarriage
Luteal phase defect (failure of the corpus luteum)	Endometrial hyperplasia
Hypothyroidism	Certain cancers, breast and endometrial

Common Causes:	Associated Risks:
Hyperprolactinemia (elevated prolactin)	Bone loss
	Anxiety

WHAT CAN HELP:

LIFESTYLE

Ditch the stress you can. Take inventory of your stress and be realistic about how it is impacting you. If you can ditch any of it, do it.

Balance your energy. Ensure your exercise and calories are balanced. You need to eat enough and not expend so much energy that your body gets tricked into thinking that the environment is not safe. Its response will be to stop ovulation or shut down sufficient progesterone production.

Get with the crew. You only need one good friend to start to bump up that progesterone, but if you're the type who enjoys a group, go for that. The key is, these people gotta fill you up, and you need to genuinely enjoy time with them.

Exercise check. If you've been pushing for a marathon or training hard and you're checking off low-progesterone symptoms, it is time to reassess that routine and perhaps dial it back.

NUTRITION

Eat sufficient carbohydrates, especially in the second half of your cycle (luteal phase) when your caloric needs are up.

Include sesame seeds and sunflower seeds in your luteal phase.

Eat foods to support progesterone. Incorporate vitamin C, vitamin B_6, and magnesium into your diet. See the table on page 369 for food sources.

SUPPLEMENTS

Vitex, 200 mg daily, can support progesterone levels and has been shown to drop prolactin levels in some cases. If you're dealing with hyper-prolactinemia, you want to chat with your doctor about the best therapy for you.

Vitamin B_6, 30-50 mg daily, can help increase progesterone levels.[25] Some research suggests much higher dosages, but toxicity can occur if used for an extended period. It's best to consult a health care provider before taking dosages beyond 100 milligrams a day.

Selenium, 40-200 mcg, is essential for progesterone production and can help PMS.

Vitamin C, 1,000 mg daily, supports ovarian production of progesterone.

Vitex, 200 mg daily, can help support progesterone production.

WHEN TO SEE A DOCTOR:

Low progesterone is associated with mood symptoms like anxiety, and sleep disorders. If you are experiencing either of those and it interrupts your life, it's time to see a provider. If you've experienced short cycles, infertility, or miscarriage, and would like to become pregnant, it is a good idea to have pre-conception care, and check your progesterone levels.

High Testosterone

Common Causes:	Associated Risks:
Chronic stress	Infertility
Insulin resistance	Depression
PCOS	Androgenic alopecia
Adrenal disorders	

WHAT CAN HELP:

LIFESTYLE

Regular exercise, especially the kind that helps you build muscles, helps the body remain sensitive to insulin, which can be a driver of high testosterone.

Reduce stress. Use the practices listed on page 310 to help manage your stress. Remember: your adrenal glands make DHEA, which can be converted into testosterone. Use the tips under the adrenal section above to care for these glands.

NUTRITION

Swap refined carbohydrates for complex carbs and nutrient-dense vegetables to manage blood sugar. See the information under high insulin on how to improve blood sugar.

Include fat and protein with your meals to support your body in blood sugar balance.

Consider drinking green tea, as it can help increase sex hormone binding globulin (SHBG), which will bind excess testosterone.

Eat ground flaxseeds during your follicular phase, which will also increase SHBG.

SUPPLEMENTS

Vitamin D, 1,000-5,000 IU daily or based on your lab results, can help support balanced testosterone.

Nettle root, 100-200 mg daily, has been shown to lower testosterone levels and improve symptoms of high testosterone like oily skin.[26]

Saw palmetto, 300-500 mg daily, can inhibit the enzyme that converts testosterone to DHT, a more potent androgen that leads to irreversible hair loss and acne.[27]

N-acetyl cysteine (NAC), 1,800 mg daily, has been shown to decrease testosterone specifically in women with PCOS.[28]

WHEN TO SEE A DOCTOR:

Acne and hair loss may not be life threatening, but they can be devastating and take a toll on our self-esteem and mental health. If you're struggling with either of these, please use the resources in this book and get extra support from your provider. If your cycles are irregular in addition, you may have PCOS, which is important to identify and treat.

Low Testosterone

Common Causes:	Associated Risks:
Inflammation	Muscle weakness
Chronic stress	Weight gain
Postmenopause	Fatigue
Oral contraceptive pill	Depression
Primary ovarian insufficiency	
Functional hypothalamic amenorrhea	

WHAT CAN HELP:

LIFESTYLE

Start strength training to build muscle mass, which is correlated with healthy testosterone levels.

Limit endocrine-disrupting chemical exposure. Check personal products, cleaning supplies, and food storage as common places in which these chemical hide.

Adrenal support. The adrenal glands are responsible for about 25 percent of testosterone production by way of DHEA. Keeping stress in check can enable your adrenals to function at their best.

Get outside. Sun exposure helps with vitamin D production, which can support healthy testosterone levels.

Have sex. Sexual activity helps modulate hormones, and testosterone is no exception.

NUTRITION

Increase anti-inflammatory foods. Take out inflammatory oils and bring in anti-inflammatory foods like ginger, turmeric, cold-water fish, olives, and berries. Follow the nutrition recommendations in the program.

Increase zinc in your diet. See the table on page 370.

Eat vitamin A, C, and E. Use the table on page 371 for guidance.

SUPPLEMENTS

Vitamin D, 1,000–5,000 IU daily, can help support healthy testosterone levels. Your dosage should be based on your lab results.

Take a daily multivitamin, which will contain zinc balanced with copper and B vitamins to support your testosterone.

Ashwagandha, 100 mg, won't push your testosterone too high; rather it will support your adrenal glands, stress levels, and the process needed to optimize testosterone.

Probiotics. They have been shown to reduce inflammation, anxiety, and depression, and HPA-axis (adrenal) stimulation.[29] Your gut microbiota plays a key role in inflammation and, as we know, inflammation can drive your testosterone into estrogen.[30]

WHEN TO SEE A DOCTOR:

Maybe you don't miss the sexual desire you once had, but I'd caution you against falling into the trap of thinking testosterone is just about libido. It is important in immune and heart health, as well as mood. If you find you're lacking motivation, feeling down, and crying easily, it is a good idea to check in with your provider.

Let's Begin!

Now that you've had a chance to go through the recommendations for the Hormone Symptom Check that you took in chapter 8, I suggest you make note of the areas you need to pull in to customize this program. We're going to start in the period phase, but again, you can jump in at any phase you're in right now. I recommend giving each phase a read-through so you understand the strategies, tools, and journal exercises involved, and then can note in your schedule when to do these. Have fun with the journal prompts, and if anything ever feels too much, you can come back to that next month. Ideally, you would complete all steps of the program, but keeping stress low and taking on what is manageable for you is an important consideration.

PHASE 1: YOUR PERIOD (DAYS 1–7)

You're starting in on that nutrient-dense style of eating we discussed in the last chapter, so make note of which foods you're focusing on this week. This is just about the easiest time in your cycle to make a dietary shift, since you've left the increase in carb, sugar, and other cravings of the luteal phase and the hormones are now in your corner. But maybe all you want to do is eat all the chocolate. I feel that. And sure, you can eat some chocolate. Opting for the 70 percent–plus cacao is going to give you that fix, plus provide you with antioxidants and the happy-making chemical release you're after. If you're having symptoms, make a note in your journal, along with what helps give you relief. Remember to follow up the next month to see the impact of this plan on your future periods. Once your period finishes, move on to the follicular phase.

SYMPTOMS

Migraine/Headache: You may notice a headache or migraine at the start of this week. Thanks, estrogen. That drop in this key cyclical hormone is behind those headache woes. If you're struggling with a headache, see the advanced protocols on page 379 to address it.

Cramps: It's normal to have light to moderate cramping the first and second day. But if cramps are disrupting your life, get those tips from page 383 to help.

Heavy periods: There's some tips for you on page 380. If it is really heavy, this may be the time to leverage ibuprofen, which seriously works and is a good temporary fix while you work on the underlying issues driving this. Remember to look at the symptoms for heavy periods discussed in chapter 10, and check for fibroids using the symptom check on page 262, so you know the information to bring to your doctor. The foods to support liver and gut health that I shared on page 308 can also help.

Period poops: Ugh. Those loose stools usually ride along with wicked cramps like I shared on page 265, which is where you'll find strategies for this. Unfortunately, there's no quick fix for this, but take heart that they won't last more than a day or two. Use the strategies in this plan specifically to address period poops and things should start to improve in one to two cycles.

NUTRITION

Blood builders. You're losing blood, so iron, B_{12}, B_6, and folate are crucial to rebuild blood cells and keep your energy up. Use the nutrient table on page 369 for the foods that contain these.

Sexy food is period food. Some of the same foods that are considered an aphrodisiac—see the box on page 306—also help with period cramps, so incorporate them.

Ginger and turmeric. Get these in your diet to help with the pain, inflammation, and digestive woes that can hit with your period. Yes, turmeric lattes count; just watch they don't sugar-bomb ya! Sip ginger tea or grate it into your food.

Flaxseeds and pumpkin seeds. From now until you reach ovulation, aim to eat 1 to 2 tablespoons of each seed, which will provide fiber, zinc, and fatty acids to support this part of your cycle.

LIFESTYLE

Bath, anyone? With that first drop of blood there is often a drop in all the PMS and mood symptoms of the luteal phase. But don't go giving up on your stress management tools just because there's no longer a sense of overwhelm. Use the list from page 310 to tend to your needs, and consider a bath, which can also help with cramps.

Sleep, nap, relax. Seems basic, but I can't even tell you how many patients are trying to get by on six hours of sleep, drinking caffeine all day to push through, and never giving themselves permission to pause. There is no shame in taking a little pampering time and recognizing that you're a cyclical creature, and you are not designed to grind all month.

Exercise. Movement is a good idea, but when the cramps come a-calling, you may feel you just want to lie in bed all day. Some gentle movement (even if just stretching in bed) can help relieve cramps and supports a sense of well-being. For some women, when their hormones drop to be more on par with men's levels, they find their athletic performance is in its prime. Ask yourself what is true for you: Do you need to dial it back or dial it up during this phase?

SUPPLEMENTS

New beginnings. If you're starting supplements on the first day of the program, put a reminder in your phone to take them. It's a new routine and, as with all things new, having reminders can really help. Be sure to also make note of them in your journal so you can track what you introduced and see how it has helped.

Vaginal health. If you struggle with yeast or BV following your period, talk to your provider about treating it directly. You can also consider a probiotic (in addition to the prebiotics you're eating) to seed the gut and support your vaginal ecology. See page 206 for details.

Take a B-complex. Extra B vitamins can help you feel more energized throughout the day. Taking them first thing in the morning with a full stomach is best. Choose a B-complex over single-B vitamins so that you get the most comprehensive array of Bs to meet your needs.

SEX

Period sex. Orgasms can offer relief from cramps, and vaginal intercourse can provide an internal massage. If intercourse doesn't sound good to you while on your period, consider all the different ways to have sex and be intimate that we discussed in chapter 5. Your hormones are at a low point, so self-lubricating and desire are often also low. Remember: lube is your friend, even while bleeding. And listen, if you're not in the mood and all you want to do is cuddle your cat and a hot water bottle, that's totally normal.

Breasts. From now until after ovulation, your breasts are their least sensitive. This may be a good time for you to begin incorporating them into erotic touch and sexual activity.

How's your desire? Remember: desire is a brain thing that then translates to a between-the-legs thing, which is why some people still get in the mood even when there's heavy bleeding, cramps, or other things some people might consider turnoffs.

Ouch! Your cervix is lower at this point in your cycle, so doggy style or any kind of deep penetration can create cervical collision. While some people enjoy this (normal), others do not, and it can hurt. This is the time in your cycle to use an Ohnut or try something like cowgirl, where you can have control of the depth of penetration.

JOURNAL

Track. Use the tracking data on page 317 to fill in your info. Is your mood better, but your energy slightly lower? Normal in those early days of your period. Be sure to make a note of it. If you're having cramps, make a note of the intensity. If it brings on other symptoms like nausea, back pain, or pain down your legs, be sure to write that down and share with your provider. It's a good idea to track your flow every day of your period and note spotting. I also recommend noting if there are clots in the menstrual blood (pea-size, dime-size, quarter-size, or bigger) and how many tampons, pads, etc., you're using, and how often you change them.

How do you feel about your period? We are inundated with messages about how dirty, icky, and shameful periods are. Believe it or not, there are people who have never once felt this way about their body. Maybe you're one of them. Either way, I encourage doing this exercise while you bleed to explore how you feel about your period. Do you dread it? Why? Are you looking forward to the day when it'll be gone forever? What would your life look like if that was the case? Do you love your period? What aspects of it make you feel joyful? I encourage you to do this while you're on your heavy days and then revisit it next month by first writing what your feelings are, and then peeking at what you wrote before. Do it again after three months since embarking on this program. What's different?

Gas and brake pedals. Building on the information you learned in chapter 3, now is the time to make a list of what gets you going and what slows you down, if not totally turns you off. The period is a time where a lot of us feel more introspective, and without progesterone in the way of our fantasies and sexual desire, it's easier to go there in our mind. In your journal, make two columns. On the left side write "Gas Pedal" and, on the right, put "Brake Pedal" as the heading. Then jot down what fits in both columns. When you're ready, share it with your partner (if you have one). See the box on page 349 with examples of common turn-ons and turnoffs. Keep in mind that while a kiss on the neck may be a turn-on, getting kissed on the neck while working on an endless pile of dishes might not get you there. It is possible to have turn-ons appear when the context is wrong and have it not work for you.

WHAT TURNS YOU ON OR OFF

GAS PEDAL

- Physical touch (specific to what you like)
- Seeing your partner excel at something
- Sharing a sexual memory or fantasy with your partner
- Watching, reading, listening to erotic media (romance novel, porn, etc.)
- Feeling wanted or desired by your partner
- Sharing a connection with your partner
- Specific partner traits
- Certain scents
- Being in a specific location
- Someone wearing a specific outfit (lingerie, suit, uniform, etc.)
- Watching someone perform a specific activity (stretching, holding a baby, etc.)
- Engaging in dirty talk, sexting, or photo sharing

BRAKE PEDAL

- Stress—any and all kinds
- Pregnancy concerns
- Feeling obligated to have sex
- Feeling "touched out" (common phenomenon for mothers who are in physical contact with their children all day)
- Body image concerns
- Anxiety about sexual performance
- Specific partner traits
- Relationship concerns (trust, honesty, respect, etc.)
- History of sexual trauma
- Concern about safety
- Fear of being discovered or someone interrupting
- Shame (about enjoying sex, having a one-night stand, not doing it to make a baby—I could fill a chapter on all the ways we are shamed)

PHASE 2: FOLLICULAR (DAYS 1-13)

Now we're getting to the good part, right? (Really, though, it's all the good part—at least that's what I want to help you recognize.) When you start feeling that energy climb, your brain and clitoris start aligning their plans, and you're feeling the pull of the ovulatory phase right ahead, things can feel amazing. It's also a good time to be mindful about skipping meals. I know there's always something that can feel more pressing than eating, but nourishing yourself now will keep both your blood sugar and adrenals happy. This tends to be a less symptom-heavy phase compared to the luteal phase, so enjoy it and make the most of that energy by getting your nutrition, lifestyle, and supplements on point. This phase begins when your period stops, so you may be starting this on day 4 of your cycle, and that's normal. Remember: the follicular phase technically includes your period, but for the purpose of this program, we are separating them.

SYMPTOMS

Acne. Estrogen and testosterone got you feeling all sexy and then . . . Damn it! Is that a zit? Acne breakouts can be common as you reach the tail end of the follicular phase. If you see signs of oily skin when your period stops, know that testosterone may be making a move that will result in breakouts. Use the Cycle Symptom Relief strategies on page 377 to make your move toward better skin.

NUTRITION

Plants. You've begun building a more nutrient-dense diet, and now is a good time to up that daily intake if you haven't already. Your body is making more estrogen, which will also be removed via the bowels (and kidneys) when your body is done with it. Plants are an excellent source of fiber, which is going to feed those helpful critters in your gut (estrobolome), help your body support vaginal health, and create epic dumps. LOL! No, but seriously, fiber will help your body stay regular, which is useful for balancing estrogen and will help come the luteal phase when estrogen excess can mess with you hard.

Appetite down? That's normal with estrogen making your cells more sensitive to insulin and slightly depressing your appetite. Heavy meals may make you feel full quickly, which is why sticking to plenty of plants with fat and protein may be the way to go. As you near ovulation, you may feel a bit hungrier before things shift into the luteal phase.

Fermented foods. Now is a good time to begin to incorporate coconut kefir, kimchi, sauerkraut, beet kvass, whole-fat plain organic yogurt (if you do dairy), and other fermented foods. Starting these now will support your microbiome and help with the bloating that can follow ovulation.

LIFESTYLE

Sleep. It's tempting not to get good sleep because, let's be honest, you could probably make it on six hours and feel fine. Don't fall for this cyclical trickery. Try to keep up your sleep routine and get the rest you need. Your luteal phase will feel so much better when you do.

Exercise. You may be able to lift more, run harder, or take on that challenging Peloton class you've been eyeing in this phase. If you're not working to get your period back, go for it. But make sure to give yourself recovery time, too. Make a note of your energy and how these activities make you feel.

Give mindfulness a go. Your mind is in a great place during this phase to try out some mindfulness activities. Start practicing now and, if you're up for it, take it to the bedroom.

SUPPLEMENTS

Plan it out. Look ahead to the luteal phase and see if there are any supplements you might want to have on hand. If headaches and cramps usually plague you, then make sure you have magnesium ready to go. Making a plan when you feel good is crucial to actually executing that plan when you don't.

If you don't take them, they won't work. Supplements only work if you take them, and if you're using herbs like vitex or rhodiola then you have to be consistent. I've had patients share that they didn't think the supplements were helping, but once I suggested that they track, we figured out pretty quickly that it wasn't working because they took them only two to four days out of the week. Track this. What you track gets your attention, and what gets your attention will enable you to reach your goals.

SEX

Vaginal lubrication. As you say buh-bye to your period, things won't be as wet just yet, but when you approach your ovulatory phase (when estrogen is higher) you may notice increased cervical fluid and an easier time producing arousal fluid. It's also normal to not have a genital response even when your brain is really ready to go. Your brain is the one to trust. Your genitals, eh, sometimes they just don't totally cooperate until you get things going, which requires lube (unless you're into the friction burn).

Nipple play, anyone? With breast tenderness absent and nipple sensitivity up, now would be a good time to try out some of the techniques covered in chapter 4.

Try a bit of spice. If you want to try out that dirty talk, role-playing, new toys, sex furniture, or anything else we covered in chapter 6, now is the adventurous time of your cycle. The rise in estrogen is also giving rise to serotonin and dopamine, which means if you're into it, you'll get reinforcement molecules to keep going and may find yourself feeling quite content after you're finished. But know that the extra serotonin may make it a little more difficult for some people to get to O as quickly as they'd like. This is where changing up the sensations and finding different paths to arrive can help.

The playlist. *Clears throat* Like *the* playlist you put on when it's time to get down. At the tail end of this phase, it can be a fun activity to build that playlist. If you hear a song and find yourself filled with the sexy feels, that's your brain telling your body, *Sexy stuff is here*. If it stirs it up and you're here for it, put it on the playlist.

JOURNAL

Track. Use the tracking data on page 317 to fill in your info. Pay special attention to changes in your energy, mood, and cervical mucus.

How's your desire? Notice where your sexual desire is. Does it feel more spontaneous? Are you finding yourself fantasizing, engaging in more physical touch, or wanting to get some more time in the bedroom (or maybe somewhere else, if that's your thing)? Is it feeling so much easier or exciting to get into sex? During this time your estrogen and testosterone are both up, which can correlate with greater interest in sex and more vaginal lubrication. Make a note in your journal about what you're experiencing.

Body scan. Remember how we talked about loving yourself despite every message you receive from society, media, and even medical professionals? That shit's hard at first. But it is made a bit easier as we near the ovulatory phase, where we're curvier, have fewer fine lines and wrinkles showing up, and most of us have a glow. (BTW, wrinkles are beautiful, too, but I recognize that it can take a bit of energy to overcome.) Stand in front of a mirror, see what you look like, and tell yourself out loud what you love. Then write down what you love, so you can remember that when things shift in the latter half of the luteal phase or any time you start to get down on yourself. Try doing this for at least two or three days out of every cycle.

PHASE 3: OVULATORY (DAYS 12–18)

This phase encompasses only a handful of days from the time your estrogen and LH levels spike to the twenty-four hours following ovulation. It's quick, but we're going to start setting the stage now for an easier luteal phase.

The temporary endocrine structure (corpus luteum) made in the ovary by ovulation will produce your progesterone through the luteal phase. Once the egg is gone (or fertilized) the progesterone begins to flow and, for some, big changes start to occur. For a lot of people, this phase is going to be the height of their sexual desire and arousal, so take advantage of it.

SYMPTOMS

Ovulatory pain. If the mittelschmerz has got ya, try applying heat to the area for about twenty minutes for comfort. You can also gently massage using your fingertips to rub in circles, or make a fist and knead your abdomen gently. If it's bad, use over-the-counter pain meds like ibuprofen. But if you do need to use a drug for the pain, chat with your doctor, because this could be a sign of a cyst or endometriosis.

Headache. At this point in your cycle, estrogen will spike to trigger the brain to release LH, and that will signal ovulation to occur. Good stuff. That is, until your head is pounding. The fluctuations in estrogen can cause headaches and migraines to occur. Use the recommendations in the Cycle Symptom Relief chart to get relief.

NUTRITION

Corpus luteum support. If you remember, this is the temporary endocrine structure made in the ovaries only after ovulation that produces your progesterone. Want a happy and uneventful (except for maybe that *bow-chickawowwow*) luteal phase? Focus on foods to support the corpus luteum in doing its job of producing progesterone. Bring vitamin B_6, vitamin C, omega-3 fatty acids, and vitamin E foods into your diet. Use the table in Appendix 2, page 369, to help you identify these foods.

How about those healthy fats? Fats support our hormones, and the quality ones are good for those ovaries, too. Now is a good time to start adding in 2 tablespoons of healthy fats at each meal if you haven't already. As we move into the luteal phase, blood sugar issues can become more apparent. Having the fats we talked about on page 309 to help blood sugar balance can make all the difference. Let's get that habit going now.

Ground sesame seeds and sunflower seeds. Aim for 1 to 2 tablespoons of each of these daily until your period comes again. Sesame seeds are anti-inflammatory and support hormone health. Sunflower seeds support estrogen detoxification and can help with balancing prostaglandins so those cramps aren't so bad.

LIFESTYLE

Make the most of movement. Exercising now while your energy and hormones are up can have a positive impact on the weeks to come and that next period. Types of exercise that you may be up for incorporating during the ovulatory phase include high-intensity interval training (HIIT), kickboxing, cycling, running, weight lifting, or swimming (just a few examples).

Meditate. If you haven't tried it out yet, now is a good time to give yourself a five-minute sesh in the day. It's a good way to drop stress and allow progesterone to do its thing, check in with your body, and get centered.

SUPPLEMENTS

Vitamin B_6. If you're not already taking a supplement that contains vitamin B_6 daily, then today is a good day to start. Aim for at least 30 milligrams daily. Some studies have shown that B_6 is even more effective when combined with calcium and magnesium.

Adaptogens. Bringing in adaptogens like rhodiola, holy basil, and ashwagandha, and adrenal-supportive nutrients like vitamin B_5 and vitamin C, can help you feel more energized, have a more even mood, and feel more resilient in the face of stress as you move into the luteal phase.

SEX

Self-lubricating and then some. Maybe it's the way they make you feel, maybe it's the estrogen, but either way, if you would describe your vagina as a Slip 'n Slide due to all the cervical fluid and vaginal lubrication, that's normal. This is the wettest time in your cycle, but if you still want lube, that's totally cool, too. Some people find "the wetter the better" is their forte, while others can pass at this time. If you're struggling with symptoms of low estrogen, know that even those with normal estrogen don't always self-lubricate like I'm describing. And just like there is stigma about being too dry, there is stigma about being too wet, because people can't just let our vaginas be.

Traverse your terrain. If there was a time to go on a pleasure exploration, this is the phase to do it. You'll be more inclined to enjoy things with your body working toward the goal of getting you laid. Your breasts are less tender and nipples more sensitive. For some, orgasms flow effortlessly at this time. For others, there's still nurturing to be done for their sexual wellness, and that's perfectly OK. But whether solo or with a partner, I encourage you to try new things (you can always say stop or change your mind) and explore other ways to find pleasure. See the box on page 357 on pleasure mapping.

How's your sexual desire? Sexual desire is generally up at this time, as is the ability to orgasm. If you've been struggling to orgasm, this is the time in your cycle where you may be more successful, so give it a try. Remember: satisfying pleasure doesn't always need to end in an orgasm. If your sexual desire isn't feeling like the spontaneous version, but rather the more responsive style we talked about, that's normal. That's a lot of people's primary mode of operation, so embrace it and indulge it if that is yours.

Try a sex fast. If you find the pressure to have sex hits the brakes for you, especially when I outline how everything is ready to go, then I recommend removing sex as an option. Maybe that sounds crazy. But if you're in a relationship and the sexpectations have got you bogged down, just make it so no one expects sex ever. You go about what you do with one rule: no one gets to touch their or anyone else's genitals, breasts, or "fun" areas in an erotic way when the other is present. For most of my patients, this melts the barrier put up by the thought of "having" to engage in sex and allows for sex to happen in a more organic way. So just because your hormones are in a place where they're greenlighting sex, it doesn't mean you actually have to have sex.

JOURNAL

Track. Use the tracking data on page 317 to fill in your info.

How's the pedals? Go back and revisit the pedals exercise you did a few weeks ago while you were still on your period. Are the brakes as sensitive right now? How are the gas pedals? It's a good time to reflect on how you were feeling then and where you're at now. Many of my patients find that the brakes are a little less touchy at this time, and they are very responsive to their turn-ons. Just know that things like trauma, shame, or relationship issues are not things that will magically resolve with your hormones. If those are stomping on brakes (or even just tapping them) be sure to meet with a qualified mental health professional to get the support you need.

PLEASURE MAPPING WITH A PARTNER

This exercise is about exploring sensations that feel good and getting to know your body and your partner's. If you really want to tune in to what you feel, consider putting on a blindfold, which will also build anticipation. You can definitely do this solo to explore on your own, too.

1. **Get naked (or at least down to your undies).** Have your partner lie down and start at the top of their head and work your way down the front of their body. You'll have them flip over once you've covered the front. The one caveat: no touching genitals.

2. **Explore.** Touch, lick, bite, pinch, massage, nibble, kiss, suck, stroke, or use whatever technique you feel inclined to do or that your partner asks for. You can pull in feathers, ice, leather, metal, polished crystals, or any other elements to offer a different sensation.
3. **Check in continuously.** "Do you like this?" "How does this feel?"
4. **The goal is not to orgasm.** So, no O. Well, not until you've mapped each other front and back, that is. Then you can both decide if you'd like to proceed with endeavors that will bring you to orgasm.
5. **Journal.** If you feel inclined, journal what this experience was like for you and what you learned.

PHASE 4: LUTEAL (DAYS 15–28)

Hi, body! What is it you need? Check in with yourself, because those symptoms aren't coming from a body that doesn't know how to function. They are coming from a body that is compensating and doing the best it can with what it's got. This is definitely the part of the cycle where most symptoms will crop up. Meet them with curiosity (even though I can totally understand why you would want to resent them). Use the Cycle Symptom Relief chart on page 377 for details on how to support your body as symptoms arise. The biggest driver of hormone symptoms in this phase is too much estrogen relative to progesterone. This is why we started supporting progesterone at ovulation and will continue to do so in this phase. Plus, we're going to make sure we've got what we need to move estrogen out.

This is the longest stretch in the program, covering about two weeks. As such, the list below may look like a lot, but I've called out the specific things to do just before your period arrives to help you get focused. It's easy to lose motivation in the 5 to 7 days before you expect your period due to shifting hormones, appetite changes, and sleep disturbances that can pop up during this phase. Keep going! It's at this point in the program where the work you're putting in will not only help those future PMS symptoms, but also that upcoming period. It's often only when the symptoms hit us that we want to remedy them immediately—the solution to your future symptoms is to tend to your needs now. Remember: your cycle may not be 28 days and you may have ovulated later, which means you're not following the exact days listed in the heading. That's OK. Honor your own cycle.

SYMPTOMS

Constipation. The solution to constipation that shows up just before your period is simple: fiber, water, move. These three things will help keep your bowels regular, which will support your body in moving estrogen out.

Acne. Not you again. Hard eye roll. With the fluctuations of sex hormones and insulin during this phase, acne can be popping up where nobody ever wanted it. I've got a protocol for you on page 381 and would encourage you to take omega-3 fatty acids, which can help with the inflammatory and IGF-1 component of acne discussed on page 240.

PMS, anxiety, sleepless nights? There's a protocol for that on page 384. This is when it likes to hit in your cycle, so get ahead of it by learning the tools now.

Cramps, poops, and headaches. Do they predictably come around for you every period? Starting the protocols for these five days before your period (if you can do nothing else, choose the magnesium) can help you keep these symptoms in check.

NUTRITION

Carbs are our friend. Serotonin can take a dip during this phase of our cycle. Carbs can help keep that dip from becoming a plummet. Remember: grains aren't the only source of carbs. This is a great time to bring on the root vegetables like sweet potatoes, turnips, beets, taro, yuca, and malanga, which will also provide diversity of fiber to tend to your microbiome and help with removing estrogen from the body. Potato chips . . . mmm . . . You may want it, but if you have trouble with water retention, skip it.

Sugar cravings up. If you need dark chocolate, then you need dark chocolate. Dark chocolate is a rich source of polyphenols, which support health, and it can boost mood. Because sugar can help bring serotonin up (at least temporarily), your cravings for it are likely to be higher now. Sugar isn't the best call for blood sugar stability, acne, and many of the other symptoms we face. Plus, it's nutrient devoid, and we want nutrient density in our meals. That said, if you eat some sugar, nobody around here is judging you, so don't judge yourself, either. If you feel you overdid it, make note of that and track it in your journal. It'll be good data to reflect on.

Cruciferous vegetables. Aim for 1/2 to 1 cup about every other day. If you have broccoli sprouts, that counts, too, and you only need a couple of tablespoons. This will help your body eliminate estrogen by supporting liver detoxification of the hormone. Be sure to use the list of liver- and gut-supporting foods on page 308, refer to the image for nutrients the liver needs for detox on page 203, and use the chart on page 369 to get those foods in your routine.

Cold-water fish. Salmon, sardines, mackerel, and anchovies are a few examples to start adding into your routine two to three days per week for added omega-3 fatty acids. They also provide iodine and selenium, which is great for thyroid health, ovarian function, and breast tenderness.

Magnesium. Use the chart on page 369 to make sure you're getting magnesium-supporting foods into your diet. It'll help with the cramps, headaches, and period poops that are on the horizon.

LIFESTYLE

Drop the stress now. You may be feeling like all is well, but trust—working on the stress-reducing techniques on page 310 and making sure they are part of your routine is going to help you keep your progesterone up, so you can maintain your chill and dread PMS so much less as you near the end of this phase.

Spend time with friends. If you know this time of the month can be an emotional one, make some plans with your inner circle to get some people time. It's not just about the support it offers, but we've also found in the research that community can help boost progesterone and is one way we can lower stress.[31] But don't worry; if your introverted self can only handle people'n with one person, that's really all it takes. Whew!

Move, even if you don't want to. Exercise has been shown to decrease fluid retention, especially if you haven't been previously very active. We know that exercise will help mood, cramps, and sleep too, so challenge yourself to get thirty minutes total of movement.

Praise yourself. Can you take five minutes to write down all the ways you rock? Can you get in front of the mirror and remind yourself of just how amazing this world is because of you? It may seem silly, and listen, most of us recoil from the thought of self-praise because we've received so many messages that tell us these practices are just all wrong. They're not. They're necessary.

Meet with a counselor. If any day of this phase starts out feeling like it's all wrong, schedule with your counselor, spiritual adviser, pastor, or close friend to make sure you'll have the mental/emotional support you'll need through the coming days. There's no shame in tending to your thoughts and mood; in fact, it's a necessary step in healing.

Sunlight. Getting out in nature or just standing in front of a window with sunlight can be an instant mood lifter. If you find you're in a dark part of the world and jonesing for some sunlight, then try an alarm clock that mimics sunlight, and definitely get your vitamin D checked.

Get your sleep. If there is any point in your cycle where sleep is going to be an issue, this is it. The corpus luteum will peak with progesterone about five to seven days following ovulation. If all is right, its metabolites will stimulate your brain just right so you can get restful sleep. But PMS be playin' with your sleep at times, and if your progesterone fails then sleep can be a real struggle. Try to go to bed earlier the week before you expect your period, and employ the sleep protocol on page 386 to help.

SUPPLEMENTS

Omega-3 fatty acids. If you haven't been including these yet, now is a good time, especially if you struggle with cramps. Omegas will also help boost your mood, keep inflammation in check (remember: inflammation can cause the enzyme that converts testosterone to estrogen to get up-regulated), and may help make your period easier. Aim for about 1,000 to 2,000 milligrams daily. If you can add cold-water fish on top of your eating routine, even better.

Estrogen and progesterone support. I recommend considering calcium D-glucarate, vitex, vitamin B_6, calcium, vitamin E, vitamin C, sulforaphane, and magnesium at this phase of your cycle to support a healthy hormone balance. If you haven't started these, it's not too late to bring them in. You can find combination supplement formulas that include all of these, so you're not bogged down taking fistfuls of pills every day.

SEX

Clitoral conundrum. How is it I can be so horny, quick to orgasm, and down for whatever one day, and then the next I could care less? Say hey to progesterone. If at any point in this phase you're like *My clit is broken* because you must put in more work, know that it's not broken, and everything is totally normal. If you were feeling like you had a little extra ally in the sexual arousal department, you may be wondering where the heck that went. As progesterone rises in the luteal phase, it's normal to need more stimulation sexually and less stimulation in the stress arena of life. Tend to your stress to help your brain pick up what your partner is putting down regarding the sex signals. Use the stress-reduction methods on page 310, or come up with your own. Finding you need more stimulation and want to bring a toy into play? That's normal during this phase. Vibrators are accomplices in pleasure (not competitors of your partner), so bring them in if that's what you need.

I'm bored. Or distracted. Or just not focused on what's going on in my pants. Your genes can definitely have a say in what happens in your jeans if you're someone who falls into the neurodivergent category. But whether it's ADHD or just me, this is a common time for all of us to need a little more mindfulness practice and, perhaps, something a little spicy. You were exploring new things around ovulation. What worked? What got you really excited? Do more of that. You can also try muting some senses with a blindfold or earplugs so you can really focus on the senses that feel the best.

Pleasure for pleasure's sake. Not every sexual encounter needs to end in intercourse. And while I've used "foreplay" in this book as it is commonly understood, foreplay is sex and can be satisfying on its own. It's this phase of our cycle where we can become more self-critical, more critical of our partner, and participate in spectatoring. But it is also in this phase of our cycle where we're in the clear for pregnancy risk, which is a common brake for those not wanting to start a family or expand it. So some brakes may be touchier and others nonexistent. Remember the pleasure mapping exercise from the ovulatory phase? You learned a lot, and what you find pleasurable may be all you need to feel satisfied in this phase. That is perfectly normal.

Lube. If it's dry down there, it's not you, it's your hormones. As you leave the ovulatory window things will progressively feel drier. That's normal. Lube is your bestie and will help keep the pleasure flowing and the pain at bay.

Cue up *the* playlist. That playlist you made a few weeks ago (you know the one) might be good to cue up in this phase if you are wanting to get intimate, but also not totally wanting to. It can start things moving in the direction you ultimately want to head to help get that desire amped up.

JOURNAL

Track. Use the tracking data on page 317 to fill in your info. This is a time in your cycle when it is normal to notice more vaginal dryness and the need for extra lube in the bedroom. The luteal phase of your cycle generally starts off with good moods and getting good sleep, but in the seven days counting down to your period, you may notice that your emotions, sleep, and physical symptoms shift.

What desire? At what point do you lose interest in your partner, masturbating, or pleasure altogether? Maybe you don't, and that's normal. But if you do, that's also normal and worth noting. I have patients who cyclically hit relationship struggles because their partner is concerned that they're not into them like they previously were. Yeah, a lot of hormone changes happen between ovulation and the next period, and those can lead to needing more stimulation of the gas pedals and a whole lot of love for releasing those brakes. You identified what those were when you were on your period. Remind your partner of those, and let them know that taking some weight off your shoulders, scheduling a date night, and being prepared to make the first move may be necessary to gain the desired outcome–pleasurable sex.

Pedals are back. The week before your period, reflect on the exercise you completed while on your previous period. What's different now? How is that different from what it was like around ovulation? For most of my patients, the brakes get touchy here, and if your hormones are taking you for a PMS or PMDD ride, well, just one poorly timed breath can make you feel livid instead of loving. It's normal when things are off-balance to feel agitated by the little things, but it's not normal to be stuck in that state. It's also normal to have more-touchy brakes and for the sexy signals to fall flat. This is where you gotta stir it up before expecting to feel the love vibes. Hello, responsive desire, my old friend.

• • •

Congratulations! You should be so proud of the work you've put in and the efforts you've made to love up your body and balance your hormones. As we discussed in chapter 8, most people struggling with symptoms will need to support themselves through multiple cycles using what is outlined in this program to get significant and lasting changes. It's my hope that you learned a lot about you and what you specifically need to feel your best. Remember: we are creating a way of life here, so please, don't throw away your excellent habits just because you reached the finish line of this program. If you find you're dealing with lingering symptoms, use the resources in the appendixes to manage those while you continue the lifestyle, nutrition, and supplement strategies you found work best for your body.

ACKNOWLEDGMENTS

Bryce Hamrick, thank you for your endless support of my work. You've lessened the mom-guilt that inevitably comes when I pour myself into a book by being an incredible partner and father.

To Bensen and Wylder, thank you for your love, your lessons, and for reminding me all the time of how important it is to have period-positive, female body–literate males in this world. I look forward to our discussions when you read this in the future.

Jaidree Braddix, you've always got my back and believe in my visions. This book wouldn't be possible without you in my corner. You are truly such a wonderful agent.

Veronica Alvarado, I am so grateful for how you see me and honor my voice. Your input helped me create a book that will serve so many and be enjoyable to read. Thank you for being such an inspiring editor.

To my mom crew: Alisa Stevens, Kim Farina, Shannon Tripp, Lisa Barba, Tarah Yee, Canay Riordan, Sidney Myer, Rose Kaiser, Cristina Guerra, Trish Leimbach, Sarah Rogers. Thanks for being my community, a listening ear when motherhood gets rough, and sometimes taking my kids off my hands so I could write.

Molly Hordos and Courtney Blankenship, you know that you sometimes are the primary reason why part of my world keeps spinning with minimal stress. Thank you! And thank you for always supporting those who seek our help.

John Lee Dumas, thanks for your support in making the audio version a low-stress endeavor so that I could both work and be with my boys.

Izabella and Michael Wentz, thank you both for being such great friends—always.

Lizzy Swick, I appreciate all your efforts and am so grateful for how you are always happy to help.

To Jen Fugo, Dr. Carrie Jones, Dr. Sarah Hill, Nicole Jardim, Dr. Lara Briden, and Dr. Amy Killen: thank you for your professional support and friendship.

To everyone at Simon & Schuster and Simon Element (including those of you I never met), thank you for all your efforts. Books are truly collaborative and without all of you, this simply could not happen.

To all my patients, readers, and social media community, thank you for trusting me with your questions and helping shape the book in your hands.

APPENDIX 1

NUTRIENT FOOD SOURCES

Nutrient	Food Source	What It Does	Signs You're Low
Magnesium	Leafy greens, black beans, edamame, lentils, almonds, flaxseeds, pumpkin seeds, avocados, cacao, tofu	Supports estrogen metabolism, improves sleep, lessens PMS, reduces menstrual cramps, aids in thyroid hormone production, regulates HPA axis, improves insulin sensitivity, supports mitochondria, supports progesterone, relieves migraines, activates vitamin D, increases bone density	Fatigue, anxiety, headaches, PMS, poor sleep, poor sleep prior to period, constipation, insulin resistance, low vitamin D, low bone density, restless legs, muscle cramps, anxiety, hypertension, HPA axis dysfunction
Calcium	Yogurt, fortified nondairy milks, dark leafy greens, figs, broccoli, oranges, almonds, tahini, sardines, anchovies, canned salmon, bone broth, tofu	Supports parathyroid hormone, bone density, electrolyte balance, nerve function, muscle contraction, uterine contraction; reduces menstrual cramps and symptoms of PMS	Low bone mineral density, headaches, low estrogen, poor blood sugar regulation, allergies, muscle pain

Nutrient	Food Source	What It Does	Signs You're Low
Potassium	Sweet potatoes, bananas, bone broth, coconut, potatoes, beans, lentils, seafood, winter squash	Supports HPA axis and adrenal glands, electrolyte balance, nervous system health; stimulates parathyroid hormone, supports growth hormone production	Tired but wired, fatigue, weakness, poor exercise recovery, muscle cramps, hypertension, frequent urination
Sodium	Sea salt, seaweed, mineral water, fermented foods, bone broth, mineral/veggie broth	Supports HPA axis and adrenal health	Low blood pressure, unbalanced thyroid
Selenium	Brazil nuts, fish and seafood, seaweed, beef, eggs, liver, sunflower seeds	Conversion of T4 to T3/thyroid hormone activation; detoxification, immunity, antioxidant, LH and FSH support, TSH support, progesterone support	Hypothyroid symptoms, poor immunity
Iodine	Seaweed, fish, seafood, dairy products, eggs	Building block of thyroid hormone; breast health, fertility	Hypothyroid, goiter, fibrocystic breasts
Zinc	Oysters, other shellfish, liver, beef/red meat, dairy, eggs, pumpkin seeds, beans	Thyroid hormone support, regulates TRH and TSH, testosterone production, supports ovulation and healthy follicles	Hypothyroid symptoms, insulin resistance, frequent colds/poor immunity, loss/reduction of taste, acne and skin issues, menstrual pain

Nutrient	Food Source	What It Does	Signs You're Low
Iron	Heme: red meat, liver, shellfish; nonheme: leafy greens, lentils, beans, dulse	Energy production/ oxygenation of all cells (including ovaries, thyroid gland, etc.)	Anemia, fatigue, headaches, poor circulation
Sulfur	Cruciferous vegetables (broccoli, cauliflower, cabbage, kale, etc.), broccoli sprouts, onions, garlic, animal proteins	Liver detoxification, phase 1 estrogen detoxification, glutathione production, adrenal production of DHEA-S	Poor detoxification, microbiome imbalance, estrogen dominance, low DHEA-S
Copper	Organ meat, cacao, shellfish, spirulina, dark leafy greens	Liver detoxification; regulates iron, blood sugar balance; fertility, thyroid function; immune support	Anemia, insulin resistance, hypothyroid symptoms, acne and skin issues
Vitamin A	Preformed vitamin A: liver, cod liver oil, egg yolks, grass-fed butter/ghee	Activation of thyroid hormone; antioxidant; fertility; HPA and HPO axis support, immune-system support, skin health	Thyroid dysfunction, insulin resistance, elevated TSH, keratosis on back of arms or upper legs, poor immunity, fertility challenges, acne and skin issues
Vitamin E	Sunflower seeds, almonds, nuts and seeds, peanuts, fish, avocado	Antioxidant, estrogen regulation, relaxes the uterus; increases progesterone; vaginal health	Migraines, acne and skin issues

Nutrient	Food Source	What It Does	Signs You're Low
Vitamin C	Strawberries, citrus fruits, bell peppers, spinach, broccoli, rose hips, tomatoes, berries, kiwi, fermented foods	Antioxidant, adrenal health, immunity, skin health, joint health, bone density, progesterone production	Poor immunity, collagen breakdown
Folate	Dark leafy greens, avocados, lentils, beans	Phase 2 estrogen detoxification, methylation, pregnancy support and fetal development, genetic expression, progesterone support, egg quality, ovulation support	Anemia, poor fertility, miscarriage, depression, shortness of breath, weakness, fatigue, headaches, irritability, high homocysteine, estrogen dominance
Vitamin B_{12}	Meat, fish, poultry, eggs, dairy–all animal foods	Phase 2 estrogen detoxification, methylation, pregnancy support and fetal development, genetic expression, egg quality, ovulation support	Anemia, poor fertility, miscarriage, neurological symptoms, depression, anxiety, neuropathy, weakness, fatigue, low stomach acid, high homocysteine, estrogen dominance
Vitamin B_1	Vegetables, whole grains, seeds, nuts, beans, lentils	Energy production, liver detoxification	Brain fog, sugar cravings, poor appetite, fatigue

Nutrient	Food Source	What It Does	Signs You're Low
Vitamin B_2	Eggs, meat, dairy, green vegetables, enriched grains	Fat metabolism, liver detoxification	Reproductive problems, thinning hair, thyroid dysfunction
Vitamin B_3	Animal products, nuts, seeds, legumes	Liver detoxification, energy production	Fatigue, skin issues, low stomach acid, mitochondrial dysfunction
Vitamin B_6	Fish, poultry, legumes, nuts, seeds	Liver detoxification, protein metabolism, supports progesterone production	Hormone imbalance, reproduction issues, low stomach acid, high homocysteine, poor energy, headaches
Choline	Liver, egg yolks, beets, dairy	Brain health, fetal development, methylation support	Nonalcoholic fatty liver disease, memory or brain fog, fatigue, mood swings, muscle pain, elevated homocysteine
Vitamin D	Sun exposure, cod liver oil, liver, fish, egg yolks, fortified dairy	Bone health, immune function, autoimmune prevention	Poor immunity, low estrogen, low testosterone, fatigue, mood swings, autoimmunity, hypothyroid, blood sugar imbalance

Nutrient	Food Source	What It Does	Signs You're Low
EPA and DHA	Fish and seafood, especially from cold water; fish oil; cod liver oil; algae oil	Anti-inflammatory, brain health, fertility	Fatigue, poor memory, dry skin, mood swings, thinning hair
CoQ_{10}	Heart, liver, and other organs; muscle meat	Liver detoxification, heart health, mitochondrial health, egg quality, energy production	Low energy, mitochondrial dysfunction, muscle pain, reproductive issues
NAC	Best supplemented, but cysteine-rich foods include seeds, legumes, dairy, and meat	Egg quality, cervical mucus	n/a
Carotenoids	Carrots, winter squash, peppers, leafy greens, tomatoes, corn, summer squash, sweet potatoes	Fertility; reducing oxidative stress; sperm health	Skin concerns and acne, reproductive issues, thyroid dysfunction
Curcumin	Turmeric	Could inhibit testosterone and estrogen signaling; anti-inflammatory; detoxification; pain relief; PMS support	n/a
Glucosinolates	Brassica veggies	Estrogen detoxification, gut support, anti-inflammatory	Hormone imbalance

Nutrient	Food Source	What It Does	Signs You're Low
Resveratrol	Red grapes, blueberries, peanuts	Increases SHBG, estrogen metabolism, antioxidant, acts as phytoestrogen	n/a
EGCG	Green tea	Modulates estrogen, testosterone, insulin; acts as antioxidant, fertility	n/a
Flavonoids	Berries, cacao, green and black tea, coffee	Liver detoxification, microbiome/ estrobolome health	n/a
Phytoestrogens	Soy, flaxseeds, other seeds, broccoli, kale, beans, peas	Support estrogen levels in menopause and perimenopause or other imbalances, counteract excess androgens	n/a
Phytoprogestins: kaempferol, luteolin, apigenin, naringenin	Kaempferol: spinach, kale cabbage, dill, chives; luteolin: celery, parsley, broccoli, carrots, cabbage; apigenin: parsley, chamomile, celery, artichokes, oregano, oranges; naringenin: grapefruit, orange, tart cherries, tomatoes	Support healthy progesterone levels, especially if low or estrogen dominance, pelvic pain, endometriosis, uterine fibroids	n/a

Nutrient	Food Source	What It Does	Signs You're Low
Probiotics and prebiotics	Probiotics: fermented foods like miso, sauerkraut, kimchi, yogurt, kefir, tempeh, kombucha, apple cider vinegar, pickles, chutneys, homemade sourdough bread; Prebiotics: green banana, onion, leek, garlic, sunchoke, jicama, dandelion, asparagus, oats, barley, lentils, kidney beans, white beans, chickpeas	Estrogen metabolism, neurotransmitter synthesis	Constipation, IBS, acne, eczema, hormone imbalance, autoimmunity, difficulty maintaining healthy weight, estrogen dominance, depression, anxiety, thyroid dysfunction

APPENDIX 2

CYCLE SYMPTOM RELIEF

These advanced protocols can be used alongside the 28-day program or added after you establish your nutrition and lifestyle routine.

Bloating

LIFESTYLE

- Exercise three times a week (aerobic is best for this) can help improve bloating and fluid retention.

NUTRITION

- Eat potassium-rich foods (see page 370).
- Reduce salty foods, as this can lead to fluid retention.
- Cook your foods to make them more easily digestible.
- Eat celery, dandelion greens, lemons, bell pepper, watermelon, garlic, and cucumber. These are all natural diuretics.

SUPPLEMENTS

- Balancing estrogen and progesterone levels, as well as supporting gut health, will help with bloating. See the foundation and solutions for high estrogen and low progesterone.

Breast Tenderness

LIFESTYLE

- See the list of medications on page 291 that can cause breast tenderness.
- Find the style of bra that fits you best, and never part ways.

NUTRITION

- Eat cruciferous vegetables like broccoli, cauliflower, kale, and Brussels sprouts, which supply diindolylmethane (DIM), which helps support estrogen metabolism.
- Seed cycle (see page 122) or be sure to eat 2 tablespoons of ground flaxseeds during your follicular phase.
- Include kelp, shrimp, and other sources of iodine found on page 370 into your diet.
- Eliminate alcohol.
- Consider eliminating caffeine.

SUPPLEMENTS

- **Diindolylmethane (DIM), 50–100 mg** daily, can help you process your estrogen more effectively.
- **Vitex, 200 mg** daily, for at least two to three cycles.
- **Calcium D-glucarate, 300–500 mg**, can help your body eliminate estrogen through the gut.
- Several studies have found that taking **vitamin E** as a supplement can help ease breast pain when you take a dose between **200 IU[1] and 1,200 IU** daily for at least two months.[2]

- **Vitamin B_6, 40 mg** daily, for at least two months may help reduce breast tenderness.[3]

Headache/Migraines

LIFESTYLE

- Keep a headache journal to help keep track of your triggers, and note when they come up in your cycle. This is great information for you and your medical provider.
- Orgasms, no matter how you arrive there, can help reduce head pain and alleviate migraines. There are rare instances in women where orgasms make migraines worse, so track what's true for you.

NUTRITION

- Avoid common triggers: aged cheese, red wine, nitrites, food additives, alcohol.
- Stay hydrated.
- Maintain stable blood sugar levels.

SUPPLEMENTS

- **Vitamin B_2, 400 mg** daily, may prevent migraines. You'll need to use it for three months to evaluate the therapy. It is not effective for acute migraines.
- **Magnesium glycinate, 300 mg** daily, for prevention, and **600 mg** at the onset of a headache.
- **Calcium, 500 mg**, may prevent headaches and menstrual migraines.
- **Feverfew, 25 mg** daily, for migraine prevention.

- **Ginger, 1,000 mg** twice daily, can reduce head pain.
- **Turmeric, 1,000–2,000 mg** daily, can reduce pain and inflammation.
- **B-complex** as directed. **Vitamins B_6, B_{12},** and **folate** taken daily may reduce migraines after six months of use.

Heavy Periods

LIFESTYLE

- Period sex can reduce the flow, the pain, and the number of days you have your period. See page 255 for tips on period sex. See chapter 6 for all things masturbation (because you don't need a partner to handle yourself).

NUTRITION

- Up the fiber in your diet, including prebiotics to help clear estrogen (see page 376).
- Eat iron-rich foods (see chart on page 371) to replace what you're losing. If you're choosing vegetarian sources, be sure to couple with vitamin C to help your body absorb it.
- Include foods to support liver metabolism of estrogen (see page 308).

SUPPLEMENTS

- **Vitex, 200 mg** daily, taken for at least two months can help slow the flow.
- **Iron, 18 mg** (you may require more) along with vitamin C to support absorption.
- **B-complex** as directed. Your body requires folate, vitamin B_{12}, and vitamin B_6 to build new red blood cells. In addition, vitamin B_6 can support estrogen and progesterone balance.

- **Turmeric** is an anti-inflammatory herb that can reduce prostaglandins (remember those from page 265?) and can keep aromatase from converting your testosterone into estrogen.
- **Ibuprofen, 200 mg** as directed. OK, I know it is technically a medication, but when it comes to heavy periods that you need to stop, this can cut the flow in half. Yes, I know all about how this can damage the gut, but two days on your period isn't going to wreck you permanently.

Hormonal Acne

LIFESTYLE

- A hydrocolloid bandage placed overnight on any zit that pops up can help reduce it significantly by morning.
- Change your pillowcase often (at least once per week).
- Check your skin care products to make sure they're not pore clogging or endocrine disrupting.
- Choose the right topical regimen by talking with a dermatologist or esthetician. For example, salicylic acid helps with inflammation and unclogs pores, while retinoids will reduce oiliness and unclogs pores. Benzoyl peroxide can work well to reduce the acne-causing bacteria *P. acnes*.
- Resist touching your face, and wash morning and night. Yes, you need to remove your makeup every night.

NUTRITION

- Cut the dairy and sugar. It's a long game, but it can make all the difference in your skin.
- Eat more fiber-rich foods.
- Omega-3-rich animal sources like salmon, sardines, and mackerel provide your skin and body with anti-inflammatory

support, which can reduce the redness associated with acne and approve the appearance of skin overall. These food sources also contain vitamin A and vitamin D, which has a bonus effect in helping your immune system keep acne in check. If you don't eat fish, aim to make freshly ground flaxseeds, algae, and walnuts part of your daily routine.

- Vitamin C is a key nutrient for supporting healthy skin and is crucial in maintaining your elasticity.
- Niacin and folate are two B vitamins that encourage increased blood flow and cell growth, and are beneficial for acne-prone skin.

SUPPLEMENTS

- **Zinc, 30–40 mg** daily, may help lower inflammation and oil production. If using zinc long term, it is important to couple it with copper, as zinc supplementation can lead to a copper deficiency.
- **Vitamin A** is best used topically for acne treatment, but there is evidence supporting oral supplementation. Aiming for **2,000-5,000 mcg** retinal activity equivalents (RAE) in a multivitamin may help support your skin.
- **DIM, 50–100 mg**, supports healthy testosterone and estrogen levels.
- **Myo-inositol, 2,000 mg** once to twice daily, can help with both androgens and insulin, which can be at the root of what is driving acne. Alone, myo-inositol can take six months to see results, which is why (like all supplements) it is better combined with nutrition and lifestyle.
- Take a **daily probiotic with *Lactobacillus rhamnosus***, which is a strain that has been shown to improve the appearance of acne and support healthy levels of insulin.
- **Omega-3 fatty acids, 1,000–2,000 mg** daily, can reduce inflammation and the effects IGF-1 has on our skin.[4]

ACNE SCARS

- For reducing acne scars, topical retinoids can help promote cell turnover, while vitamin C helps brighten skin and reduce dark spots. It's important to note that reducing and eliminating acne scars is something you'll have to be consistent with treating, and patient with its progress.
- Azelaic acid can also help fade dark marks on the skin and is another to consider putting into your routine. In the morning after you wash your face, apply azelaic acid followed by sunscreen. When you get ready for bed, wash your face again and apply retinol, followed by a moisturizer with niacinamide, a vitamin B_3 derivative.
- Niacinamide can help even your skin tone and reduce hyperpigmentation. If you've got really stubborn or deep scars, make an appointment with your dermatologist to discuss laser treatments, chemical peels, and microneedling.

Menstrual Cramps

LIFESTYLE

- Hot water bottle or heating pad applied to abdomen and/or lower back. No more than twenty minutes per area.
- Warm bath with 1 cup Epsom salt.
- Gentle walking, stretching, and movement can help relieve cramps.
- External massage: Make a fist and gently press into lower abdomen with a kneading motion.
- Vaginal sex with a penis or a toy can provide an internal massage.
- Orgasms release hormones and feel-good chemicals that relieve pain.

- Topical cannabidiol (CBD) may help reduce menstrual cramps and pain. Hummingway Cycle Soother patches can be placed for twenty-four hours and can reduce pain as well as bloating.

NUTRITION

- Eat foods rich in magnesium, thiamine (B_1), calcium, vitamin E, and omega-3 fatty acids.
- Increase fiber intake by eating a variety of plants.
- Incorporate ginger and turmeric into the diet.

SUPPLEMENTS

- **Magnesium glycinate, 300 mg** twice daily five days before your period. You may benefit from **300 mg** daily ongoing.
- **Omega-3 fatty acids, 1,500–2,000 mg** daily. Generally, they need to be used for at least two cycles for noticeable improvement.
- **Vitamin E, 400 IU**, daily.
- **Cramp bark, 1 to 2 droppers full of tincture**, at the start of your cycle.
- **Ginger root, 1,000 mg**, has been shown in small studies to be as effective as ibuprofen for menstrual cramps.

PMS

LIFESTYLE

- Exercise most days of the week for thirty to sixty minutes.
- Expose yourself to sunlight upon waking, or use a light box. Bonus if you can get out into nature.
- Ditch the alcohol and cigarettes. Short term they may feel like a win, but long term they are a big-time loss.

- Do more things that bring you joy and avoid (if you can) those things that aren't a "hell yes."
- Set your boundaries during the follicular phase and honor them in the luteal phase, when PMS crops up.
- Cognitive behavioral therapy can help with the symptoms of PMS.
- Use the recommendations found on page 333 to optimize high estrogen and low progesterone.
- Spend time with friends and people you feel close to. This can help increase your progesterone levels.[5]

NUTRITION

- Eat foods that contain iron, vitamin C, vitamin B_6, magnesium, and calcium, which can help PMS and the period that follows. See appendix 1 for suggestions.
- Include whole foods, including unrefined carbohydrates, in the diet, like sweet potatoes, oats, chickpeas, quinoa, and squash, to support serotonin and caloric needs.
- Aim for 2 tablespoons each of sunflower seeds and ground sesame seeds as part of seed cycling.
- I know how good a donut sounds before your period, but sugar and refined carbs can make PMS (and blood sugar roller coasters) worse. Reach for dark chocolate instead, which is full of antioxidants and can improve mood.
- Avoid alcohol. It messes with your hormones and can make your sleep, moods, boobs, and periods regret every single drop.
- Cuddle a human, pet a dog, hug hard, or get orgasms in. All of these will boost oxytocin and serotonin, and help improve your mood.
- Eat turmeric, which is anti-inflammatory and can help with physical and mood symptoms of PMS.

SUPPLEMENTS

- **Vitex (chasteberry), 200 mg**, can help optimize progesterone and can help improve mood.
- **Vitamin B_6, 30–50 mg**, can help improve PMS and may yield enhanced benefit when combined with calcium and magnesium.[6]
- **Calcium, 200–500 mg**, can reduce moodiness, cravings, and headaches.
- **Vitamin D_3, 2,000 IU** (or the dose based on lab testing), can help with the physical symptoms of PMS.
- **Myo-inositol, 2,000 mg**, helps stabilize blood sugar, supports ovarian function, and can help with symptoms of PMS.
- **Selenium, 40–200 mcg**, is essential for progesterone production and can help PMS.
- **Magnesium glycinate, 150–300 mg**, can help improve symptoms of PMS.
- **Omega-3 fatty acids, 2,000 mg**, provides anti-inflammatory support and has been shown to offer relief for depression, anxiety, nervousness, lack of concentration, headaches, bloating, and breast tenderness.[7]

Sleep Disturbance

LIFESTYLE

- See the sleep tips on page 313.
- Supporting healthy adrenal function can help with the natural decline of cortisol that is supposed to happen in the evening.
- Optimizing progesterone can help with sleep. See page 337 for details on how to do that.

NUTRITION

- Eat tart cherries, goji berries, mushrooms, and pistachios—all of which contain melatonin.
- Avoid alcohol. Even a small amount can hijack sleep.
- Consider a snack of healthy fat, protein, and carbohydrates two hours before bed if blood sugar spikes have you waking at night.

SUPPLEMENTS

- **Phosphatidylserine, 50 mg nightly**, helps gently lower cortisol.
- **Ashwagandha, 100 mg**, is an apoptogenic herb that has a calming effect and promotes restorative sleep.
- **Valerian, passionflower, lemon balm at 100 mg** are all herbs that can help you get restful sleep and promote a sense of calm.
- **Melatonin, 1-3 mg**, may help you get to sleep when jet-lagged, traveling across time zones, dealing with dreaded time changes, or when you just plain can't sleep.
- **L-theanine, 200 mg**, can help your body wind down for a good night's sleep.
- **Vitamin B_6, 20-50 mg**, supports the production of serotonin, and **magnesium glycinate, 150-300 mg,** plus **zinc, 8-11 mg**, supports the conversion of serotonin to melatonin (the sleep hormone) within the brain.[8]

NOTES

Introduction

1. "Sex and HIV Education," Guttmacher Institute, July 1, 2022, https://www.guttmacher.org/state-policy/explore/sex-and-hiv-education.

Chapter 1: Sex

What's Normal for Getting It On?

1. Anna Duff, " What Is Adultery, Is It the Same as Cheating, Is It Illegal in the UK and Is It Grounds For Divorce?," *Sun*, September 18, 2018, https://www.thesun.co.uk/fabulous/7247548/adultery-same-as-cheating-illegal-uk-grounds-for-divorce/.
2. "United Nations Agencies Call for Ban on Virginity Testing," World Health Organization, October 17, 2018, https://www.who.int/news/item/17-10-2018-united-nations-agencies-call-for-ban-on-virginity-testing.
3. United Nations, "'Virginity Testing': A Human Rights Violation, with No Scientific Basis—UN," UN News, October 17, 2018, https://news.un.org/en/story/2018/10/1023401.
4. EJ Dickson, "It Isn't Just T.I.—Virginity Testing is a Worldwide Problem," *Rolling Stone*, November 6, 2019, https://www.rollingstone.com/culture/culture-news/ti-gynecologist-virginity-test-908990/.
5. "Virginity Testing," American College of Obstetricians and Gynecologists, January 2020, https://www.acog.org/clinical-information/policy-and-position-statements/statements-of-policy/2020/virginity-testing.
6. Keum Hwa Lee et al., "Imperforate Hymen: A Comprehensive Sys-

tematic Review," *Journal of Clinical Medicine* 8, no. 1 (January 2019): 56, https://doi.org/10.3390/jcm8010056.

7. Ranit Mishori et al., "The Little Tissue That Couldn't—Dispelling Myths about the Hymen's Role in Determining Sexual History and Assault," *Reproductive Health* 16 (2019): 74, https://doi.org/10.1186/s12978-019-0731-8.
8. Centers for Disease Control and Prevention, "Key Statistics from the National Survey of Family Growth," https://www.cdc.gov/nchs/nsfg/key_statistics/s-keystat.htm#vaginalsexual.
9. "Sexual Journeys," DrEd, 2018, https://www.zavamed.com/uk/sexual-journeys.html.
10. Bethy Squires, "How Lesbians Lose Their Virginity," *Vice*, June 15, 2016, https://www.vice.com/en/article/pg77e9/how-lesbians-lose-their-virginity.
11. Esther D. Rothblum et al., "Asexual and Non-Asexual Respondents from a U.S. Population-Based Study of Sexual Minorities," *Archives of Sexual Behavior* 49, no. 2 (2020): 757–67, https://doi.org/10.1007/s10508-019-01485-0.
12. Susan Estrich, "Rape," *Yale Law Journal* 95, no. 6 (May 1986): 1087–184, https://doi.org/10.2307/796522.
13. "Sexual Consent," Planned Parenthood, 2020, https://www.plannedparenthood.org/learn/relationships/sexual-consent.
14. "Sexual Assault," United States Department of Justice, https://www.justice.gov/ovw/sexual-assault.
15. "An Updated Definition of Rape," United States Department of Justice blog, January 6, 2012, https://www.justice.gov/archives/opa/blog/updated-definition-rape.
16. "About the National Sexual Assault Telephone Hotline," Rape, Abuse & Incest National Network, https://rainn.org/about-national-sexual-assault-telephone-hotline.
17. "Q&A on 'Blue Ball' Syndrome," Sexual Medicine Society of North America, https://www.smsna.org/patients/did-you-know/q-a-on-blue-ball-syndrome.
18. "Virile," Dictionary.com, https://www.dictionary.com/browse/virile.
19. "Slut," Thesaurus.com, https://www.thesaurus.com/browse/slut.
20. Michael J. Marks, Tara M. Young, and Yuliana Zaikman, "The Sex-

ual Double Standard in the Real World," *Social Psychology* 50, no. 2 (March 2019): 67–79, https://doi.org/10.1027/1864-9335/a000362.

21. Kirstin R. Mitchell et al., "Why Do Men Report More Opposite-Sex Sexual Partners than Women? Analysis of the Gender Discrepancy in a British National Probability Survey," *Journal of Sex Research* 56, no. 1 (2018): 1–8, https://doi.org/10.1080/00224499.2018.1481193.
22. Kim Parker, Juliana Menasce Horowitz, and Renee Stepler, "2. Americans See Different Expectations for Men and Women," Pew Research Center, December 5, 2017, https://www.pewresearch.org/social-trends/2017/12/05/americans-see-different-expectations-for-men-and-women/.
23. "What's Risky Sex?," WebMD, 2020, https://www.webmd.com/sex-relationships/features/promiscuity-differs-by-gender.
24. "Key Statistics from the National Survey of Family Growth—N Listing," National Center for Health Statistics, Centers for Disease Control and Prevention, November 8, 2021, https://www.cdc.gov/nchs/nsfg/key_statistics/n-keystat.htm.
25. "What's Your Number?," Superdrug Online Doctor, https://onlinedoctor.superdrug.com/whats-your-number/.
26. Jean M. Twenge, Ryne A. Sherman, and Brooke E. Wells, "Declines in Sexual Frequency among American Adults, 1989–2014," *Archives of Sexual Behavior* 46, no. 8 (2017): 2389–401, https://doi.org/10.1007/s10508-017-0953-1.
27. David Farley Hurlbert and Karen Elizabeth Whittaker, "The Role of Masturbation in Marital and Sexual Satisfaction: A Comparative Study of Female Masturbators and Nonmasturbators," *Journal of Sex Education and Therapy* 17, no. 4 (1991): 272–82, https://doi.org/10.1080/01614576.1991.11074029.
28. "The Global Sex Index," From Mars, 2021, https://www.frommars.com/the-global-sex-index.
29. Hayden Chakra, "The Way Sexual Acts Were Treated in the Medieval Ages Will Make You Feel Free Today," *About History*, February 12, 2021, https://about-history.com/sex-in-medieval-ages/.
30. "What Is Kama Sutra?," WebMD, 2021, https://www.webmd.com/sex/what-is-kama-sutra.
31. Debby Herbenick, et al., "Sexual Diversity in the United States: Re-

sults from a Nationally Representative Probability Sample of Adult Women and Men," *PLoS ONE* 12, no. 7 (2017): e0181198, https://doi.org/10.1371/journal.pone.0181198.

32. "Sexual Diversity in the United States: Results from a Nationally Representative Probability Sample of Adult Women and Men," *PLOS One* 12, no. 7 (2017), https://doi.org/10.1371/journal.pone.0181198.
33. Christian C. Joyal and Julie Carpentier, "The Prevalence of Paraphilic Interests and Behaviors in the General Population: A Provincial Survey," *Journal of Sex Research* 54, no. 2 (2017): 161–71, https://doi.org/10.1080/00224499.2016.1139034;Christian C. Joyal et al., "What Exactly Is an Unusual Sexual Fantasy?," *Journal of Sexual Medicine* 12, no. 2 (February 2015): 328–40, https://doi.org/10.1111/jsm.12734.
34. Heidi Stevens, "Americans' No. 1 Sexual Fantasy? Survey Says . . ." *Chicago Tribune*, July 30, 2018, https://www.chicagotribune.com/columns/heidi-stevens/ct-life-stevens-Monday-americans-sexual-fantasies-0730-story.html.
35. Herbenick et al., "Sexual Diversity in the United States."
36. Tyler Schmall, "Your Partner Probably Wants a Kinkier Sex Life," *New York Post*, January 31, 2018, https://nypost.com/2018/01/31/your-partner-probably-wants-a-kinkier-sex-life/.
37. Lien Holvoet et al., "Fifty Shades of Belgian Gray: The Prevalence of BDSM-Related Fantasies and Activities in the General Population," *Journal of Sexual Medicine* 14, no. 9 (September 2017): 1152–59, https://doi.org/10.1016/j.jsxm.2017.07.003.
38. Wendy Rose Gould, "How BDSM Might Benefit Your Health and Improve Your Relationship," Verywell Mind, April 28, 2021, https://www.verywellmind.com/how-bdsm-might-benefit-your-health-and-your-relationship-4846462.

Chapter 2: Is Down There Normal?

Too Hairy, Too Long, Too Big, Too Small (We'll Cover It All)

1. Victoria Waldersee, "Half of Brits Don't Know Where the Vagina Is—And It's Not Just the Men," YouGov, March 8, 2019, https://

yougov.co.uk/topics/health/articles-reports/2019/03/08/half-brits-don't-know-where-vagina-and-its-not-just.

2. "25% of Women Can't Correctly Identify Vagina (Infographic)," Intimina blog, November 10, 2020, https://www.intimina.com/blog/women-and-their-bodies/.
3. "'Sexist' Sex Ed: The Teachers Who Won't Say 'Vagina,'" *Tes Magazine*, August 29, 2019, https://www.tes.com/magazine/archive/sexist-sex-ed-teachers-who-wont-say-vagina.
4. Calla Wahlquist, "The Sole Function of the Clitoris Is Female Orgasm. Is That Why It's Ignored by Medical Science?," *Guardian*, October 31, 2020, https://www.theguardian.com/lifeandstyle/2020/nov/01/the-sole-function-of-the-clitoris-is-female-orgasm-is-that-why-its-ignored-by-medical-science.
5. Rachel E. Gross, "The Clitoris, Uncovered: An Intimate History," *Scientific American*, March 4, 2020, https://www.scientificamerican.com/article/the-clitoris-uncovered-an-intimate-history/.
6. Lucy Bellerby, "If You Can't Say the Word 'Vagina,' How Are You Ever Going to Own One Responsibly?," *Independent*, August 17, 2015, https://www.independent.co.uk/voices/if-you-can-t-say-the-word-vagina-how-are-you-ever-going-to-own-one-responsibly-10459493.html.
7. Benjamin VanHoose, "Ellen Pompeo Recalls Not Being Allowed to Say 'Vagina' on *Grey's Anatomy*: 'There Was a Big Fight,'" *People*, November 13, 2020, https://people.com/tv/ellen-pompeo-recalls-greys-anatomy-censorship/.
8. "Saying the Word Vagina Is Not Brave, It's Normal," Eve Appeal blog, 2019, https://eveappeal.org.uk/blog/saying-word-vagina-not-brave-normal/.
9. Franny White, "Pleasure-Producing Human Clitoris Has More than 10,000 Nerve Fibers," OHSU News, October 27, 2022, https://news.ohsu.edu/2022/10/27/peasure-producing-human-clitoris-has-more-than-10-000-nerve-fibers.
10. Theresa M. Wizemann and Mary Lou Pardue, *Exploring the Biological Contributions to Human Health: Does Sex Matter?* (Washington, DC: National Academies Press, 2001); Mary Jane Sherfey, "Some Biology of Sexuality," *Journal of Sex & Marital Therapy* 1, no. 2 (1974): 97–109, https://doi.org/10.1080/00926237408405278.

11. Jillian Lloyd et al., "Female Genital Appearance: 'Normality' Unfolds," *BJOG: An International Journal of Obstetrics & Gynaecology* 112, no. 5 (May 2005): 643–46, https://doi.org/10.1111/j.1471-0528.2004.00517.x; "Clitoris," Topics, ScienceDirect, https://www.sciencedirect.com/topics/medicine-and-dentistry/clitoris; Joseph A. Kelling et al., "Anatomical Dissection of the Dorsal Nerve of the Clitoris," *Aesthetic Surgery Journal* 40, no. 5 (May 2020): 541–47, https://doi.org/10.1093/asj/sjz330.
12. Susan H. Oakley et al., "Clitoral Size and Location in Relation to Sexual Function Using Pelvic MRI," *Journal of Sexual Medicine* 11, no. 4 (April 2014): 1013–22, https://doi.org/10.1111/jsm.12450.
13. G. E. Tagatz et al., "The Clitoral Index: A Bioassay of Androgenic Stimulation," *Obstetrics and Gynecology* 54, no. 5 (November 1979): 562–64, https://pubmed.ncbi.nlm.nih.gov/503381/.
14. Naomi Russo, "The Still-Misunderstood Shape of the Clitoris," *Atlantic*, March 9, 2017, https://www.theatlantic.com/health/archive/2017/03/3d-clitoris/518991/.
15. Pedro Vieira-Baptista et al., "Women without Vulvodynia Can Have a Positive 'Q-Tip Test': A Cross Sectional Study," *Journal of Psychosomatic Obstetrics & Gynecology* 38, no. 4 (2017): 256–59, https://doi.org/10.1080/0167482x.2017.1327519.
16. E. J. Dickson, "The Dangerous Rise of Vaginal Lightening," *Vox*, December 6, 2018, https://www.vox.com/the-goods/2018/12/6/18127154/vaginal-bleaching-lightening-creams.
17. Miranda Farage and Howard Maibach, "Lifetime Changes in the Vulva and Vagina," *Archives of Gynecology and Obstetrics* 273, no. 4 (2006): 195–202, https://doi.org/10.1007/s00404-005-0079-x.
18. "18 U.S.C. 116—Female Genital Mutilation," GovInfo.gov, https://www.gpo.gov/fdsys/granule/USCODE-2011-title18/USCODE-2011-title18-partI-chap7-sec116.
19. Sara Ramsey et al., "Pubic Hair and Sexuality: A Review," *Journal of Sexual Medicine* 6, no. 8 (2009): 2102–10, https://doi.org/10.1111/j.1743-6109.2009.01307.x.
20. Jesse Bering, "A Bushel of Facts about the Uniqueness of Human Pubic Hair," *Scientific American*, March 1, 2010, https://blogs.scientificamerican.com/bering-in-mind/a-bushel-of-facts-about-the-uniqueness-of-human-pubic-hair/.

21. P. B. Pendergrass et al., "The Shape and Dimensions of the Human Vagina as Seen in Three-Dimensional Vinyl Polysiloxane Casts," *Gynecologic and Obstetric Investigation* 42, no. 3 (February 1996): 178–82, https://doi.org/10.1159/000291946.
22. Elizabeth Siegel, "Vaginal Rejuvenation Is on the Rise, but the Results Don't Always Live Up to the Hype," *Allure*, March 27, 2019, https://www.allure.com/story/vaginal-rejuvenation-treatment-results-efficacy.
23. "Vaginal Rejuvenation Market Size, Share & Trends Analysis by Treatment Type (Reconstructive Vaginal Rejuvenation, Cosmetic Vaginal Rejuvenation) and Segment Forecasts, 2022–2030," Grand View Research, June 3, 2022, https://www.grandviewresearch.com/industry-analysis/vaginal-rejuvenation-market.
24. Heather Grey, "Why Do Some Women Undergo Vaginal Rejuvenation?," Healthline, September 15, 2017, https://www.healthline.com/health-news/why-some-women-undergo-vaginal-rejuvenation#Frank-discussion-is-needed.
25. Turkia Abbed et al., "Labiaplasty: Current Trends of ASAPS Members," *Aesthetic Surgery Journal* 38, no. 8 (August 2018): 114–17, https://academic.oup.com/asj/article/38/8/NP114/5009390.
26. Annemette Wildfang Lykkebo et al., "The Size of Labia Minora and Perception of Genital Appearance: A Cross-Sectional Study," *Journal of Lower Genital Tract Disease* 21, no. 3 (July 2017): 198–203, https://doi.org/10.1097/lgt.0000000000000308.
27. Devan Stahl and Christian J. Vercler, "What Should Be the Surgeon's Role in Defining 'Normal' Genital Appearance?," *AMA Journal of Ethics* 20, no. 4 (2018): 384–91, https://doi.org/10.1001/journalofethics.2018.20.4.msoc4-1804.
28. "Vaginal Rejuvenation, Labiaplasty, and Other Female Genital Cosmetic Surgery," American College of Obstetricians and Gynecologists, April 2021, https://www.acog.org/womens-health/faqs/vaginal-rejuvenation-labiaplasty-and-other-female-genital-cosmetic-surgery.
29. Aesthetic Society, https://www.theaestheticsociety.org/.
30. A. Dubinskaya et al., "Female Genitalia in Pornography: The Source of Labiaplasty Trends?," *Journal of Sexual Medicine* 19, no. 4 (April 2022): 21–22, https://doi.org/10.1016/j.jsxm.2022.01.051.
31. Kristin Hall, "Selling Sexual Certainty? Advertising Lysol as a Con-

traceptive in the United States and Canada, 1919–1939," *Enterprise & Society* 14, no. 1 (March 2013): 71–98, https://doi.org/10.1093/es/khs041.

32. Nicole Pasulka, "When Women Used Lysol as Birth Control," *Mother Jones*, March 8, 2012, https://www.motherjones.com/media/2012/03/when-women-used-lysol-birth-control/.
33. "An Updated Review of Evidence to Discourage Douching," *MCN: The American Journal of Maternal/Child Nursing* 35, no. 2 (March 2010): 108–9, https://doi.org/10.1097/01.nmc.0000369403.02659.2b.
34. Erkan Alataş et al., "Laparoscopic Management of a Primary Ectopic Ovarian Pregnancy and Vaginal Douching as a Possible Cause," *Archives of Gynecology and Obstetrics* 277, no. 4 (September 2008): 363–65, https://doi.org/10.1007/s00404-007-0464-8.
35. Julie Morse, "Why Douching Won't Die," *Atlantic*, April 21, 2015, https://www.theatlantic.com/health/archive/2015/04/why-douching-wont-die/390198/.
36. "Douching," Office on Women's Health, US Department of Health & Human Services, February 22, 2021, https://www.womenshealth.gov/a-z-topics/douching.
37. Michelle Ferranti, "An Odor of Racism: Vaginal Deodorants in African-American Beauty Culture and Advertising," *Advertising & Society Review* 11, no. 4 (2011), https://doi.org/10.1353/asr.2011.0003; M. Diane McKee et al., "Vaginal Douching among Latinas: Practices and Meaning," *Maternal and Child Health Journal* 13 (2009): 98–106, https://doi.org/10.1007/s10995-008-0327-3.

Chapter 3: Is My Libido Normal?

Why It's Normal to Be in the Mood, Not in the Mood, and in the Mood for Chocolate

1. "Queering Reproductive Health, Rights & Justice," National LGBTQ Task Force, May 5, 2022, https://www.thetaskforce.org/reproductive-justice/.
2. Rosemary Basson et al., "Assessment and Management of Women's Sexual Dysfunctions: Problematic Desire and Arousal," *Journal of*

Sexual Medicine 2, no. 3 (May 2005): 291–300, https://pubmed.ncbi.nlm.nih.gov/16422860/.

3. "Sexual Violence Is Preventable," Centers for Disease Control and Prevention, July 5, 2022, https://www.cdc.gov/injury/features/sexual-violence/index.html; and Rebecca L. Stotzer, "Violence against Transgender People: A Review of United States Data," *Aggression and Violent Behavior* 14, no. 3 (May–June 2009): 170–79, https://doi.org/10.1016/j.avb.2009.01.006.
4. Rakibul M. Islam et al., "Safety and Efficacy of Testosterone for Women: A Systematic Review and Meta-Analysis of Randomised Controlled Trial Data," *Lancet Diabetes & Endocrinology* 7, no. 10 (October 2019): 754–66, https://doi.org/10.1016/s2213-8587(19)30189-5.
5. "The Dual Control Model of Sexual Response," Kinsey Institute, 2020, https://kinseyinstitute.org/research/dual-control-model.php.
6. Deanna Carpenter et al., "The Sexual Inhibition/Sexual Excitation Scales—Short Form (SIS/SES-SF)," in Terri D. Fisher et al., eds., *Handbook of Sexuality-Related Measures*, 4th ed. (New York: Routledge, 2019); Robin R. Milhausen et al., "Sexual Excitation/Sexual Inhibition Inventory for Women and Men," *Archives of Sexual Behavior* 39, no. 5 (2010): 1091–104, https://doi.org/10.1037/t70809-000; Cynthia A. Graham, Stephanie A. Sanders, and Robin R. Milhausen, "The Sexual Excitation/Sexual Inhibition Inventory for Women: Psychometric Properties," *Archives of Sexual Behavior* 35, no. 4 (2006): 397–409, https://doi.org/10.1007/s10508-006-9041-7.
7. "Allostatic Load," Topics, ScienceDirect, https://www.sciencedirect.com/topics/neuroscience/allostatic-load.
8. Susan R. Davis et al., "Circulating Androgen Levels and Self-Reported Sexual Function in Women," *Journal of the American Medical Association* 294, no. 1 (2005): 91–96, https://doi.org/10.1001/jama.294.1.91.
9. Kwangsung Park, et al., "Diabetes Induced Alteration of Clitoral Hemodynamics and Structure in the Rabbit," *Journal of Urology* 168, no. 3 (September 2002): 1269–72, https://pubmed.ncbi.nlm.nih.gov/12187280/.
10. "General Information/Press Room," American Thyroid Association, 2018, https://www.thyroid.org/media-main/press-room
11. Sarah Wåhlin-Jacobsen et al., "Is There a Correlation between Andro-

gens and Sexual Desire in Women?," *Journal of Sexual Medicine* 12, no. 2 (February 2015): 358–73, https://doi.org/10.1111/jsm.12774.

12. Laura Mernone, Serena Fiacco, and Ulrike Ehlert, "Psychobiological Factors of Sexual Functioning in Aging Women—Findings from the Women 40+ Healthy Aging Study," *Frontiers in Psychology* 10 (2019): 546, https://doi.org/10.3389/fpsyg.2019.00546.
13. Carola S. Scheffers et al., "Dehydroepiandrosterone for Women in the Peri- or Postmenopausal Phase," *Cochrane Database of Systematic Reviews* 2015, no. 1: CD011066, https://doi.org/10.1002/14651858.cd011066.pub2.
14. Bennink Coelingh et al., "Maintaining Physiological Testosterone Levels by Adding Dehydroepiandrosterone to Combined Oral Contraceptives: I. Endocrine Effects," *Contraception* 96, no. 5 (2017): 322–29, https://doi.org/10.1016/j.contraception.2016.06.022.
15. B. A. Arnow et al., "Women with Hypoactive Sexual Desire Disorder Compared to Normal Females: A Functional Magnetic Resonance Imaging Study," *Neuroscience* 158, no. 2 (2009): 484–502, https://doi.org/10.1016/j.neuroscience.2008.09.044.

Chapter 4: Are My Orgasms Normal?

Putting the "O" in Oh, Uh-Oh, and OMG

1. Siofra Brennan, "Revealed: The Most Googled Sex Question Involves Locating the G-Spot," Daily Mail, Associated Newspapers, September 21, 2017, https://www.dailymail.co.uk/femail/article-4906366/Most-googled-sex-question-involves-finding-G-spot.html.
2. Zahra Salmani et al., "The Existing Therapeutic Interventions for Orgasmic Disorders: Recommendations for Culturally Competent Services, Narrative Review," *Iranian Journal of Reproductive Medicine* 13, no. 7 (July 2015), https://www.ncbi.nlm.nih.gov/pmc/articles/PMC4609319/.
3. Jennifer E. Frank, Patricia Mistretta, and Joshua Will, "Diagnosis and Treatment of Female Sexual Dysfunction," *American Family Physician* 77, no. 5 (2008), https://www.aafp.org/afp/2008/0301/p635.html.

4. Bangshowbiz.com, "Nicki Minaj Demands Orgasms," *Washington Post*, May 29, 2015, https://www.washingtonpost.com/entertainment/nicki-minaj-demands-orgasms/2015/05/29/1978abcc-0668-11e5-93f4-f24d4af7f97d_story.html.
5. David A. Frederick et al., "Differences in Orgasm Frequency among Gay, Lesbian, Bisexual, and Heterosexual Men and Women in a U.S. National Sample," *Archives of Sexual Behavior* 47, no. 1 (2018): 273–88, https://doi.org/10.1007/s10508-017-0939-z.
6. "Defining Sexual Health," 2020, World Health Organization, https://www.who.int/teams/sexual-and-reproductive-health-and-research/key-areas-of-work/sexual-health/defining-sexual-health; "The Pleasure Project," The Pleasure Project, https://thepleasureproject.org/.
7. Mirela Zaneva et al., "What Is the Added Value of Incorporating Pleasure in Sexual Health Interventions? A Systematic Review and Meta-Analysis," *PLOS One* 17, no. 2 (2022): e0261034, https://doi.org/10.1371/journal.pone.0261034.
8. Kathrin F. Stanger-Hall and David W. Hall, "Abstinence-Only Education and Teen Pregnancy Rates: Why We Need Comprehensive Sex Education in the U.S.," *PLOS One* 6, no. 10 (2011): e24658, https://doi.org/10.1371/journal.pone.0024658.
9. Cindy M. Meston et al., "Women's Orgasm," *Annual Review of Sex Research* 15, no. 1 (2004): 173–257, https://kinseyinstitute.org/pdf/womens%20orgasm%20annual%20review.pdf.
10. "Should Men Worry about Dry Orgasms?," Sexual Medicine Society of North America, March 15, 2016. https://www.smsna.org/patients/blog/should-men-worry-about-dry-orgasms.
11. Ellen Belle Vance and Nathaniel N. Wagner, "Written Descriptions of Orgasm: A Study of Sex Differences," *Archives of Sexual Behavior* 5, no. 1 (1976): 87–98, https://doi.org/10.1007/bf01542242.
12. Lynsey Hope, "Women's Orgasms Last 51 Seconds & Men Think about Sex 19 Times a Day—Sex Drive Differences Revealed," *U.S. Sun*, April 13, 2021. https://www.the-sun.com/lifestyle/2697001/women-orgasms-51-seconds-men-think-19-times/; "Everything You Need to Know about Orgasms," Medical News Today, January 7, 2022, International, https://www.medicalnewstoday.com/articles/232318.
13. "25 Facts about Orgasms," *Cosmopolitan*, April 19, 2022, https://www

.cosmopolitan.com/uk/love-sex/sex/tips/g1709/25-facts-about-orgasms-101542/?slide=2.

14. Stanislav Kratochvíl, "Trvání zenského orgasmu [The Duration of Female Orgasm]," *Ceskoslovenska Psychiatrie* 89, no. 5 (1993): 296–99, https://pubmed.ncbi.nlm.nih.gov/8269524/.
15. Antti Dahlberg et al., "Sexual Activity and Satisfaction in Men with Traumatic Spinal Cord Lesion," *Journal of Rehabilitation Medicine* 39, no. 2 (2007): 152–55, https://pubmed.ncbi.nlm.nih.gov/17351698/.
16. Stephen Matthews, "7 In 10 Women Can Climax More than Once during Sex." Daily Mail Online. Associated Newspapers, April 10, 2017. https://www.dailymail.co.uk/health/article-4397674/7-10-women-climax-sex.html.
17. Gayle Brewer and Colin A. Hendrie, "Evidence to Suggest That Copulatory Vocalizations in Women Are Not a Reflexive Consequence of Orgasm," *Archives of Sexual Behavior* 40, no. 3 (2011): 559–64, https://link.springer.com/article/10.1007/s10508-010-9632-1.
18. Erin B. Cooper, Allan Fenigstein, and Robert L. Fauber, "The Faking Orgasm Scale for Women: Psychometric Properties," *Archives of Sexual Behavior* 43, no. 3 (April 2014): 423–35, https://doi.org/10.1007/s10508-013-0212-z.
19. Erin B. Cooper, Allan Fenigstein, and Robert L. Fauber, "The Faking Orgasm Scale for Women: Psychometric Properties," *Archives of Sexual Behavior* 43, no. 3 (2013): 423–35, https://doi.org/10.1007/s10508-013-0212-z.
20. David A. Frederick et al. "Differences in Orgasm Frequency among Gay, Lesbian, Bisexual, and Heterosexual Men and Women in a U.S. National Sample," *Archives of Sexual Behavior* 47, no. 1 (2017): 273–88, https://doi.org/10.1007/s10508-017-0939-z.
21. Lisa Wade, Emily Kremer, and Jessica Brown, "The Incidental Orgasm: The Presence of Clitoral Knowledge and the Absence of Orgasm for Women," *Women & Health* 42, no. 1 (2017): 117–38, https://pubmed.ncbi.nlm.nih.gov/16418125/.
22. Ian Kerner, *The Cliterate Male: A Primer on Pleasuring Women* (Good in Bed Guides, 2018). https://www.goodreads.com/book/show/18920564-the-cliterate-male.
23. Shere Hite. *The Hite Report* (Australia: Summit Books, 1977).

24. Alfred C. Kinsey et al., *Sexual Behavior in the Human Female* (Philadelphia: W.B. Saunders, 1953).
25. Justin J. Lehmiller, *Tell Me What You Want: The Science of Sexual Desire and How It Can Help You Improve Your Sex Life* (New York: Hachette Go, 2020).
26. David Rowland and Brittany R. Gutierrez, "Phases of the Sexual Response Cycle," *Psychology Faculty Publications (2007)*, 62, https://scholar.valpo.edu/psych_fac_pub/62/.
27. Cesare Battaglia et al., "Menstrual Cycle-Related Morphometric and Vascular Modifications of the Clitoris," *Journal of Sexual Medicine* 5, no. 12 (2008): 2853–61, https://doi.org/10.1111/j.1743-6109.2008.00972.x.
28. David L. Rowland et al., "Orgasmic Latency and Related Parameters in Women during Partnered and Masturbatory Sex," *Journal of Sexual Medicine* 15, no. 10 (2018): 1463–71, https://doi.org/10.1016/j.jsxm.2018.08.003.
29. Marika J. Hess and Sigmund Hough, "Impact of Spinal Cord Injury on Sexuality: Broad-Based Clinical Practice Intervention and Practical Application," *Journal of Spinal Cord Medicine* 35, no. 4 (2012): 211–18, https://doi.org/10.1179/2045772312y.0000000025.
30. Kinsey et al., *Sexual Behavior in the Human Female.*
31. Mary Burleson, Wenda R. Trevathan, and W. Larry Gregory, "Sexual Behavior in Lesbian and Heterosexual Women: Relations with Menstrual Cycle Phase and Partner Availability," *Psychoneuroendocrinology* 27, no. 4 (May 2002):489–503, https://asu.pure.elsevier.com/en/publications/sexual-behavior-in-lesbian-and-heterosexual-women-relations-with-; Susan B. Bullivant et al., "Women's Sexual Experience During the Menstrual Cycle: Identification of the Sexual Phase by Noninvasive Measurement of Luteinizing Hormone," *Journal of Sex Research* 41, no. 1 (2004):82–93, https://www.tandfonline.com/doi/abs/10.1080/00224490409552216; James R. Roney and Zachary L. Simmons, "Hormonal Predictors of Sexual Motivation in Natural Menstrual Cycles," *Hormones and Behavior* 63, no. 4 (2013): 636–45, https://labs.psych.ucsb.edu/roney/james/roneysimmons.published.pdf.
32. Kim Wallen and Elisabeth A. Lloyd, "Female Sexual Arousal: Genital

Anatomy and Orgasm in Intercourse," *Hormones and Behavior* 59, no. 5 (May 2011): 780–92, https://doi.org/10.1016/j.yhbeh.2010.12.004.

33. Michael Castleman, "The Truth about Vaginal Orgasms," *Psychology Today*, May 2, 2021, https://www.psychologytoday.com/us/blog/all-about-sex/202105/the-truth-about-vaginal-orgasms.
34. Pedro Vieira-Baptista et al., "G-Spot: Fact or Fiction? A Systematic Review," *Sexual Medicine* 9, no. 5 (2021): 100435, https://doi.org/10.1016/j.esxm.2021.100435.
35. Barry R. Komisaruk et al., "Women's Clitoris, Vagina, and Cervix Mapped on the Sensory Cortex: fMRI Evidence," *Journal of Sexual Medicine* 8, no. 10 (2011): 2822–30, https://doi.org/10.1111/j.1743-6109.2011.02388.x; Louisa Thompson, "The Uterus," TeachMeAnatomy, May 12, 2019, https://teachmeanatomy.info/pelvis/female-reproductive-tract/uterus/.
36. Komisaruk et al., "Women's Clitoris."
37. Barbara L. Wells, "Predictors of Female Nocturnal Orgasms: A Multivariate Analysis," *Journal of Sex Research* 22, no. 4 (1986): 421–37, http://www.jstor.org/stable/3812289.
38. Debra Herbenick and J. Dennis Fortenberry, "Exercise-Induced Orgasm and Pleasure among Women," *Sexual and Relationship Therapy* 26, no. 4 (2011): 373–88, https://doi.org/10.1080/14681994.2011.647902.
39. Gabby Landsverk, "As Many as 1 in 10 Women Have Accidentally Orgasmed during a Workout. A Sex Researcher Reveals Which Exercises Are the Most Arousing," *Insider*, August 1, 2019, https://www.insider.com/crunches-climbing-and-other-core-exercises-can-cause-orgasms-2019-7.
40. Beverly Whipple, Gina Ogden, and Barry R. Komisaruk. "Physiological Correlates of Imagery-Induced Orgasm in Women," *Archives of Sexual Behavior* 21, no. 2 (1992): 121–33, https://doi.org/10.1007/bf01542589.
41. William H. Masters and Virginia E. Johnson, *Human Sexual Response* (Boston: Little, Brown, 1976).
42. Ina May Gaskin, *Ina May's Guide to Childbirth* (New York: Bantam, 2003).
43. Denise Bijlenga et al., "Prevalence of Sexual Dysfunctions and Other

Sexual Disorders in Adults with Attention-Deficit/Hyperactivity Disorder Compared to the General Population," *ADHD Attention Deficit and Hyperactivity Disorders* 10, no. 1 (2018): 87–96, https://pubmed.ncbi.nlm.nih.gov/28831742/.

44. "Orgasmic Dysfunction in Women," MedlinePlus, U.S. National Library of Medicine, https://medlineplus.gov/ency/article/001953.htm; Raymond C. Rosen, "Prevalence and Risk Factors of Sexual Dysfunction in Men and Women," *Current Psychiatry Reports* 2, no. 3 (June 2000): 189–95, https://doi.org/10.1007/s11920-996-0006-2.
45. "Elective Female Genital Cosmetic Surgery," American College of Obstetricians and Gynecologists, January 2020, https://www.acog.org/clinical/clinical-guidance/committee-opinion/articles/2020/01/elective-female-genital-cosmetic-surgery; "Labiaplasty," Cleveland Clinic, https://my.clevelandclinic.org/health/treatments/21953-labiaplasty#risks--benefits.
46. Erica Marchand, "Psychological and Behavioral Treatment of Female Orgasmic Disorder," *Sexual Medicine Reviews* 9, no. 2 (April 2021): 194–211, https://doi.org/10.1016/j.sxmr.2020.07.007.
47. Rachel Baxter, "What Is Postcoital Dysphoria ('Post-Sex Blues')?," International Society for Sexual Medicine, December 1, 2015, https://www.issm.info/sexual-health-qa/what-is-postcoital-dysphoria-post-sex-blues/.
48. Arielle Tschinkel, "12 Unexpected Health Benefits of Orgasms," *Insider*, March 1, 2019, https://www.insider.com/orgasm-health-benefits-2018-11.
49. Nan J. Wise, Eleni Frangos, and Barry R. Komisaruk. "Brain Activity Unique to Orgasm in Women: An fMRI Analysis," *Journal of Sexual Medicine* 14, no. 11 (2017): 1380–91, https://doi.org/10.1016/j.jsxm.2017.08.014.
50. Michele Lastella et al., "Sex and Sleep: Perceptions of Sex as a Sleep Promoting Behavior in the General Adult Population," *Frontiers in Public Health* 7 (2019), https://doi.org/10.3389/fpubh.2019.00033.
51. Merissa Nathan Gerson, "How Orgasm Could Dull Pain," *Atlantic*, May 12, 2014, https://www.theatlantic.com/health/archive/2014/05/how-orgasm-could-dull-pain/361470/.

52. George Davey Smith and Stephen Frankel, "Sex and Death: Are They Related? Findings from the Caerphilly Cohort Study," in George Davey Smith, ed., *Health Inequalities* (Bristol, UK: Policy Press, 2003), 369–80, https://doi.org/10.51952/9781447342229.ch029.
53. Jessica DeFino, "Can You Orgasm Your Way to Better Skin? I Tried," *Marie Claire*, October 18, 2018, https://www.marieclaire.com/beauty/a23727184/orgasm-skin-effects/.
54. "Sex 'Key' to Staying Young," BBC News,October 10, 2000, http://news.bbc.co.uk/2/hi/uk_news/scotland/965045.stm.
55. Winnifred B. Cutler, Celso R. Garcia, and Abba M. Krieger, "Sexual Behavior Frequency and Menstrual Cycle Length in Mature Premenopausal Women," *Psychoneuroendocrinology* 4, no. 4 (1979): 297–309, https://doi.org/10.1016/0306-4530(79)90014-3.
56. Anke Hambach et al., "The Impact of Sexual Activity on Idiopathic Headaches: An Observational Study," *Cephalalgia* 33, no. 6 (2013): 384–89, https://doi.org/10.1177/0333102413476374.
57. Mariana C. Biermann et al., "Reasons to Pretend Orgasm, Mate Retention, and Relationship Satisfaction in Brazilian Women," *Evolutionary Psychology* 19, no. 3 (2021): 147470492110329, https://doi.org/10.1177/14747049211032939.
58. Kerstin Uvnäs-Moberg and Maria Petersson, "Oxytocin, ein Vermittler von Antistress, Wohlbefinden, sozialer Interaktion, Wachstum und Heilung [Oxytocin, a Mediator of Anti-Stress, Well-Being, Social Interaction, Growth and Healing]," *Zeitschrift für Psychosomatische Medizin und Psychotherapie* 51, no. 1 (2005): 57–80, https://doi.org/10.13109/zptm.2005.51.1.57; Shari Young Kuchenbecker et al. "Oxytocin, Cortisol, and Cognitive Control during Acute and Naturalistic Stress," *Stress* 24, no. 4 (2021): 370–83, https://doi.org/10.1080/10253890.2021.1876658.
59. Stuart Brody and Tillmann H. C. Krüger, "The Post-Orgasmic Prolactin Increase following Intercourse Is Greater than Following Masturbation and Suggests Greater Satiety," *Biological Psychology* 71, no. 3 (2006): 312–15, https://doi.org/10.1016/j.biopsycho.2005.06.008.
60. Sari M. van Anders et al., "Associations between Testosterone Secretion and Sexual Activity in Women," *Hormones and Behavior* 51, no. 4 (2007): 477–82, https://pubmed.ncbi.nlm.nih.gov/17320881/.

61. Debra Herbenick et al., "Women's Experiences with Genital Touching, Sexual Pleasure, and Orgasm: Results from a U.S. Probability Sample of Women Ages 18 to 94," *Journal of Sex & Marital Therapy* 44, no. 2 (2017): 201–12, https://doi.org/10.1080/0092623x.2017.1346530.
62. Zlatko Pastor, "Female Ejaculation Orgasm vs. Coital Incontinence: A Systematic Review," *Journal of Sexual Medicine* 10, no. 7 (2013): 1682–91, https://doi.org/10.1111/jsm.12166.
63. "Orgasms," Planned Parenthood, 2020, https://www.plannedparenthood.org/learn/sex-pleasure-and-sexual-dysfunction/sex-and-pleasure/orgasms.
64. Samuel Salama et al., "Nature and Origin of 'Squirting' in Female Sexuality," *Journal of Sexual Medicine* 12, no. 3 (2015): 661–66, https://doi.org/10.1111/jsm.12799.
65. Kelly Gonsalves, "Yes, Squirting Is Real: The Research on Female Ejaculation & What Squirt Is," *MindBodyGreen*, June 25, 2021, https://www.mindbodygreen.com/articles/is-squirting-real-research.
66. Zlatko Pastor and Roman Chmel, "Differential Diagnostics of Female 'Sexual' Fluids: A Narrative Review," *International Urogynecology Journal* 29, no. 5 (2017): 621–29, https://doi.org/10.1007/s00192-017-3527-9.
67. Florian Wimpissinger, Christopher Springer, and Walter Stackl, "International Online Survey: Female Ejaculation Has a Positive Impact on Women's and Their Partners' Sexual Lives," *BJU International* 112, no. 2 (2013), https://doi.org/10.1111/j.1464-410x.2012.11562.x.
68. R. Robin Baker and Mark A. Bellis, "Human Sperm Competition: Ejaculate Manipulation by Females and a Function for the Female Orgasm," in Todd K. Shackelford and Nicholas Pound, eds., *Sperm Competition in Humans* (Boston: Springer, 1993), 177–210, https://doi.org/10.1007/978-0-387-28039-4_11.
69. Joseph Lindberg, *Kama Sutra: 100 Sex Positions with Photos and Explanations* (self-pub, 2017).
70. Jill Hamilton, "37 Truly Mind-Blowing Lesbian Sex Positions," *Cosmopolitan*, June 16, 2021, https://www.cosmopolitan.com/sex-love/positions/g4090/mind-blowing-lesbian-sex-positions/.
71. Debby Herbenick, "Women's Experiences with Genital Touching, Sexual Pleasure, and Orgasm: Results from a U.S. Probability Sample

of Women Ages 18 to 94," *Journal of Sex & Marital Therapy* 44, no. 2 (2018): 201–212, https://doi.org/10.1080/0092623X.2017.1346530.

72. Jessica Wood et al., "A Cross-Sectional Survey of Sex Toy Use, Characteristics of Sex Toy Use Hygiene Behaviours and Vulvovaginal Health Outcomes in Canada," *Canadian Journal of Human Sexuality* 26, no. 3 (2017): 196–204, https://doi.org/10.3138/cjhs.2017-0016.
73. "Vibrator Use Common, Linked to Sexual Health," *ScienceDaily*, June 29, 2009, https://www.sciencedaily.com/releases/2009/06/090629100643.htm.
74. Pascal de Sutter, James Day, and François Adam, "Who Are the Orgasmic Women? Exploratory Study among a Community Sample of French-Speaking Women," *Sexologies* 23, no. 3 (2014), https://doi.org/10.1016/j.sexol.2014.05.003.
75. Matthew Wills, "The Strange Story Behind Your Breakfast Cereal," *JSTOR Daily*, February 26, 2019, https://daily.jstor.org/the-strange-backstory-behind-your-breakfast-cereal/.
76. Kristine Fellizar, "What 46% Of Women Fantasize About During Sex," *Bustle*, June 5, 2015, https://www.bustle.com/articles/88057-46-percent-of-women-think-about-someone-else-during-sex-new-british-survey-says-plus-5.
77. Taylor Kohut et al., "But What's Your Partner Up To? Associations between Relationship Quality and Pornography Use Depend on Contextual Patterns of Use within the Couple," *Frontiers in Psychology*, July 30, 2021. https://doi.org/10.3389/fpsyg.2021.661347.

Chapter 5: Sex of All Kinds

Getting Down and Dirty with Vaginal, Oral, Anal, Outercourse, and Everything In Between

1. "When Sex Is Painful," American College of Obstetricians and Gynecologists, September 2017, https://www.acog.org/womens-health/faqs/when-sex-is-painful.
2. Dan Abramov et al., "The Influence of Gender on the Outcome of Coronary Artery Bypass Surgery," *Annals of Thoracic Surgery* 70, no. 3 (2000): 800–805, https://doi.org/10.1016/s0003-4975(00)01563-0;

Diane E. Hoffmann and Anita J. Tarzian, "The Girl Who Cried Pain: A Bias against Women in the Treatment of Pain," *Journal of Law, Medicine & Ethics* 29 (2003), https://doi.org/10.2139/ssrn.383803; Zhang Lanlan et al., "Gender Biases in Estimation of Others' Pain," *Journal of Pain* 22, no. 9 (2021): 1048–59, https://doi.org/10.1016/j.jpain.2021.03.001; "Vulvodynia: Get the Facts," National Vulvodynia Association, 2015, https://www.nva.org/media-center/.

3. Esther H. Chen et al., "Gender Disparity in Analgesic Treatment of Emergency Department Patients with Acute Abdominal Pain," *Academic Emergency Medicine* 15, no. 5 (2008): 414–18, https://doi.org/10.1111/j.1553-2712.2008.00100.x.
4. Elizabeth G. Nabel, "Coronary Heart Disease in Women—an Ounce of Prevention," *New England Journal of Medicine* 343, no. 8 (2000): 572–74, https://doi.org/10.1056/nejm200008243430809.
5. Kelly M. Hoffman et al., "Racial Bias in Pain Assessment and Treatment Recommendations, and False Beliefs about Biological Differences between Blacks and Whites," *Proceedings of the National Academy of Sciences* 113, no. 16 (2016): 4296–301, https://doi.org/10.1073/pnas.1516047113.
6. Bernard Harlow and Elizabeth Stewart, "A Population-Based Assessment of Chronic Unexplained Vulvar Pain: Have We Underestimated the Prevalence of Vulvodynia?," *Journal of the American Medical Women's Association* 58 (1972): 82–88, https://pubmed.ncbi.nlm.nih.gov/12744420/.
7. J. S. Dungan, "Oral Desipramine and Topical Lidocaine for Vulvodynia: A Randomized Controlled Trial," *Yearbook of Obstetrics, Gynecology and Women's Health* (2011): 279–80, https://doi.org/10.1016/j.yobg.2011.05.132.
8. "Vulvodynia: Get the Facts," National Vulvodynia Association.
9. Parveen Parasar, Pinar Ozcan, and Kathryn L. Terry, "Endometriosis: Epidemiology, Diagnosis and Clinical Management," *Current Obstetrics and Gynecology Reports* 6, no. 1 (2017): 34–41, https://doi.org/10.1007/s13669-017-0187-1.
10. Sanjay K.Agarwal, "Clinical Diagnosis of Endometriosis: A Call to Action." *American Journal of Obstetrics and Gynecology* 220, no. 4 (2019), https://doi.org/10.1016/j.ajog.2018.12.039.

11. Christina Rei, Thomas Williams, and Michael Feloney, "Endometriosis in a Man as a Rare Source of Abdominal Pain: A Case Report and Review of the Literature," *Case Reports in Obstetrics and Gynecology* 2018 (January 31, 2018): 1–6, https://doi.org/10.1155/2018/2083121.
12. Ivan Urits et al., "Cognitive Behavioral Therapy for the Treatment of Chronic Pelvic Pain," *Best Practice & Research Clinical Anaesthesiology* 34, no. 3 (2020): 409–26, https://doi.org/10.1016/j.bpa.2020.08.001.
13. Denny Wall, "Female Sexual Pain," Association for Behavioral and Cognitive Therapies, April 8, 2021, https://www.abct.org/fact-sheets/female-sexual-pain/.
14. Sam Hostettler, "Acupuncture Could Ease Women's Vulvar Pain," UIC Today, University of Illinois Chicago, October 11, 2017, https://today.uic.edu/acupuncture-could-ease-womens-vulvar-pain.
15. Tatiane Regina de Sousa et al., "The Effect of Acupuncture on Pain, Dyspareunia, and Quality of Life in Brazilian Women with Endometriosis: A Randomized Clinical Trial," *Complementary Therapies in Clinical Practice* 25 (2016): 114–21, https://doi.org/10.1016/j.ctcp.2016.09.006.
16. Rui Miguel Costa, Geoffrey F. Miller, and Stuart Brody, "Women Who Prefer Longer Penises Are More Likely to Have Vaginal Orgasms (but Not Clitoral Orgasms): Implications for an Evolutionary Theory of Vaginal Orgasm," *Journal of Sexual Medicine* 9, no. 12 (2012): 3079–88, https://doi.org/10.1111/j.1743-6109.2012.02917.x.
17. David Veale et al., "Am I Normal? A Systematic Review and Construction of Nomograms for Flaccid and Erect Penis Length and Circumference in up to 15,521 Men," *BJU International* 115, no. 6 (2015): 978–86, https://doi.org/10.1111/bju.13010.
18. "Vaginal Dryness," Mayo Clinic, December 4, 2020, https://www.mayoclinic.org/symptoms/vaginal-dryness/basics/causes/sym-20151520.
19. "Vaginal Dryness," Mayo Clinic.
20. Sheryl A. Kingsberg et al., "The Women's EMPOWER Survey: Identifying Women's Perceptions on Vulvar and Vaginal Atrophy and Its Treatment," *Journal of Sexual Medicine* 14, no. 3 (2017): 413–24, https://doi.org/10.1016/j.jsxm.2017.01.010.
21. L. Elaine Waetjen et al., "Factors Associated with Developing Vaginal Dryness Symptoms in Women Transitioning through Menopause: A

Longitudinal Study," *Menopause* 25, no. 10 (2018): 1094–104, https://doi.org/10.1097/gme.0000000000001130.

22. Anna Jenczura et al., "Sexual Function of Postmenopausal Women Addicted to Alcohol," *International Journal of Environmental Research and Public Health* 15, no. 8 (2018): 1629, https://www.ncbi.nlm.nih.gov/pmc/articles/PMC6121656/.
23. Jeanette Norris, "Alcohol and Female Sexuality: A Look at Expectancies and Risks," *Alcohol Health and Research World* 18, no. 3 (1994): 197–201, https://www.ncbi.nlm.nih.gov/pmc/articles/PMC6876398/pdf/arhw-18-3-197.pdf.
24. Parnan Emamverdikhan et al., "A Survey of the Therapeutic Effects of Vitamin E Suppositories on Vaginal Atrophy in Postmenopausal Women," *Iranian Journal of Nursing and Midwifery Research* 21, no. 5 (2016): 475–81, https://doi.org/10.4103/1735-9066.193393.
25. Guaraldi Dinicola et al., "Hyaluronic Acid and Vitamins Are Effective in Reducing Vaginal Atrophy in Women Receiving Radiotherapy," *Minerva Ginecologica* 67, no. 6 (December 2015), https://pubmed.ncbi.nlm.nih.gov/26788875/.
26. Nafiseh Saghafi et al., "Effects of Phytoestrogens in Alleviating the Menopausal Symptoms: A Systematic Review and Meta-Analysis," *Iranian Journal of Pharmaceutical Research* 16 (2017), https://www.ncbi.nlm.nih.gov/pmc/articles/PMC5963651/.
27. "Vaginal Dryness," Mayo Clinic.
28. Chandler Jarvis, "The Effect of Omega 3 Fatty Acids on Atrophic Vaginitis in Breast Cancer Survivors" (undergraduate thesis, College of Nursing, Ohio State University, 2012), https://kb.osu.edu/handle/1811/51959.
29. Fernand Labrie et al., "Efficacy of Intravaginal Dehydroepiandrosterone (DHEA) on Moderate to Severe Dyspareunia and Vaginal Dryness, Symptoms of Vulvovaginal Atrophy." *Maturitas* 82, no. 3 (2015): 315–16, https://doi.org/10.1016/j.maturitas.2015.06.010.
30. Valentina Lucia La Rosa et al., "Treatment of Genitourinary Syndrome of Menopause: The Potential Effects of Intravaginal Ultralow-Concentration Oestriol and Intravaginal Dehydroepiandrosterone on Quality of Life and Sexual Function," *Przegląd Menopauzalny* [*Menopausal Review*] 18, no. 2 (June 2019): 116–22, https://doi.org/10.5114/pm.2019.86836.

31. Cecilia M. Shing et al., "Acute Protease Supplementation Effects on Muscle Damage and Recovery across Consecutive Days of Cycle Racing," *European Journal of Sport Science* 16, no. 2 (2016): 206–12, https://doi.org/10.1080/17461391.2014.1001878.
32. Emmanuel Amabebe and Dilly O. Anumba, "Female Gut and Genital Tract Microbiota-Induced Crosstalk and Differential Effects of Short-Chain Fatty Acids on Immune Sequelae," *Frontiers in Immunology* 11 (2020), https://doi.org/10.3389/fimmu.2020.02184.
33. "Naturally Moisturizing Vaginal Melts," Femallay, 2020, https://www.femallay.com/collections/suppositories-moisture-lubrication.
34. Alok Semwal et al., "Pheromones and Their Role as Aphrodisiacs: A Review," *Journal of Acute Disease* 2, no. 4 (2013): 253–61, https://doi.org/10.1016/s2221-6189(13)60140-7.
35. Aly Walansky, "10 Men Share Their Unfiltered Thoughts on the Taste of Your Vagina," *YourTango*, March 24, 2017, https://www.yourtango.com/2017300517/men-share-their-unfiltered-thoughts-your-vagina-taste.
36. Xiaodi Chen et al., "The Female Vaginal Microbiome in Health and Bacterial Vaginosis," *Frontiers in Cellular and Infection Microbiology* 11 (April 2021): 631972, https://doi.org/10.3389/fcimb.2021.631972; "Lesbians Explain: What Vagina Tastes Like," YouTube, 2016, https://www.youtube.com/watch?v=OcwNXylqAVM.
37. Barton F. Hill and Jeffrey S. Jones, "Venous Air Embolism following Orogenital Sex during Pregnancy," *American Journal of Emergency Medicine* 11, no. 2 (1993): 155–57, https://doi.org/10.1016/0735-6757(93)90111-n.
38. Brian J. Morris, "Estimation of Country-Specific and Global Prevalence of Male Circumcision," *Population Health Metrics* 14, no. 1 (2016): 4, https://doi.org/10.1186/s12963-016-0073-5; Maria Owings, Sayeedha Uddin, and Sonja Williams, "Trends in Circumcision among Male Newborns Born in U.S. Hospitals: 1979–2010," National Center for Health Statistics, Centers for Disease Control and Prevention, November 6, 2015, https://www.cdc.gov/nchs/data/hestat/circumcision_2013/circumcision_2013.htm.
39. Helena Smith, "Laid Bare: The Sex Life of the Ancient Greeks in

All Its Physical Glory," *Guardian*, December 9, 2009, https://www.theguardian.com/culture/2009/dec/09/museums-greece.

40. Frederick Mansfield Hodges, "The Ideal Prepuce in Ancient Greece and Rome: Male Genital Aesthetics and Their Relation to Lipodermos, Circumcision, Foreskin Restoration, and the Kynodesme," *Bulletin of the History of Medicine* 75, no. 3 (2001): 375–405, https://doi.org/10.1353/bhm.2001.0119.
41. Z. Mukandavire, K. Bowa, and W. Garira, "Modelling Circumcision and Condom Use as HIV/AIDS Preventive Control Strategies," *Mathematical and Computer Modelling* 46, nos. 11–12 (2007): 1353–72, https://doi.org/10.1016/j.mcm.2007.01.001; Brian J. Morris et al., "Estimation of Country-Specific and Global Prevalence of Male Circumcision," *Population Health Metrics* 14, no. 1 (2016), https://doi.org/10.1186/s12963-016-0073-5.
42. Erik Betjes, "What Factors Determine Semen Volume?," International Society for Sexual Medicine, May 25, 2015, https://www.issm.info/sexual-health-qa/what-factors-determine-semen-volume/.
43. "Low Sperm Count," Mayo Clinic, October 30, 2020, https://www.mayoclinic.org/diseases-conditions/low-sperm-count/diagnosis-treatment/drc-20374591.
44. Patricio C. Gargollo, "Sperm: How Long Do They Live after Ejaculation?," Mayo Clinic, May 5, 2022, https://www.mayoclinic.org/healthy-lifestyle/getting-pregnant/expert-answers/pregnancy/faq-20058504.
45. John L. Fitzpatrick et al., "Chemical Signals from Eggs Facilitate Cryptic Female Choice in Humans," *Proceedings of the Royal Society B: Biological Sciences* 287, no. 1928 (2020): 20200805, https://doi.org/10.1098/rspb.2020.0805.
46. Stephen R. Killick et al., "Sperm Content of Pre-Ejaculatory Fluid," *Human Fertility* 14, no. 1 (2011): 48–52, https://doi.org/10.3109/14647273.2010.520798.
47. "What Is Pre-Ejaculatory Fluid (Also Known as Pre-Cum), and Can It Cause Pregnancy?," International Planned Parenthood Federation, February 13, 2019, https://www.ippf.org/blogs/what-pre-ejaculatory-fluid-also-known-pre-cum-and-can-it-cause-pregnancy.

48. "Yellow Semen," Cleveland Clinic, 2021, https://my.clevelandclinic.org/health/symptoms/21600-yellow-semen.
49. Tim Jewell, "Yellow, Clear, Brown, and More: What Does Each Semen Color Mean?," Healthline, May 2, 2022, https://www.healthline.com/health/mens-health/semen-color-chart.
50. Hannah Smothers, "Is His Semen Normal?" *Cosmopolitan*, December 2, 2016, https://www.cosmopolitan.com/sex-love/a8459063/semen-is-it-normal/.
51. "How Many Nutrients Are in Semen?," WebMD, 2021, https://www.webmd.com/sex-relationships/how-many-nutrients-are-in-semen.
52. Jesse Bering, "An Ode to the Many Evolved Virtues of Human Semen," *Scientific American*, September 22, 2010, https://blogs.scientificamerican.com/bering-in-mind/an-ode-to-the-many-evolved-virtues-of-human-semen/.
53. "It's All Coming Up Anal," Pornhub, November 7, 2015, https://www.pornhub.com/insights/anal-searches-increase.
54. "Sodomy Laws Are Still Being Used to Persecute Queer People," *LGBTQ Nation*, December 29, 2021, https://www.lgbtqnation.com/2021/12/sodomy-laws-still-used-persecute-queer-people/.
55. Kristen L. Hess et al., "Prevalence and Correlates of Heterosexual Anal Intercourse among Men and Women, 20 U.S. Cities," *AIDS and Behavior* 20, no. 12 (2016): 2966–75, https://doi.org/10.1007/s10461-016-1295-z.

Chapter 6: Is Masturbation Normal?

Why Parties of One Are Fun and Good for You

1. "Toys (Adult)," Transportation Security Administration, 2018, https://www.tsa.gov/travel/security-screening/whatcanibring/items/toys-adult.
2. Nell Frizzell, "Ridin' Dirty: A Sweeping Look at Witches Mounting Their Broomsticks," *Vice*, October 27, 2015, https://www.vice.com/en/article/gvze93/ridin-dirty-a-sweeping-look-at-witches-and-their-broomsticks.
3. Lesley A. Hall, "Masturbation," *Encyclopedia.com*, 2020, https://www

.encyclopedia.com/international/encyclopedias-almanacs-transcripts-and-maps/masturbation.

4. *Human Sexuality* (Chicago: American Medical Association, 1975).
5. Cecilia Tasca et al., "Women and Hysteria in the History of Mental Health," *Clinical Practice & Epidemiology in Mental Health* 8, no. 1 (2012): 110–19, https://doi.org/10.2174/1745017901208010110.
6. John Roberts, "Surgeon General Resigns in Masturbation Row," *British Medical Journal* 1994, no. 309: 1604, https://doi.org/10.1136/bmj.309.6969.1604.
7. "Is Masturbation Healthy?," Planned Parenthood, 2020, https://www.plannedparenthood.org/learn/sex-pleasure-and-sexual-dysfunction/masturbation/masturbation-healthy.
8. Marika J. Hess and Sigmund Hough, "Impact of Spinal Cord Injury on Sexuality: Broad-Based Clinical Practice Intervention and Practical Application," *Journal of Spinal Cord Medicine* 35, no. 4 (2012): 211–18, https://doi.org/10.1179/2045772312y.0000000025.
9. Debra Herbenick et al., "Prevalence and Characteristics of Vibrator Use by Women in the United States: Results from a Nationally Representative Study," *Journal of Sexual Medicine* 6, no. 7 (2009), 1857–66.
10. Martin Dahlberg et al., "Retained Sex Toys: An Increasing and Possibly Preventable Medical Condition," *International Journal of Colorectal Disease* 34 (2019): 181–183, https://link.springer.com/article/10.1007/s00384-018-3125-4
11. Varinder Kaur and Sylvia Lindinger-Sternart, "Masturbation: Gender Stigmatized Sexual Behavior Affecting Women's Sexual Wellness," *Journal of Counseling Sexology & Sexual Wellness* (Fall 2020), 7–11.
12. Herbenick et al., "Prevalence and Characteristics of Vibrator Use."
13. Herbenick et al., "Prevalence and Characteristics of Vibrator Use."
14. Christina McGrath Fair, "Will Masturbation Hurt your Relationship?," American Counseling Association blog, July 25, 2019, https://www.counseling.org/news/aca-blogs/aca-counseling-corner/aca-member-blogs/2019/07/25/will-masturbation-hurt-your-relationship.
15. Nick Hoffman, "Count Dracula and Victorian Sexual Identities," Methods of Literary and Cultural Studies blog, February 18, 2015, https://blogs.commons.georgetown.edu/engl-090-02-spring2015/2015/02/18/count-dracula-and-victorian-sexual-identities/.

16. "Tenga Self-Pleasure Report 2020," Tenga, 2020, https://usstore.tenga.co/pages/globalreport
17. "The United State(s) of Masturbation 2016," Tenga, September 23, 2016, https://www.tenga.co/press/TENGA_2016_US_Full_Report.pdf.
18. Sarah Boxer, "Truth or Lies? In Sex Surveys, You Never Know," *New York Times*, July 22, 2000, https://www.nytimes.com/2000/07/22/arts/truth-or-lies-in-sex-surveys-you-never-know.html.
19. Andrew Gurza, "Sex Toy and Disability Survey Findings," May 28, 2018, https://webcache.googleusercontent.com/search?q=cache:https://static1.squarespace.com/static/5b23884f5ffd20276dafbbfb/t/5b238ffd352f530edd130f34/1529057429349/sex%2Btoy%2Bresearch%2Bsurvey%2Bresults.pdf
20. Marcalee Alexander et al., "Improving Sexual Satisfaction in Persons with Spinal Cord Injuries: Collective Wisdom," *Topics in Spinal Cord Injury Rehabilitation* 23, no. 1 (2017): 57–70, https://doi.org/10.1310/sci2301-57; Marika J. Hess and Sigmund Hough, "Impact of Spinal Cord Injury on Sexuality: Broad-Based Clinical Practice Intervention and Practical Application," *Journal of Spinal Cord Medicine* 35, no. 4 (2012): 211–18, https://doi.org/10.1179/2045772312y.0000000025.
21. S. M. Yasir Arafat et al., "Sex During Pandemic: Panic Buying of Sext Toys During COVID-19 Lockdown," *Journal of Psychosexual Health* 3, no 2 (2021), https://journals.sagepub.com/doi/pdf/10.1177/26318318211013347; S. A. Qalati et al., "A Review Study of the Effects of the COVID-19 Pandemic on Individual Sexual Behavoir, Purchasing Sex Toys, and Related Consequences," *Sexologies* (2022), https://www.sciencedirect.com/science/article/pii/S1158136022000603.
22. Tong Li et al., "Approaches Mediating Oxytocin Regulation of the Immune System," *Frontiers in Immunology* 7 (2017), https://doi.org/10.3389/fimmu.2016.00693; Philip Haake et al., "Effects of Sexual Arousal on Lymphocyte Subset Circulation and Cytokine Production in Man," *Neuroimmunomodulation* 11, no. 5 (2004): 293–98, https://doi.org/10.1159/000079409.
23. "Tenga Self-Pleasure Report 2020," Tenga.
24. Caitlyn Hitt, "From the Ancient Greeks to Bluetooth Vibrators: The

History of Sex Toys," *Thrillist*, June 30, 2021, https://www.thrillist.com/news/nation/history-of-sex-toys.

25. Alexandra Klausner, "The Ancient Chinese Were Pretty Kinky," *New York Post*, January 26, 2017, https://nypost.com/2017/01/26/the-ancient-chinese-were-pretty-kinky/.
26. Debbie Josefson, "FDA Approves Device for Female Sexual Dysfunction," *British Medical Journal* 2000, no. 320: 1427, https://www.bmj.com/content/320/7247/1427.3.
27. "CPSC Prohibits Certain Phthalates in Children's Toys and Child Care Products," US Consumer Product Safety Commission, October 20, 2017, https://www.cpsc.gov/content/CPSC-Prohibits-Certain-Phthalates-in-Children%E2%80%99s-Toys-and-Child-Care-Products.

Chapter 7: Is My Discharge Normal?

The Good, the Green, the Gooey

1. "Vaginal Dryness," MedlinePlus, U.S. National Library of Medicine, https://medlineplus.gov/ency/article/000892.htm.
2. Luciene Setsuko Gunther et al., "Prevalence of *Candida albicans* and Non-*albicans* Isolates from Vaginal Secretions: Comparative Evaluation of Colonization, Vaginal Candidiasis and Recurrent Vaginal Candidiasis in Diabetic and Non-Diabetic Women," Sao Paulo Medical Journal 132, no. 2 (2014): 116–20, https://doi.org/10.1590/1516-3180.2014.1322640; Mehmet Emre Atabek, Nesibe Akyürek, and Beray Selver Eklioglu, "Frequency of Vagınal *Candida* Colonization and Relationship between Metabolic Parameters in Children with Type 1 Diabetes Mellitus," *Journal of Pediatric & Adolescent Gynecology* 26, no. 5 (2013): 257–60, https://doi.org/10.1016/j.jpag.2013.03.016.
3. Lubna Mohammed et al., "The Interplay between Sugar and Yeast Infections: Do Diabetics Have a Greater Predisposition to Develop Oral and Vulvovaginal Candidiasis?," *Cureus* 13, no. 2 (2021), https://doi.org/10.7759/cureus.13407.
4. Nathan A. Thompson, "Why Does BO Sometimes Smell like Weed?," *Vice*, February 1, 2016, https://www.vice.com/en/article/5gjedd/why-does-my-bo-smell-like-weed-420.

5. "Vaginal Discharge," Sutter Health, October 2019, https://www.sutterhealth.org/health/teens/female/vaginal-discharge.
6. Filipa de Castro Coelho and Cremilda Barros, "The Potential of Hormonal Contraception to Influence Female Sexuality," *International Journal of Reproductive Medicine* 2019: 1–9, https://doi.org/10.1155/2019/9701384.
7. "Vaginal Yeast Infection (Thrush): Overview," InformedHealth.org, US National Library of Medicine, June 19, 2019, https://www.ncbi.nlm.nih.gov/books/NBK543220/
8. "Vaginal Yeast Infection (Thrush): Overview," InformedHealth.org.
9. "Boric Acid (Vaginal)," University of Michigan Medicine, August 8, 2016, https://www.uofmhealth.org/health-library/d01225a1.
10. Melinda Zeron Mullins and Konia M. Trouton, "BASIC Study: Is Intravaginal Boric Acid Non-Inferior to Metronidazole in Symptomatic Bacterial Vaginosis? Study Protocol for a Randomized Controlled Trial," Trials 16 (2015): 315, https://doi.org/10.1186/s13063-015-0852-5.
11. K. M. Khameneie et al., "Fluconazole and Boric Acid for Treatment of Vaginal Candidiasis—New Words about Old Issue," *East African Medical Journal* 90, no. 4 (April 2013): 117–23, https://pubmed.ncbi.nlm.nih.gov/26866095/.
12. Debarti Ray et al., "Prevalence of *Candida glabrata* and Its Response to Boric Acid Vaginal Suppositories in Comparison with Oral Fluconazole in Patients with Diabetes and Vulvovaginal Candidiasis," *Diabetes Care* 30, no. 2 (2007): 312–17, https://doi.org/10.2337/dc06-1469.
13. Douglas J. Fort et al., "Boric Acid Is Reproductively Toxic to Adult *Xenopus laevis*, but Not Endocrine Active," *Toxicological Sciences* 154, no. 1 (2016): 16–26, https://doi.org/10.1093/toxsci/kfw138.
14. D. O. Ogbolu et al., "In Vitro Antimicrobial Properties of Coconut Oil on *Candida* Species in Ibadan, Nigeria," *Journal of Medicinal Food* 10, no. 2 (2007): 384–87, https://doi.org/10.1089/jmf.2006.1209.
15. Darshna Yagnik, Vlad Serafin, and Ajit J. Shah, "Antimicrobial Activity of Apple Cider Vinegar against *Escherichia coli*, *Staphylococcus aureus* and *Candida albicans*; Downregulating Cytokine and Microbial Protein Expression," *Scientific Reports* 8, no. 1 (2018): 1732, https://doi.org/10.1038/s41598-017-18618-x.

16. Maryam Darvishi et al., "The Comparison of Vaginal Cream of Mixing Yogurt, Honey and Clotrimazole on Symptoms of Vaginal Candidiasis," *Global Journal of Health Science* 7, no. 6 (2015): 108–16, https://doi.org/10.5539/gjhs.v7n6p108.
17. Safaa Fares et al., "Effect of Ingestion of Yogurt Containing *Lactobacillus acidophilus* on Vulvovaginal Candidiasis among Women Attending a Gynecological Clinic," *Egyptian Nursing Journal* 14, no. 1 (2017): 41–49, https://doi.org/10.4103/enj.enj_8_17.
18. Maura Di Vito et al., "In Vitro Activity of Tea Tree Oil Vaginal Suppositories against Candida Spp. And Probiotic Vaginal Microbiota," *Phytotherapy Research* 29, no. 10 (October 2015): 1628–33, https://doi.org/10.1002/ptr.5422.
19. K. A. Hammer, C. F. Carson, and T. V. Riley, "In Vitro Susceptibilities of Lactobacilli and Organisms Associated with Bacterial Vaginosis to *Melaleuca alternifolia* (Tea Tree) Oil," *Antimicrobial Agents and Chemotherapy* 43, no. 1 (January 1999): 196, https://doi.org/10.1128/aac.43.1.196.
20. "Bacterial Vaginosis," Cleveland Clinic, 2020, https://my.clevelandclinic.org/health/diseases/3963-bacterial-vaginosis.
21. "Bacterial Vaginosis," Cleveland Clinic.
22. R. Russo, E. Karadja, and F. De Seta, "Evidence-Based Mixture Containing Lactobacillus Strains and Lactoferrin to Prevent Recurrent Bacterial Vaginosis: A Double Blind, Placebo Controlled, Randomised Clinical Trial," *Beneficial Microbes* 10, no. 1 (2019): 19–26; R. Russo et al., "Randomised Clinical Trial in Women with Recurrent Vulvovaginal Candidiasis: Efficacy of Probiotics and Lactoferrin as Maintenance Treatment," *Mycoses* 62, no. 4 (2019): 328–35; Davide De Alberti et al., "Lactobacilli Vaginal Colonisation after Oral Consumption of Respecta Complex: A Randomised Controlled Pilot Study," *Archives of Gynecology and Obstetrics* 292, no. 4 (October 2015): 861–67.
23. N. El-Saied et al., "Efficacy of Vitamin C Vaginal Suppository in Treatment of Bacterial Vaginosis: A Randomized Controlled Trial," *Journal of Gynecology Research* 2, no. 1 (2016), https://doi.org/10.15744/2454-3284.2.103.
24. A. Cardone et al., "Utilisation of Hydrogen Peroxide in the Treatment of Recurrent Bacterial Vaginosis," *Minerva Ginecologica* 55, no. 6 (December 2003): 483–92, https://pubmed.ncbi.nlm.nih.gov/14676737/.

25. Orna Reichman and Jack Sobel, "Desquamative Inflammatory Vaginitis," *Best Practice & Research Clinical Obstetrics & Gynaecology* 28, no. 7 (2014): 1042–50, https://doi.org/10.1016/j.bpobgyn.2014.07.003; Paul Nyirjesy et al., "Causes of Chronic Vaginitis," *Obstetrics & Gynecology* 108, no. 5 (2006): 1185–91, https://doi.org/10.1097/01.aog.0000239103.67452.1a.
26. Jack D. Sobel et al., "Prognosis and Treatment of Desquamative Inflammatory Vaginitis," Obstetrics & Gynecology 117, no. 4 (2011): 850–55, https://doi.org/10.1097/aog.0b013e3182117c9e.
27. Oluwatosin Goje, "Three Difficult-to-Diagnose Forms of Chronic Vaginitis," Consult QD, Cleveland Clinic, April 9, 2019, https://consultqd.clevelandclinic.org/three-difficult-to-diagnose-forms-of-chronic-vaginitis/.
28. "Lichen Planus," University of Iowa Hospitals & Clinics, May 2020, https://uihc.org/health-topics/lichen-planus.
29. Rachel Baxter, "What Is a Sperm Allergy?," International Society for Sexual Medicine, November 19, 2016, https://www.issm.info/sexual-health-qa/what-is-a-sperm-allergy/.
30. Baxter, "What Is a Sperm Allergy?"
31. "Sexually Transmitted Infections Prevalence, Incidence, and Cost Estimates in the United States," Centers for Disease Control and Prevention, 2021, https://www.cdc.gov/std/statistics/prevalence-incidence-cost-2020.htm.
32. "Expedited Partner Therapy," Centers for Disease Control and Prevention, April 19, 2021, https://www.cdc.gov/std/ept/default.htm.
33. R. Scott McClelland et al., "Infection with *Trichomonas vaginalis* Increases the Risk of HIV-1 Acquisition," *Journal of Infectious Diseases* 195, no. 5 (2007): 698–702, https://doi.org/10.1086/511278; Barbara Van Der Pol et al., "Trichomonas Vaginalis Infection and Human Immunodeficiency Virus Acquisition in African Women," *Journal of Infectious Diseases* 197, no. 4 (2008): 548–54, https://doi.org/10.1086/526496.
34. S. J. Reynolds, "High Rates of Syphilis among STI Patients Are Contributing to the Spread of HIV-1 in India," *Sexually Transmitted Infections* 82, no. 2 (2006): 121–26, https://doi.org/10.1136/sti.2005.015040; D. T. Fleming and J. N. Wasserheit, "From Epidemi-

ological Synergy to Public Health Policy and Practice: The Contribution of Other Sexually Transmitted Diseases to Sexual Transmission of HIV Infection," *Sexually Transmitted Infections* 75, no. 1 (1999): 3–17, https://doi.org/10.1136/sti.75.1.3.

35. "Genital Herpes—CDC Basic Fact Sheet," Centers for Disease Control and Prevention, January 3, 2022, https://www.cdc.gov/std/herpes/stdfact-herpes.htm.
36. Jennifer A. Lee and Cat J. Pausé, "Stigma in Practice: Barriers to Health for Fat Women," *Frontiers in Psychology* 7 (2016), https://doi.org/10.3389/fpsyg.2016.02063.

Chapter 8: Are My Hormones Normal?

Stress, PMS, and Other Not Fun Things

1. Lee and Pausé, "Stigma in Practice."
2. John D. Meeker and Kelly K. Ferguson, "Urinary Phthalate Metabolites Are Associated with Decreased Serum Testosterone in Men, Women, and Children from NHANES 2011–2012," *Journal of Clinical Endocrinology & Metabolism* 99, no. 11 (November 2014): 4346–52, https://doi.org/10.1210/jc.2014-2555.
3. Pauline Vabre et al., "Environmental Pollutants, a Possible Etiology for Premature Ovarian Insufficiency: A Narrative Review of Animal and Human Data," *Environmental Health* 16, no. 1 (2017), https://doi.org/10.1186/s12940-017-0242-4.
4. Ting Ding et al., "Endocrine Disrupting Chemicals Impact on Ovarian Aging: Evidence from Epidemiological and Experimental Evidence," *Environmental Pollution* 305 (2022): 119269, https://doi.org/10.1016/j.envpol.2022.119269.
5. Jelonia T. Rumph et al., "Environmental Endocrine Disruptors and Endometriosis," in *Animals Models for Endometriosis*, Advances in Anatomy, Embryology and Cell Biology, vol. 232 (Springer, Cham; 2020), 57–78, https://doi.org/10.1007/978-3-030-51856-1_4; Diksha Sirohi, Ruqaiya Al Ramadhani, and Luke D. Knibbs, "Environmental Exposures to Endocrine Disrupting Chemicals (EDCs) and Their Role in Endometriosis: A Systematic Literature Review," *Re-*

views on Environmental Health 36, no. 1 (2020): 101–15, https://doi.org/10.1515/reveh-2020-0046.

6. Eleni Palioura and Evanthia Diamanti-Kandarakis, "Polycystic Ovary Syndrome (PCOS) and Endocrine Disrupting Chemicals (EDCs)," *Reviews in Endocrine and Metabolic Disorders* 16, no. 4 (2015): 365–71, https://doi.org/10.1007/s11154-016-9326-7; Aleksandra Konieczna et al., "Serum Bisphenol A Concentrations Correlate with Serum Testosterone Levels in Women with Polycystic Ovary Syndrome," *Reproductive Toxicology* 82 (December 2018): 32–37, https://doi.org/10.1016/j.reprotox.2018.09.006.
7. Maria Victoria Bariani et al., "The Role of Endocrine-Disrupting Chemicals in Uterine Fibroid Pathogenesis," *Current Opinion in Endocrinology, Diabetes and Obesity* 27, no. 6 (2020): 380–87, https://doi.org/10.1097/med.0000000000000578.
8. L. Yu et al., "Bisphenol A Induces Human Uterine Leiomyoma Cell Proliferation through Membrane-Associated Erα36 via Nongenomic Signaling Pathways," *Molecular and Cellular Endocrinology* 484 (2019): 59–68, https://doi.org/10.1016/j.mce.2019.01.001.
9. Partha Roy et al., "Screening of Some Anti-Androgenic Endocrine Disruptors Using a Recombinant Cell-Based In Vitro Bioassay," *Journal of Steroid Biochemistry and Molecular Biology* 88, no. 2 (2004): 157–66, https://pubmed.ncbi.nlm.nih.gov/15084347/; Li-Chun Xu et al., "Evaluation of Androgen Receptor Transcriptional Activities of Bisphenol A, Octylphenol and Nonylphenol In Vitro," *Toxicology* 216, no. 2–3 (2005): 197–203, https://pubmed.ncbi.nlm.nih.gov/16169144/.
10. Shigeyuki Kitamura et al., "Thyroid Hormonal Activity of the Flame Retardants Tetrabromobisphenol A and Tetrachlorobisphenol A," *Biochemical and Biophysical Research Communications* 293, no. 1 (2002): 554–59, https://doi.org/10.1016/S0006-291X(02)00262-0.
11. Z. Lazúrová and I. Lazúrová, "[The Environmental Estrogen Bisphenol A and Its Effects on the Human Organism]," *Vnitrni Lekarstvi* 59, no. 6 (2013), https://pubmed.ncbi.nlm.nih.gov/23808741/.
12. Xiaona Huo et al., "Bisphenol-A and Female Infertility: A Possible Role of Gene-Environment Interactions," *International Journal of Environmental Research and Public Health* 12 (2015): 11101–16, https://www.ncbi.nlm.nih.gov/pmc/articles/PMC4586663/; Angela Si-

monelli et al., "Environmental and Occupational Exposure to Bisphenol A and Endometriosis: Urinary and Peritoneal Fluid Concentration Levels," *International Archives of Occupational and Environmental Health* 90 (2017): 49–61, https://link.springer.com/article/10.1007/s00420-016-1171-1; Frederick S.vom Saal et al., "The Estrogenic Endocrine Disrupting Chemical Bisphenol A (BPA) and Obesity," *Molecular and Cellular Endocrinology* 354, nos. 1–2 (2012): 74–84, https://doi.org/10.1016/j.mce.2012.01.001; Mihi Yang et al., "Effects of Bisphenol A on Breast Cancer and Its Risk Factors," *Archives of Toxicology* 83, no. 3 (2009): 281–85, https://doi.org/10.1007/s00204-008-0364-0.

13. Tengteng Wang et al., "Urinary Estrogen Metabolites and Long-Term Mortality Following Breast Cancer," *JNCI Cancer Spectrum* 4, no. 3 (June 2020): pkaa014, https://doi.org/10.1093/jncics/pkaa014; Joshua N. Sampson et al., "Association of Estrogen Metabolism with Breast Cancer Risk in Different Cohorts of Postmenopausal Women," *Cancer Research* 77, no. 4 (2017): 918–25, https://doi.org/10.1158/0008-5472.can-16-1717.
14. Roberto Flores et al., "Fecal Microbial Determinants of Fecal and Systemic Estrogens and Estrogen Metabolites: A Cross-Sectional Study," *Journal of Translational Medicine* 10, no. 1 (2012): 253, https://doi.org/10.1186/1479-5876-10-253.
15. Claudia S. Plottel and Martin J. Blaser, "Microbiome and Malignancy," *Cell Host & Microbe* 10, no. 4 (2011): 324–35, https://doi.org/10.1016/j.chom.2011.10.003.
16. Michael T. Bailey and Christoper L. Coe, "Endometriosis Is Associated with an Altered Profile of Intestinal Microflora in Female Rhesus Monkeys," *Human Reproduction* 17, no. 7 (2002): 1704–8, https://doi.org/10.1093/humrep/17.7.1704; Mary E. Salliss et al., "The Role of Gut and Genital Microbiota and the Estrobolome in Endometriosis, Infertility and Chronic Pelvic Pain," *Human Reproduction Update* 28, no. 1 (2021): 92–131, https://doi.org/10.1093/humupd/dmab035.
17. Lisa Lindheim et al., "Alterations in Gut Microbiome Composition and Barrier Function Are Associated with Reproductive and Metabolic Defects in Women with Polycystic Ovary Syndrome (PCOS): A Pilot Study," *PLOS One* 12, no. 1 (2017), https://doi.org/10.1371/journal.pone.0168390; Yanjie Guo et al., "Association between Poly-

cystic Ovary Syndrome and Gut Microbiota," *PLOS One* 11, no. 4 (2016), https://doi.org/10.1371/journal.pone.0153196.

18. Sheetal Parida and Dipali Sharma, "The Microbiome–Estrogen Connection and Breast Cancer Risk," *Cells* 8, no. 12 (2019): 1642, https://doi.org/10.3390/cells8121642.
19. James M. Baker, Layla Al-Nakkash, and Melissa M. Herbst-Kralovetz, "Estrogen–Gut Microbiome Axis: Physiological and Clinical Implications," *Maturitas* 103 (2017): 45–53, https://doi.org/10.1016/j.maturitas.2017.06.025.
20. Madeline E. Graham et al., "Gut and Vaginal Microbiomes on Steroids: Implications for Women's Health," *Trends in Endocrinology & Metabolism* 32, no. 8 (2021): 554–65, https://doi.org/10.1016/j.tem.2021.04.014.
21. Rosario Russo, Antoine Edu, and Francesco De Seta, "Study on the Effects of an Oral Lactobacilli and Lactoferrin Complex in Women with Intermediate Vaginal Microbiota," *Archives of Gynecology and Obstetrics* 298, no. 1 (2018): 139–45, https://doi.org/10.1007/s00404-018-4771-z.
22. R. Russo, E. Karadja, and F. De Seta, "Evidence-Based Mixture Containing *Lactobacillus* Strains and Lactoferrin to Prevent Recurrent Bacterial Vaginosis: A Double Blind, Placebo Controlled, Randomised Clinical Trial," *Beneficial Microbes* 10, no. 1 (2019): 19–26, https://doi.org/10.3920/BM2018.0075, Rosario Russo et al., "Randomised Clinical Trial in Women with Recurrent Vulvovaginal Candidiasis: Efficacy of Probiotics and Lactoferrin as Maintenance Treatment," *Mycoses* 62, no. 4 (2019): 328–35, https://doi.org/10.1111/myc.12883; Davide De Alberti et al., "Lactobacilli Vaginal Colonisation after Oral Consumption of Respecta Complex: A Randomised Controlled Pilot Study," *Archives of Gynecology and Obstetrics* 292, no. 4 (2015): 861–67, https://link.springer.com/article/10.1007/s00404-015-3711-4.
23. Y. A. Dound et al., "The Effect of Probiotic *Bacillus subtilis* HU58 on Immune Function in Healthy Human," *Indian Practitioner* 70, no. 9 (2017): 15–20, http://articles.theindianpractitioner.com/index.php/tip/article/view/293.
24. Kushal Gandhi et al., "Lactobacillus Species and Inflammatory Cytokine Profile in the Vaginal Milieu of Pre-Menopausal and Post-Menopausal

Women," *Gynecological and Reproductive Endocrinology & Metabolism* (March 2020):180–87, https://doi.org/10.53260/GREM.201038; Jolien F. van Nimwegen et al., "Vaginal Dryness in Primary Sjögren's Syndrome: A Histopathological Case–Control Study," *Rheumatology* 59, no. 10 (2020): 2806–15, https://doi.org/10.1093/rheumatology/keaa017.

25. Pipat Piewngam et al., "Pathogen Elimination by Probiotic *Bacillus* via Signalling Interference," *Nature* 562, no. 7728 (2018): 532–37, https://doi.org/10.1038/s41586-018-0616-y.
26. Haiyan Xu, "Obesity and Metabolic Inflammation," *Drug Discovery Today: Disease Mechanisms* 10, nos. 1–2 (June 2013), https://doi.org/10.1016/j.ddmec.2013.03.006.
27. Klaudia Barabás, Edina Szabó-Meleg, and István M. Ábrahám, "Effect of Inflammation on Female Gonadotropin-Releasing Hormone (GnRH) Neurons: Mechanisms and Consequences," *International Journal of Molecular Sciences* 21, no. 2 (2020): 529, https://doi.org/10.3390/ijms21020529.
28. Céline Gérard and Kristy A. Brown, "Obesity and Breast Cancer—Role of Estrogens and the Molecular Underpinnings of Aromatase Regulation in Breast Adipose Tissue," *Molecular and Cellular Endocrinology* 466 (2018): 15–30, https://doi.org/10.1016/j.mce.2017.09.014.
29. Marc J. Gunter et al., "Breast Cancer Risk in Metabolically Healthy but Overweight Postmenopausal Women," *Cancer Research* 75, no. 2 (2015): 270–74, https://doi.org/10.1158/0008-5472.can-14-2317; Agathocles Tsatsoulis and Stavroula A. Paschou, "Metabolically Healthy Obesity: Criteria, Epidemiology, Controversies, and Consequences," *Current Obesity Reports* 9, no. 2 (2020): 109–20, https://doi.org/10.1007/s13679-020-00375-0; Gordon I. Smith, Bettina Mittendorfer, and Samuel Klein, "Metabolically Healthy Obesity: Facts and Fantasies," *Journal of Clinical Investigation* 129, no. 10 (2019): 3978–89, https://doi.org/10.1172/jci129186.
30. Meng-Ting Tsou et al., "Visceral Adiposity, Pro-Inflammatory Signaling and Vasculopathy in Metabolically Unhealthy Non-Obesity Phenotype," *Diagnostics* 11, no. 1 (2020): 40, https://doi.org/10.3390/diagnostics11010040.
31. Jenny Guidi et al., "Allostatic Load and Its Impact on Health: A System-

atic Review," *Psychotherapy and Psychosomatics* 90, no. 1 (2020): 11–27, https://doi.org/10.1159/000510696.

32. Adrienne A. Taren, J. David Creswell, and Peter J. Gianaros, "Dispositional Mindfulness Co-Varies with Smaller Amygdala and Caudate Volumes in Community Adults," *PLOS One* 8, no. 5 (2013), https://doi.org/10.1371/journal.pone.0064574.
33. Thomas G. Guilliams, *The Role of Stress and the HPA Axis in Chronic Disease Management* (Stevens Point, Wis.: The Point Institute, 2015).
34. "Circadian Rhythms," National Institute of General Medical Sciences, US Department of Health and Human Services, 2020, https://www.nigms.nih.gov/education/fact-sheets/Pages/circadian-rhythms.aspx; Aritro Sen, and Hanne M. Hoffmann, "Role of Core Circadian Clock Genes in Hormone Release and Target Tissue Sensitivity in the Reproductive Axis," *Molecular and Cellular Endocrinology* 501 (February 2020): 110655, https://doi.org/10.1016/j.mce.2019.110655.
35. Jason Brainard et al., "Health Implications of Disrupted Circadian Rhythms and the Potential for Daylight as Therapy," *Anesthesiology* 122, no. 5 (2015): 1170–75, https://doi.org/10.1097/aln.0000000000000596.
36. Michael T. Sellix, "Circadian Clock Function in the Mammalian Ovary," *Journal of Biological Rhythms* 30, no. 1 (2015): 7–19, https://doi.org/10.1177/0748730414554222.
37. Olubodun Michael Lateef and Michael Olawale Akintubosun, "Sleep and Reproductive Health," *Journal of Circadian Rhythms* 18, no. 1 (2020), https://doi.org/10.5334/jcr.190.
38. Anna Merklinger-Gruchala et al., "Low Estradiol Levels in Women of Reproductive Age Having Low Sleep Variation," *European Journal of Cancer Prevention* 17, no. 5 (2008): 467–72, https://doi.org/10.1097/cej.0b013e3282f75f67.

Chapter 9: Is My Menstrual Cycle Normal?

Is Your Flow Going with the Flow?

1. Tamaki Matsumoto, Hiroyuki Asakura, and Tatsuya Hayashi, "Biopsychosocial Aspects of Premenstrual Syndrome and Premenstrual

Dysphoric Disorder," *Gynecological Endocrinology* 29, no. 1 (2013): 67–73, https://doi.org/10.3109/09513590.2012.705383.

2. Sandra Zárate, Tinna Stevnsner, and Ricardo Gredilla, "Role of Estrogen and Other Sex Hormones in Brain Aging. Neuroprotection and DNA Repair," *Frontiers in Aging Neuroscience* 9 (2017), https://doi.org/10.3389/fnagi.2017.00430; Belinda Pletzer et al., "The Cycling Brain: Menstrual Cycle Related Fluctuations in Hippocampal and Fronto-Striatal Activation and Connectivity during Cognitive Tasks," *Neuropsychopharmacology* 44, no. 11 (2019): 1867–75, https://doi.org/10.1038/s41386-019-0435-3.
3. "The Hormones of Desire," HealthyWomen, September 22, 2009, https://www.healthywomen.org/content/article/hormones-desire.
4. Inger Sundström Poromaa and Malin Gingnell, "Menstrual Cycle Influence on Cognitive Function and Emotion Processing—from a Reproductive Perspective," *Frontiers in Neuroscience* 8 (2014): 380, https://doi.org/10.3389/fnins.2014.00380; Syed Suhail Andrabi, Suhel Parvez, and Heena Tabassum, "Neurosteroids and Ischemic Stroke: Progesterone a Promising Agent in Reducing the Brain Injury in Ischemic Stroke," *Journal of Environmental Pathology Toxicology and Oncology* 36, no. 3 (January 2017), https://doi.org/10.3389/fnins.2014.00380.
5. Hsiu-Wei Su et al., "Detection of Ovulation, a Review of Currently Available Methods," *Bioengineering & Translational Medicine* 2, no. 3 (September 2017): 238–46, https://doi.org/10.1002/btm2.10058.
6. S. Parenteau-Carreau and C. Infante-Rivard, "Self-Palpation to Assess Cervical Changes in Relation to Mucus and Temperature," *International Journal of Fertility* 33, Suppl. (1988): 10–16, https://pubmed.ncbi.nlm.nih.gov/2902020/.
7. Nathan R. Brott and Jacqueline K. Le, "Mittelschmerz," in *Statpearls* (Treasure Island, Fla.: StatPearls Publishing, 2022).
8. Talia N. Shirazi et al.,"Menstrual Cycle Phase Predicts Women's Hormonal Responses to Sexual Stimuli," *Hormones and Behavior* 103 (July 2018): 45–53, https://doi.org/10.1016/j.yhbeh.2018.05.023; Mary H. Burleson, Wenda R. Trevathan, and W. Larry Gregory, "Sexual Behavior in Lesbian and Heterosexual Women: Relations with Menstrual Cycle Phase and Partner Availability," *Psychoneuroendocrinology* 27, no. 4 (2002): 489–503, https://doi.org/10.1016/s0306-4530(01)00066-x.

9. Susan B. Bullivant et al., "Women's Sexual Experience during the Menstrual Cycle: Identification of the Sexual Phase by Noninvasive Measurement of Luteinizing Hormone," *Journal of Sex Research* 41, no. 1 (2004): 82–93, https://doi.org/10.1080/00224490409552216.
10. Dimitra Mantzou et al., "Impaired Sexual Function in Young Women with PCOS: The Detrimental Effect of Anovulation," *Journal of Sexual Medicine* 18, no. 11 (2021): 1872–79, https://doi.org/10.1016/j.jsxm.2021.09.004.
11. Angela Kerchner et al., "Risk of Depression and Other Mental Health Disorders in Women with Polycystic Ovary Syndrome: A Longitudinal Study," *Fertility and Sterility* 91, no. 1 (2009): 207–12, https://doi.org/10.1016/j.fertnstert.2007.11.022; D. W. Stovall et al., "Sexual Function in Women with Polycystic Ovary Syndrome," *Journal of Sexual Medicine* 9, no. 1 (2009): 224–30, https://www.jsm.jsexmed.org/article/S1743-6095(15)33738-3/fulltext.
12. J. E. Robinson and R. V. Short, "Changes in Breast Sensitivity at Puberty, during the Menstrual Cycle, and at Parturition," *British Medical Journal* 1977, no. 1: 1188–89, https://doi.org/10.1136/bmj.1.6070.1188.
13. Samantha J. Dawson, Kelly D. Suschinsky, and Martin L. Lalumière, "Sexual Fantasies and Viewing Times across the Menstrual Cycle: A Diary Study," *Archives of Sexual Behavior* 41, no. 1 (2012): 173–83, https://doi.org/10.1007/s10508-012-9939-1.
14. Kelly D. Suschinsky, Jennifer A. Bossio, and Meredith L. Chivers, "Women's Genital Sexual Arousal to Oral versus Penetrative Heterosexual Sex Varies with Menstrual Cycle Phase at First Exposure," *Hormones and Behavior* 65, no. 3 (2014): 319–27, https://doi.org/10.1016/j.yhbeh.2014.01.006.
15. Cesare Battaglia et al., "Menstrual Cycle-Related Morphometric and Vascular Modifications of the Clitoris," *Journal of Sexual Medicine* 5, no. 12 (2008): 2853–61, https://doi.org/10.1111/j.1743-6109.2008.00972.x.
16. Jonathan R. Bull et al., "Real-World Menstrual Cycle Characteristics of More than 600,000 Menstrual Cycles," *NPJ Digital Medicine* 2, no. 1 (2019): 83, https://doi.org/10.1038/s41746-019-0152-7.
17. Kirstine Münster, Lone Schmidt, and Peter Helm, "Length and Vari-

ation in the Menstrual Cycle: A Cross-Sectional Study from a Danish County," *BJOG: An International Journal of Obstetrics and Gynaecology* 99, no. 5 (1992): 422–29, https://doi.org/10.1111/j.1471-0528.1992.tb13762.x; Ian S. Fraser et al., "Can We Achieve International Agreement on Terminologies and Definitions Used to Describe Abnormalities of Menstrual Bleeding?," *Human Reproduction* 22, no. 3 (2007): 635–43, https://doi.org/10.1093/humrep/del478.

18. Paula J. Adams Hillard, "Menstruation in Adolescents: What Do We Know? And What Do We Do with the Information?," *Journal of Pediatric and Adolescent Gynecology* 27, no. 6 (2014): 309–19, https://doi.org/10.1016/j.jpag.2013.12.001.
19. Practice Committees of the American Society for Reproductive Medicine and the Society for Reproductive Endocrinology and Infertility, "Diagnosis and Treatment of Luteal Phase Deficiency: A Committee Opinion," *Fertility and Sterility* 115, no. 6 (2021): 1416–23, https://doi.org/10.1016/j.fertnstert.2021.02.010.
20. Elinor C. Vogt et al., "Primary Ovarian Insufficiency in Women with Addison's Disease," *Journal of Clinical Endocrinology & Metabolism* 106, no. 7 (July 2021): e2656–63, https://doi.org/10.1210/clinem/dgab140.
21. Ritu Deswal et al., "The Prevalence of Polycystic Ovary Syndrome: A Brief Systematic Review," *Journal of Human Reproductive Sciences* 13, no. 4 (2020): 261–71, https://doi.org/10.4103/jhrs.JHRS_95_18.
22. "Two Years, Multiple Doctors Often Needed to Diagnose Polycystic Ovary Syndrome, Study Shows," January 9, 2017, *ScienceDaily*, https://www.sciencedaily.com/releases/2017/01/170109191555.htm.
23. Stephanie Watson, "Polycystic Ovary Syndrome (PCOS) and Weight Gain," WebMD, 2020, https://www.webmd.com/women/polycystic-ovary-syndrome-pcos-and-weight-gain.
24. Renato Pasquali and Alessandra Gambineri, "Cortisol and the Polycystic Ovary Syndrome," *Expert Review of Endocrinology & Metabolism* 7, no. 5 (2012): 555–66, https://doi.org/10.1586/eem.12.42.
25. Holly R. Harris et al., "Polycystic Ovary Syndrome, Oligomenorrhea, and Risk of Ovarian Cancer Histotypes: Evidence from the Ovarian Cancer Association Consortium," *Cancer Epidemiology Biomarkers &*

Prevention 27, no. 2 (2018): 174–82, https://doi.org/10.1158/1055-9965.epi-17-0655.

26. Małgorzata Szczuko et al., "Nutrition Strategy and Life Style in Polycystic Ovary Syndrome—Narrative Review," *Nutrients* 13, no. 7 (2021): 2452, https://doi.org/10.3390/nu13072452.
27. Nelson Prager et al., "A Randomized, Double-Blind, Placebo-Controlled Trial to Determine the Effectiveness of Botanically Derived Inhibitors of 5-Alpha-Reductase in the Treatment of Androgenetic Alopecia," *Journal of Alternative and Complementary Medicine* 8, no. 2 (November 2006): 199, https://doi.org/10.1089/acm.2002.8.143; Rumi Fujita et al., "Anti-Androgenic Activities of *Ganoderma lucidum*," *Journal of Ethnopharmacology* 102, no. 1 (October 2005): 107–112, https://doi.org/10.1016/j.jep.2005.05.041; Hamid Reza Moradi, "The Histological and Histometrical Effects of *Urtica dioica* Extract on Rat's Protate Hyperplasia," *Vetinary Research Forum* 6, no. 1 (Winter 2015): 23–29, https://pubmed.ncbi.nlm.nih.gov/25992248/; A. Nahata and V. K. Dixit, "Ameliorative Effects of Stinging Nettle (*Urtica dioica*) on Testosterone-Induced Prostatic Hyperplasia in Rats," *Andrologia* 44, suppl. 1 (May 2012): 396–409, https://doi.org/10.1111/j.1439-0272.2011.01197.x.
28. Rotterdam ESHRE/ASRM-Sponsored PCOS Consensus Workshop Group, "Revised 2003 Consensus on Diagnostic Criteria and Long-Term Health Risks Related to Polycystic Ovary Syndrome (PCOS)," *Human Reproduction* 19, no. 1 (2004): 41–47, https://doi.org/10.1093/humrep/deh098.
29. "Premenstrual Syndrome (PMS)," Office on Women's Health, US Department of Health & Human Services, March 16, 2018, https://www.womenshealth.gov/menstrual-cycle/premenstrual-syndrome.
30. Lori M. Dickerson, Pamela J. Mazyck, and Melissa H. Hunter, "Premenstrual Syndrome," *American Family Physician* 67, no. 8 (2003): 1743–52, https://www.aafp.org/pubs/afp/issues/2003/0415/p1743.html.
31. "Feeling Close to a Friend Increases Progesterone, Boosts Well-Being and Reduces Anxiety and Stress," June 3, 2009, *ScienceDaily*, https://www.sciencedaily.com/releases/2009/06/090602171941.htm.
32. Patrick Michael Shaughn O'Brien et al., , "Towards a Consensus

on Diagnostic Criteria, Measurement and Trial Design of the Premenstrual Disorders: The ISPMD Montreal Consensus," *Archives of Women's Mental Health* 14, no. 1 (2011): 13–21, https://doi.org/10.1007/s00737-010-0201-3.

33. Wendy S. Biggs and Robin H. Demuth, "Premenstrual Syndrome and Premenstrual Dysphoric Disorder," *American Family Physician* 84, no. 8 (2011): 918–24, https://www.aafp.org/pubs/afp/issues/2011/1015/p918.html; Kazuo Yamada and Eiichiro Kamagata, "Reduction of Quality-Adjusted Life Years (QALYs) in Patients with Premenstrual Dysphoric Disorder (PMDD)," *Quality of Life Research* 26, no. 11 (2017): 3069–73, https://doi.org/10.1007/s11136-017-1642-1.

34. N. Dubey et al., "The ESC/E(Z) Complex, an Effector of Response to Ovarian Steroids, Manifests an Intrinsic Difference in Cells from Women with Premenstrual Dysphoric Disorder," *Molecular Psychiatry* 22, no. 8 (2017): 1172–84, https://doi.org/10.1038/mp.2016.229.

35. "Premenstrual Dysphoric Disorder (PMDD)," Johns Hopkins Medicine, 2019, https://www.hopkinsmedicine.org/health/conditions-and-diseases/premenstrual-dysphoric-disorder-pmdd.

36. American Psychiatric Association, *Diagnostic and Statistical Manual of Mental Disorders*, 5th ed. (Washington, DC: American Psychiatric Association, 2013): 171–172.

37. "Premenstrual Dysphoric Disorder (PMDD)," Johns Hopkins Medicine.

38. Farangis Dorani et al., "Prevalence of Hormone-Related Mood Disorder Symptoms in Women with ADHD," *Journal of Psychiatric Research* 133 (January 2021): 10–15, https://doi.org/10.1016/j.jpsychires.2020.12.005.

39. Anne G. Lever and Hilde M. Geurts, "Psychiatric Co-Occurring Symptoms and Disorders in Young, Middle-Aged, and Older Adults with Autism Spectrum Disorder," *Journal of Autism and Developmental Disorders* 46, no. 6 (2016): 1916–30, https://doi.org/10.1007/s10803-016-2722-8.

40. "Self-Diagnosis-Friendly Resources and Communities," University of Washington Autism Center, May 2021, https://depts.washington.edu/uwautism/wp-content/uploads/2021/05/Self-Diagnosed-Adult-Autism-Resources-handout-04.05.21.pdf; Alexandra Leed-

ham et al., "'I Was Exhausted Trying to Figure It Out': The Experiences of Females Receiving an Autism Diagnosis in Middle to Late Adulthood," *Autism* 24, no. 1 (2019): 135–46, https://doi.org/10.1177/1362361319853442; Kayla N. Anderson et al., "Attention-Deficit/Hyperactivity Disorder Medication Prescription Claims among Privately Insured Women Aged 15–44 Years—United States, 2003–2015," *Morbidity and Mortality Weekly Report* 67, no. 2 (2018): 66–70, https://doi.org/10.15585/mmwr.mm6702a3.

41. Asmaa Zki Bin Mahmoud et al., "Association between Menstrual Disturbances and Habitual Use of Caffeine," *Journal of Taibah University Medical Sciences* 9, no. 4 (December 2014): 341–44, https://doi.org/10.1016/j.jtumed.2014.03.012.
42. J. S. Sisti et al., "Caffeine, Coffee, and Tea Intake and Urinary Estrogens and Estrogen Metabolites in Premenopausal Women," *Cancer Epidemiology Biomarkers & Prevention* 24, no. 8 (2015): 1174–83, https://doi.org/10.1158/1055-9965.epi-15-0246.
43. Amanda Daley, "Exercise and Premenstrual Symptomatology: A Comprehensive Review," *Journal of Women's Health* 18, no. 6 (2009): 895–99, https://doi.org/10.1089/jwh.2008.1098.
44. Kimberly Albert et al., "Estrogen Enhances Hippocampal Gray-Matter Volume in Young and Older Postmenopausal Women: A Prospective Dose-Response Study," *Neurobiology of Aging* 56 (August 2017): 1–6, https://doi.org/10.1016/j.neurobiolaging.2017.03.033.
45. "For Women, Greater Exposure to Estrogen in Life May Protect Brain Regions That Are Vulnerable to Alzheimer's," *ScienceDaily*, November 4, 2021, https://www.sciencedaily.com/releases/2021/11/211104140355.htm.
46. Francisco Núñez, María J. Maraver, and Lorenza S. Colzato, "Sex Hormones as Cognitive Enhancers?," *Journal of Cognitive Enhancement* 4 (December 2020), https://doi.org/10.1007/s41465-019-00156-1.
47. Colin P. White et al., "Fluid Retention over the Menstrual Cycle: 1-Year Data from the Prospective Ovulation Cohort," *Obstetrics and Gynecology International* 2011 (2011): 138451, https://doi.org/10.1155/2011/138451.
48. Sam Murphy, "Seven Ways to Boost Your Metabolism," *Guardian*, January 27, 2006, https://www.theguardian.com/lifeandstyle/2006/jan/28/healthandwellbeing.features1.

49. Angelica Lindén Hirschberg, "Sex Hormones, Appetite and Eating Behaviour in Women," *Maturitas* 71, no. 3 (2012): 248–56, https://doi.org/10.1016/j.maturitas.2011.12.016.
50. Claudia Barth, Arno Villringer, and Julia Sacher, "Sex Hormones Affect Neurotransmitters and Shale the Adult Female Brain During Hormonal Transition Periods," *Frontiers in Neuroscience* 9 (2015): 37, https://doi.org/10.3389/fnins.2015.00037.
51. Q. U. Inam et al., "Effects of Sugar Rich Diet on Brain Serotonin, Hyperphagia and Anxiety in Animal Model of Both Genders," *Pakistan Journal of Pharmaceutical Sciences* 29, no. 3 (2016), 757–63, https://pubmed.ncbi.nlm.nih.gov/27166525/.
52. Lynnette Leidy Sievert, Carla Makhlouf Obermeyer, and Kim Price, "Determinants of Hot Flashes and Night Sweats," *Annals of Human Biology* 33, no. 1 (2006): 4–16, https://doi.org/10.1080/03014460500421338; Karen C. Schliep et al., "Alcohol Intake, Reproductive Hormones, and Menstrual Cycle Function: A Prospective Cohort Study," *American Journal of Clinical Nutrition* 102, no. 4 (2015): 933–42, https://doi.org/10.3945/ajcn.114.102160; Jinju Bae, Susan Park, and Jin-Won Kwon, "Factors Associated with Menstrual Cycle Irregularity and Menopause," *BMC Women's Health* 18, no. 1 (2018), https://doi.org/10.1186/s12905-018-0528-x.
53. "General Information/Press Room," American Thyroid Association, 2016, https://www.thyroid.org/media-main/press-room/; Luca Chiovato et al., "Hypothyroidism in Context: Where We've Been and Where We're Going," *Advances in Therapy* 36, Suppl. 2 (2019): 47–58, https://www.ncbi.nlm.nih.gov/pmc/articles/PMC6822815/; Maja Sulejmanovic et al., "Annual Incidence of Thyroid Disease in Patients Who First Time Visit Department for Thyroid Diseases in Tuzla Canton," *Materia Socio-Medica* 31, no. 2 (2019): 130–134, https://www.ncbi.nlm.nih.gov/pmc/articles/PMC6690314/.
54. Barbara Brody, "PMS and Sleep: What's the Connection?," WebMD, 2022, https://www.webmd.com/women/pms/features/why-pms-gives-you-insomnia.

Chapter 10: Is My Period Normal?

Red, Brown, Spotting, Clotting, and More

1. Samuel Lurie, "Does Intercourse during Menses Increase the Risk for Sexually Transmitted Disease?," *Archives of Gynecology and Obstetrics* 282, no. 6 (2010): 627–30, https://doi.org/10.1007/s00404-010-1564-4.
2. Anke Hambach et al., "The Impact of Sexual Activity on Idiopathic Headaches: An Observational Study," *Cephalalgia* 33, no. 6 (2013): 384–89, https://doi.org/10.1177/0333102413476374; Navneet Magon and Sanjay Kalra, "The Orgasmic History of Oxytocin: Love, Lust, and Labor," Indian Journal of Endocrinology and Metabolism 15, (2011): 156, https://doi.org/10.4103/2230-8210.84851.
3. "What to Know about Oxytocin Hormone," 2021, WebMD, https://www.webmd.com/sex-relationships/what-to-know-about-oxytocin.
4. Susan Wolters and Heli Kurjanen, "The Menstrubation Study," Womanizer and Lunette, 2021, archived at https://webcache.googleusercontent.com/search?q=cache:ORbG732oy8YJ:https://menstrubation.com/wp-content/uploads/2021/03/WMZ_Menstruba tion-Results_Report_UK.pdf.
5. Eleanor Jones, "11 Things to Know about Having Sex on Your Period," *Cosmopolitan*, April 23, 2021, https://www.cosmopolitan.com/uk/love-sex/sex/news/a40295/things-know-period-sex/.
6. Alice Broster, "Stigma Attached to Period Sex May Be a Thing of the Past, Research Suggests," *Forbes* Sites, July 10, 2020, https://www.forbes.com/sites/alicebroster/2020/07/10/stigma-attached-to-period-sex-may-be-a-thing-of-the-past-research-suggests/.
7. Amanda MacMillan, "6 Things You Should Know About Having Sex during Your Period," *Time*, August 7, 2017, https://time.com/4890156/sex-during-period/.
8. Olivia Goldhill, "Period Pain Can Be 'Almost as Bad as a Heart Attack.' Why Aren't We Researching How to Treat It?," *Quartz*, February 15, 2016, https://qz.com/611774/period-pain-can-be-as-bad-as-a-heart-attack-so-why-arent-we-researching-how-to-treat-it/.

9. T. I. Hillen et al., "Primary Dysmenorrhea in Young Western Australian Women: Prevalence, Impact, and Knowledge of Treatment," *Journal of Adolescent Health* 25, no. 1 (1999): 40–45, https://doi.org/10.1016/s1054-139x(98)00147-5; Hong Ju, Mark Jones, and Gita Mishra, "The Prevalence and Risk Factors of Dysmenorrhea," *Epidemiologic Reviews* 36, no. 1 (2014): 104–13, https://doi.org/10.1093/epirev/mxt009; Mark E. Schoep et al., "The Impact of Menstrual Symptoms on Everyday Life: A Survey among 42,879 Women," *American Journal of Obstetrics & Gynecology* 220, no. 6 (June 2019), 569.E1–569.E7, https://doi.org/10.1016/j.ajog.2019.02.048.
10. Nadia A. Khan et al., "Sex Differences in Acute Coronary Syndrome Symptom Presentation in Young Patients," *JAMA Internal Medicine* 173, no. 20 (2013): 1863–71, https://doi.org/10.1001/jamainternmed.2013.10149.
11. M. Yusoff Dawood, "Primary Dysmenorrhea: Advances in Pathogenesis and Management," *Obstetrics and Gynecology* 108, no. 2 (2006): 428–41, https://doi.org/10.1097/01.aog.0000230214.26638.0c.
12. Dilprit Bagga et al., "Differential Effects of Prostaglandin Derived from Omega-6 and Omega-3 Polyunsaturated Fatty Acids on COX-2 Expression and IL-6 Secretion," *Proceedings of the National Academy of Sciences* 100, no. 4 (2003): 1751–6, https://doi.org/10.1073/pnas.0334211100.
13. B. Seifert et al., "[Magnesium—A New Therapeutic Alternative In Primary Dysmenorrhea]," *Zentralblatt fur Gynakologie* 111, no. 11 (1989): 755–60, https://pubmed.ncbi.nlm.nih.gov/2675496/; Fabio Parazzini et al., "Magnesium in the Gynecological Practice: A Literature Review," *Magnesium Research* 30, no. 1 (2017): 1–7, https://doi.org/10.1684/mrh.2017.0419.
14. "Safety Considerations for Mirena," Bayer Pharmaceuticals, 2022.
15. David A. Grimes et al., "Oral Contraceptives for Functional Ovarian Cysts," *Cochrane Database of Systematic Reviews* 2014, no. 4: CD006134, https://doi.org/10.1002/14651858.cd006134.pub5.
16. "Menstrual Cycle: What's Normal, What's Not," Mayo Clinic, April 29, 2021, https://www.mayoclinic.org/healthy-lifestyle/womens-health/in-depth/menstrual-cycle/art-20047186.

17. "Heavy Menstrual Bleeding," Centers for Disease Control and Prevention, 2012, https://www.cdc.gov/ncbddd/blooddisorders/women/menorrhagia.html.
18. Donna Day Baird, "High Cumulative Incidence of Uterine Leiomyoma in Black and White Women: Ultrasound Evidence," *American Journal of Obstetrics & Gynecology* 188, no. 1 (2003): 100–107, https://doi.org/10.1067/mob.2003.99
19. Elizabeth A. Stewart et al., "The Burden of Uterine Fibroids for African-American Women: Results of a National Survey," *Journal of Women's Health* 22, no. 10 (2013): 807–16, https://doi.org/10.1089/jwh.2013.4334.
20. Renée Boynton-Jarrett et al., "Abuse in Childhood and Risk of Uterine Leiomyoma: The Role of Emotional Support In Biologic Resilience," *Epidemiology* 22, no. 1 (2011): 6–14, https://doi.org/10.1097/ede.0b013e3181ffb172; Lauren A. Wise and Shannon K. Laughlin-Tommaso, "Epidemiology of Uterine Fibroids: From Menarche to Menopause," *Clinical Obstetrics and Gynecology* 59, no. 1 (2016): 2–24, https://doi.org/10.1097%2FGRF.0000000000000164; Anissa I. Vines, Myduc Ta, Denise A. Esserman, "The Association between Self-Reported Major Life Events and the Presence of Uterine Fibroids," *Women's Health Issues* 20, no. 4 (2010): 294–98, https://doi.org/10.1016/j.whi.2010.03.009; Donna Baird and Lauren Wise, "Childhood Abuse and Fibroids," *Epidemiology* 22, no. 1 (2011): 15–17, https://doi.org/10.1097%2FEDE.0b013e3181fe1fbe; Lauren A. Wise, Julie R. Palmer, and Lynn Rosenberg, "Lifetime Abuse Victimization and Risk of Uterine Leiomyomata in Black Women," *American Journal of Obstetrics and Gynecology* 208, no. 4 (April 2013): 272.E1–272.E13, https://doi.org/10.1016/j.ajog.2012.12.034; Lauren A. Wise et al., "Perceived Racial Discrimination and Risk of Uterine Leiomyomata," *Epidemiology* 18, no. 6 (2007):747, 747–57, https://doi.org/10.1097%2FEDE.0b013e3181567e92.
21. Lauren A. Wise et al., "Intake of Fruit, Vegetables, and Carotenoids in Relation to Risk of Uterine Leiomyomata," *American Journal of Clinical Nutrition* 94, no. 6 (2011): 1620–31, https://doi.org/10.3945/ajcn.111.016600.

22. Rose G. Radin et al., "Dietary Glycemic Index and Load in Relation to Risk of Uterine Leiomyomata in the Black Women's Health Study," *American Journal of Clinical Nutrition* 91, no. 5 (2010): 1281–88, https://doi.org/10.3945/ajcn.2009.28698.
23. Lauren A. Wise, "Risk of Uterine Leiomyomata in Relation to Tobacco, Alcohol and Caffeine Consumption in the Black Women's Health Study," *Human Reproduction* 19, no. 8 (2004): 1746–54, https://doi.org/10.1093/humrep/deh309.
24. F. Chiaffarino et al., "Diet and Uterine Myomas," *Obstetrics and Gynecology* 94 (3): 395–98, https://doi.org/10.1016/s0029-7844(99)00305-1.
25. Mostafa A. Borahay et al., "Estrogen Receptors and Signaling in Fibroids: Role in Pathobiology and Therapeutic Implications," *Reproductive Sciences* 24, no. 9 (2017): 1235–44, https://doi.org/10.1177/1933719116678686.
26. "Overview—Heavy Periods," NHS, 2019, https://www.nhs.uk/conditions/heavy-periods/.
27. "Heavy Menstrual Bleeding," Centers for Disease Control and Prevention.
28. Danielle Wehn, "Are Blood Clots Normal during Your Period?," Cleveland Clinic, October 30, 2018, https://health.clevelandclinic.org/menstrual-clots-during-heavy-periods-whats-normal-whats-not/.
29. Janet Michel et al., "Period Poverty: Why It Should Be Everybody's Business," *Journal of Global Health Reports* 6 (2022), https://www.joghr.org/article/32436-period-poverty-why-it-should-be-everybody-s-business.
30. "'Period Poverty' Sanitary Products 'Improve School Attendance,'" BBC News, November 28, 2018, https://www.bbc.com/news/av/uk-england-hampshire-46361899.
31. Lauren F. Cardoso et al., "Period Poverty and Mental Health Implications among College-Aged Women in the United States," *BMC Women's Health* 21, no. 14 (2020), https://doi.org/10.1186/s12905-020-01149-5.
32. "What to Know About Period Poverty," Medical News Today, September 6, 2021, https://www.medicalnewstoday.com/articles/period-poverty.

33. Magnesium Glycinate," Topics, ScienceDirect, https://www.sciencedirect.com/topics/nursing-and-health-professions/magnesium-glycinate.
34. Magnesium Citrate," Topics, ScienceDirect, https://www.sciencedirect.com/topics/medicine-and-dentistry/magnesium-citrate.
35. W. A. Fogel, "Diamine Oxidase (DAO) and Female Sex Hormones," *Agents and Actions* 18 (1986): 44–45, https://doi.org/10.1007/bf01987978.
36. M. Vasiadi et al., "Progesterone Inhibits Mast Cell Secretion," *International Journal of Immunopathology and Pharmacology* 19, no. 4 (2006): 787–94, https://doi.org/10.1177/039463200601900408.
37. "Pandemic Periods: Why Women's Menstrual Cycles Have Gone Haywire," *Guardian*, March 25, 2021, https://www.theguardian.com/society/2021/mar/25/pandemic-periods-why-womens-menstrual-cycles-have-gone-haywire.
38. Kezhen Li et al., "Analysis of Sex Hormones and Menstruation in COVID-19 Women of Child-Bearing Age," *Reproductive BioMedicine Online* 42, no. 1 (2021): 260–67, https://doi.org/10.1016/j.rbmo.2020.09.020.
39. Victoria Male, "Menstrual Changes after Covid-19 Vaccination," *British Medical Journal* 2021, no. 375: n2211, https://doi.org/10.1136/bmj.n2211.
40. "Yes Dear, Tonight! I Have a Headache," Premier Health, January 8, 2017, https://www.premierhealth.com/your-health/articles/women-wisdom-wellness-/yes-dear-tonight!-i-have-a-headache.
41. Michal Fila et al., "Nutrients to Improve Mitochondrial Function to Reduce Brain Energy Deficit and Oxidative Stress in Migraine," *Nutrients* 13, no. 12 (2021): 4433, https://doi.org/10.3390/nu13124433.
42. "Historical Perspectives Reduced Incidence of Menstrual Toxic-Shock Syndrome—United States, 1980–1990," *Morbidity and Mortality Weekly Report* 39, no. 25 (1990): 421–23, https://www.cdc.gov/mmwr/preview/mmwrhtml/00001651.htm.
43. "Menopause," Mayo Clinic, https://www.mayoclinic.org/diseases-conditions/menopause/symptoms-causes/syc-20353397.
44. Adi Gasner and Anis Rehman, "Primary Amenorrhea," in *Statpearls* (Treasure Island, Fla.: StatPearls Publishing, 2022).

45. Gasner and Rehman, "Primary Amenorrhea."
46. David A. Klein and Merrily A. Poth, "Amenorrhea: An Approach to Diagnosis and Management," *American Family Physician* 87, no. 11 (2013): 781–88, https://www.aafp.org/afp/2013/0601/p781.html.
47. Klein and Poth, "Amenorrhea."
48. Laureen M. Lopez et al., "Hormonal Contraceptives and Bone Health in Women," Cochrane, June 24, 2014, https://www.cochrane.org/CD006033/FERTILREG_hormonal-contraceptives-and-bone-health-in-women.
49. "No Easy Answers: New Functional Hypothalamic Amenorrhea Treatment Guidelines Released," Endocrine News, June 2017, https://endocrinenews.endocrine.org/no-easy-answers-new-hypothalamic-amenorrhea-treatment-guidelines/.
50. Maria Phylactou et al., "Clinical and Biochemical Discriminants between Functional Hypothalamic Amenorrhoea (FHA) and Polycystic Ovary Syndrome (PCOS)," *Clinical Endocrinology* 95, no. 2 (August 2021): 239–52, https://doi.org/10.1111/cen.14402.

Chapter 11: Are My Breasts Normal?

Big, Small, Pointy, Round, and Everything In Between

1. Frances E. Mascia-Lees, John H. Relethford, and Tom Sorger, "Evolutionary Perspectives on Permanent Breast Enlargement in Human Females," *American Anthropologist* 88, no. 2 (June 1986): 423–28, https://doi.org/10.1525/aa.1986.88.2.02a00090.
2. Mascia-Lees, Relethford, and Sorger, "Evolutionary Perspectives on Permanent Breast Enlargement."
3. Viren Swami et al., "The Breast Size Satisfaction Survey (BSSS): Breast Size Dissatisfaction and Its Antecedents and Outcomes in Women from 40 Nations," *Body Image* 32 (March 2020): 199–217, https://doi.org/10.1016/j.bodyim.2020.01.006.
4. "Does Breast Size Matter?," Zava, 2018, https://www.zavamed.com/uk/does-breast-size-matter.html.
5. "Breast Reduction in Young Women Improves Quality of Life Decades Later," American Society of Plastic Surgeons, October 28, 2019, https://

www.plasticsurgery.org/news/press-releases/breast-reduction-in-young-women-improves-quality-of-life-decades-later.

6. Norma I. Cruz, "Breast Asymmetry in Women Requesting Plastic Surgery of the Breast," *Plastic and Reconstructive Surgery—Global Open* 4, no. 9S (September 2016): 195–96, https://doi.org/10.1097/01.gox.0000503151.64989.00.
7. Miriam Brennan, Mike Clarke, and Declan Devane, "The Use of Anti Stretch Marks' Products by Women in Pregnancy: A Descriptive, Cross-Sectional Survey," *BMC Pregnancy and Childbirth* 16, no. 1 (2016): 276, https://doi.org/10.1186/s12884-016-1075-9.
8. Rao D. Nagaraja and R. Winters, "Inverted Nipple," in *Statpearls* (Treasure Island, Fla.: StatPearls Publishing, 2022).
9. Edward P. Miranda, "Congenital Defects of the Skin and Hands," in Arnold G. Coran et al. eds., *Pediatric Surgery*, 7th ed. (Mosby: 2012): 1711–24, https://doi.org/10.1016/b978-0-323-07255-7.00138-0.
10. Tom Connick, "Watch Mark Wahlberg Reveal He Has a Third Nipple to a Shocked Will Ferrell," *NME*, November 17, 2017, https://www.nme.com/news/film/watch-mark-wahlberg-reveal-third-nipple-shocked-will-ferrell-2160546.
11. Barry R. Komisaruk et al., "Women's Clitoris, Vagina, and Cervix Mapped on the Sensory Cortex: fMRI Evidence," *Journal of Sexual Medicine* 8, no. 10 (October 2011): 2822–30, https://doi.org/10.1111/j.1743-6109.2011.02388.x.
12. Roy Levin and Cindy Meston, "Nipple/Breast Stimulation and Sexual Arousal in Young Men and Women," Journal of Sexual Medicine 3, no. 3 (May 2006): 450–54, https://doi.org/10.1111/j.1743-6109.2006.00230.x.
13. Komisaruk et al., "Women's Clitoris, Vagina, and Cervix Mapped."
14. Swami et al., "The Breast Size Satisfaction Survey."
15. Tunc Eren et al., "Factors Effecting Mastalgia," *Breast Care* 11, no. 3 (2016): 188–93, https://doi.org/10.1159/000444359.
16. "Breast Pain (Mastalgia)," Johns Hopkins Medicine, 2021, https://www.hopkinsmedicine.org/health/conditions-and-diseases/mastalgia-breast-%20pain.
17. "Breast Pain (Mastalgia)," Johns Hopkins Medicine.
18. Dana Seidlova-Wuttke and Wolfgang Wuttke, "The Premenstrual Syndrome, Premenstrual Mastodynia, Fibrocystic Mastopathy and

Infertility Have Often Common Roots: Effects of Extracts of Chasteberry (*Vitex agnus castus*) as a Solution," *Clinical Phytoscience* 3, no. 1 (2017), https://doi.org/10.1186/s40816-016-0038-z.

19. "Fibrocystic Breasts," Mayo Clinic, https://www.mayoclinic.org/diseases-conditions/fibrocystic-breasts/symptoms-causes/syc-20350438.
20. "Fibrocystic Breast Changes," Cleveland Clinic, 2019, https://my.clevelandclinic.org/health/diseases/4185-fibrocystic-breast-.
21. Gholamali Godazandeh, "The Comparison of the Effect of Flaxseed Oil and Vitamin E on Mastalgia and Nodularity of Breast Fibrocystic: A Randomized Double-Blind Clinical Trial," *Journal of Pharmaceutical Health Care and Sciences* 7, no. 1 (2021): 4, https://doi.org/10.1186/s40780-020-00186-4.
22. Lyn Patrick, "Review of Iodine: Deficiency and Therapeutic Considerations," *Alternative Medicine Review* 13, no. 2 (2008): 116–27, http://www.encognitive.com/files/Iodine:%20Deficiency%20and%20Therapeutic%20Considerations_0.pdf.
23. "Breast Pain," Breast Cancer Now, November 2018, https://breastcancernow.org/information-support/have-i-got-breast-cancer/benign-breast-conditions/breast-pain.
24. "Breast Pain (Mastalgia)," Johns Hopkins Medicine.
25. "Breast Pain (Mastalgia)," Cleveland Clinic, https://my.clevelandclinic.org/health/diseases/15469-breast-pain-mastalgia.
26. "Inflammatory Breast Cancer," March 1, 2022, American Cancer Society, https://www.cancer.org/cancer/breast-cancer/about/types-of-breast-cancer/inflammatory-breast-cancer.html.
27. "Common Benign Lumps," Johns Hopkins Medicine, 2021, https://www.hopkinsmedicine.org/health/conditions-and-diseases/common-benign-%20lumps.
28. "Common Benign Lumps," Johns Hopkins Medicine.
29. Tunc Eren et al., "Factors Effecting Mastalgia."
30. "What Is Breast Implant Illness?," Breastcancer.org, July 27, 2022, https://www.breastcancer.org/treatment/surgery/breast-reconstruction/types/implant-reconstruction/illness/breast-implant-illness.
31. "What Is Breast Implant Illness?," Breastcancer.org.
32. "What Is Breast Implant Illness?," Breastcancer.org.
33. "What Is Breast Implant Illness?," Breastcancer.org.

Chapter 12: Welcome to the 28-Day Program

Let's Get Down to Business (Not *That* Kind, but Helpful for That Kind, Too!)

1. V. Lobo et al., "Free Radicals, Antioxidants and Functional Foods: Impact on Human Health," *Pharmacognosy Reviews* 4, no. 8 (2010): 118–26, https://doi.org/10.4103/0973-7847.70902; Ullah Asmat, Khan Abad, and Khan Ismail, "Diabetes Mellitus and Oxidative Stress—A Concise Review," *Saudi Pharmaceutical Journal* 24, no. 5 (2016): 547–53; https://doi.org/10.1016%2Fj.jsps.2015.03.013; Kashif M. Munir et al., "Mechanisms for Food Polyphenols to Ameliorate Insulin Resistance and Endothelial Dysfunction: Therapeutic Implications for Diabetes and Its Cardiovascular Complications," *American Journal of Physiology—Endocrinology and Metabolism* 305, no. 6 (September 2013): E679–86, https://doi.org/10.1152/ajpendo.00377.2013; Gabriela Radulian et al., "Metabolic Effects of Low Glycaemic Index Diets," *Nutrition Journal* 8, no. 1 (2009), https://doi.org/10.1186/1475-2891-8-5.
2. Kashif M. Munir et al., "Mechanisms for Food Polyphenols to Ameliorate Insulin Resistance and Endothelial Dysfunction: Therapeutic Implications for Diabetes and Its Cardiovascular Complications," *American Journal of Physiology—Endocrinology and Metabolism* 305, no. 6 (2013): E679–86, https://doi.org/10.1152/ajpendo.00377.2013.
3. Gabriela Radulian et al., "Metabolic Effects of Low Glycaemic Index Diets," *Nutrition Journal* 8, no. 1 (2009): 5, https://doi.org/10.1186/1475-2891-8-5.
4. Russell J. de Souza et al., "Intake of Saturated and Trans Unsaturated Fatty Acids and Risk of All Cause Mortality, Cardiovascular Disease, and Type 2 Diabetes: Systematic Review and Meta-Analysis of Observational Studies," *British Medical Journal* 2015, no. 351: h3978, https://doi.org/10.1136/bmj.h3978.
5. Andrea G. Izquierdo et al., "Leptin, Obesity, and Leptin Resistance: Where Are We 25 Years Later?," *Nutrients* 11, no. 11 (2019): 2704, https://doi.org/10.3390/nu11112704.
6. Jordi Salas-Salvadó et al., "Effect of Two Doses of a Mixture of Soluble Fibres on Body Weight and Metabolic Variables in Over-

weight or Obese Patients: A Randomised Trial," *British Journal of Nutrition* 99, no. 6 (June 2008): 1380–87, https://doi.org/10.1017/s0007114507868528; Husam Ghanim et al., "Increase in Plasma Endotoxin Concentrations and the Expression of Toll-like Receptors and Suppressor of Cytokine Signaling-3 in Mononuclear Cells after a High-Fat, High-Carbohydrate Meal: Implications for Insulin Resistance," *Diabetes Care* 32, no. 12 (December 2009): 2281–87, https://doi.org/10.2337/dc09-0979; Karine Spiegel et al., "Leptin Levels Are Dependent on Sleep Duration: Relationships with Sympathovagal Balance, Carbohydrate Regulation, Cortisol, and Thyrotropin," *Journal of Clinical Endocrinology & Metabolism* 89, no. 11 (November 2004): 5762–71, https://doi.org/10.1210/jc.2004-1003; David S. Weigle et al., "A High-Protein Diet Induces Sustained Reductions in Appetite, Ad Libitum Caloric Intake, and Body Weight despite Compensatory Changes in Diurnal Plasma Leptin and Ghrelin Concentrations," *American Journal of Clinical Nutrition* 82, no. 1 (July 2005): 41–48, https://doi.org/10.1093/ajcn.82.1.41; Janne E. Reseland et al., "Effect of Long-Term Changes in Diet and Exercise on Plasma Leptin Concentrations," *American Journal of Clinical Nutrition* 73, no. 2 (February 2001): 240–45, https://doi.org/10.1093/ajcn/73.2.240.

7. Ladan Kashani et al., "Saffron for Treatment of Fluoxetine-Induced Sexual Dysfunction in Women: Randomized Double-Blind Placebo-Controlled Study." *Human Psychopharmacology: Clinical & Experimental* 28, no. 1 (January 2013): 54–60, https://doi.org/10.1002/hup.2282.
8. Hossein Ranjbar and Akram Ashrafizaveh, "Effects of Saffron (*Crocus sativus*) on Sexual Dysfunction among Men and Women: A Systematic Review and Meta-Analysis," *Avicenna Journal of Phytomedicine* 9, no. 5 (September–October 2019): 419–27, https://www.ncbi.nlm.nih.gov/pmc/articles/PMC6727438/.
9. Hajime Fukui, Kumiko Toyoshima, and Ryoichi Komaki, "Psychological and Neuroendocrinological Effects of Odor of Saffron (*Crocus Sativus*)," *Phytomedicine* 18, nos. 8–9 (June 2011): 726–30, https://doi.org/10.1016/j.phymed.2010.11.013.
10. Agnes M. Rimando and Penelope M. Perkins-Veazie, "Determination of Citrulline in Watermelon Rind," *Journal of Chromatography A* 1078, nos. 1–2 (2005): 196–200, https://doi.org/10.1016/j.chroma.2005.05.009.

11. Vedat Cinar et al., "Effects of Magnesium Supplementation on Testosterone Levels of Athletes and Sedentary Subjects at Rest and after Exhaustion," *Biological Trace Element Research* 140, no. 1 (2010): 18–23, https://doi.org/10.1007/s12011-010-8676-3.
12. Ioannis Mykoniatis et al., "Sexual Dysfunction among Young Men: Overview of Dietary Components Associated with Erectile Dysfunction," *Journal of Sexual Medicine* 15, no. 2 (2018): 176–82, https://doi.org/10.1016/j.jsxm.2017.12.008.
13. L. E. Pelayo, "PNM-06 Capsaicin Improves Sexual Behavior in Male Rat," *Journal of Sexual Medicine* 14, no. 12 (2007): e384–85, https://doi.org/10.1016/j.jsxm.2017.10.053.
14. Christina M. Dording et al., "A Double-Blind, Randomized, Pilot Dose-Finding Study of Maca Root (*L. Meyenii*) for the Management of SSRI-Induced Sexual Dysfunction," *CNS Neuroscience & Therapeutics* 14, no. 3 (Fall 2008): 182–91, https://doi.org/10.1111/j.1755-5949.2008.00052.x.
15. Nicole A. Brooks et al., "Beneficial Effects of *Lepidium Meyenii* (Maca) on Psychological Symptoms and Measures of Sexual Dysfunction in Postmenopausal Women Are Not Related to Estrogen or Androgen Content," *Menopause* 15, no. 6 (2008): 1157–62, https://doi.org/10.1097/gme.0b013e3181732953.
16. Bernadette M. Marriott, ed., *Food Components to Enhance Performance: An Evaluation of Potential Performance-Enhancing Food Components for Operational Rations* (Washington, DC: National Academies Press, 1994); A. Holmäng and P. Björntorp, "The Effects of Cortisol on Insulin Sensitivity in Muscle," *Acta Physiologica Scandinavica* 144, no. 4 (1992): 425–31, https://onlinelibrary.wiley.com/doi/10.1111/j.1748-1716.1992.tb09316.x.
17. Lisa Dawn Hamilton, Alessandra H. Rellini, and Cindy M. Meston, "Cortisol, Sexual Arousal, and Affect in Response to Sexual Stimuli," *Journal of Sexual Medicine* 5, no. 9 (September 2008): 2111–18, https://doi.org/10.1111/j.1743-6109.2008.00922.x; Lisa Dawn Hamilton and Cindy M. Meston, "Chronic Stress and Sexual Function in Women," *Journal of Sexual Medicine* 10, no. 10 (2013): 2443–54, https://doi.org/10.1111/jsm.12249.

18. J. Kabat-Zinn et al., "Effectiveness of a Meditation-Based Stress Reduction Program in the Treatment of Anxiety Disorders," *American Journal of Psychiatry* 149, no. 7 (1992): 936–43, https://doi.org/10.1176/ajp.149.7.936.
19. Ravindra P. Nagendra, Nirmala Maruthai, and Bindu M. Kutty, "Meditation and Its Regulatory Role on Sleep," *Frontiers in Neurology* 3 (2012), https://doi.org/10.3389/fneur.2012.00054.
20. Nagendra, Maruthai, and Kutty, "Meditation and Its Regulatory Role on Sleep."
21. Troels W. Kjaer et al., "Increased Dopamine Tone during Meditation-Induced Change of Consciousness," *Cognitive Brain Research* 13, no. 2 (April 2002): 255–59, https://doi.org/10.1016/s0926-6410(01)00106-9.
22. Iulia Dascalu and Lori A. Brotto, "Sexual Functioning in Experienced Meditators," *Journal of Sex & Marital Therapy* 44, no. 5 (2018): 459–67, https://doi.org/10.1080/0092623x.2017.1405311.
23. Julia Velten et al., "Effects of a Mindfulness Task on Women's Sexual Response," *Journal of Sex Research* 55, no. 6 (2017): 747–57, https://doi.org/10.1080/00224499.2017.1408768.
24. Ronald S. Duman and Lisa M. Monteggia, "A Neurotrophic Model for Stress-Related Mood Disorders," *Biological Psychiatry* 59, no. 12 (2006): 1116–27, https://doi.org/10.1016/j.biopsych.2006.02.013.
25. Pradeep C. Bollu et al., "Sleep Medicine: Parasomnias," *Missouri Medicine* 115, no. 2 (2018): 169–75, https://www.omagdigital.com/publication/?m=11307&i=490187&p=78&ver=html5.
26. M. González-Ortiz et al., "Effect of Sleep Deprivation on Insulin Sensitivity and Cortisol Concentration in Healthy Subjects," *Diabetes, Nutrition & Metabolism* 13, no. 2 (April 2000), 80–83, https://pubmed.ncbi.nlm.nih.gov/10898125/; Esther Donga et al. "A Single Night of Partial Sleep Deprivation Induces Insulin Resistance in Multiple Metabolic Pathways in Healthy Subjects," *Journal of Clinical Endocrinology and Metabolism* 95, no. 6 (2010): 2963–68, https://doi.org/10.1210/jc.2009-2430.
27. Danielle Pacheco, "The Best Temperature for Sleep," Sleep Foundation, OneCare Media, March 11, 2022, https://www.sleepfoundation.org/bedroom-environment/best-temperature-for-sleep.

Chapter 13: The 28-Day Program

One Cycle to Change Them All

1. Michael A. Starks et al., "The Effects of Phosphatidylserine on Endocrine Response to Moderate Intensity Exercise," *Journal of the International Society of Sports Nutrition* 5 (July 2008): 11, https://doi.org/10.1186/1550-2783-5-11; D. Benton et al., "The Influence of Phosphatidylserine Supplementation on Mood and Heart Rate When Faced with an Acute Stressor." *Nutritional Neuroscience* 4, no. 3 (2001): 169–78, https://doi.org/10.1080/1028415x.2001.11747360.
2. Etienne Pouteau et al., "Superiority of Magnesium and Vitamin B_6 over Magnesium Alone on Severe Stress in Healthy Adults with Low Magnesemia: A Randomized, Single-Blind Clinical Trial," *PLOS One* 13, no. 12 (2018): e0208454, https://doi.org/10.1371/journal.pone.0208454.
3. Siegfried Kasper and Angelika Dienel, "Multicenter, Open-Label, Exploratory Clinical Trial with *Rhodiola Rosea* Extract in Patients Suffering from Burnout Symptoms," *Neuropsychiatric Disease and Treatment* 2017, no. 13: 889–98, https://doi.org/10.2147/NDT.S120113.
4. Alex B. Speers et al., "Effects of *Withania Somnifera* (Ashwagandha) on Stress and the Stress-Related Neuropsychiatric Disorders Anxiety, Depression, and Insomnia," *Current Neuropharmacology* 19, no. 9 (2021), https://doi.org/10.2174/1570159x19666210712151556.
5. Jackson L. Williams, "The Effects of Green Tea Amino Acid L-Theanine Consumption on the Ability to Manage Stress and Anxiety Levels: A Systematic Review," *Plant Foods for Human Nutrition* 75 (November 2019): 1468–95, https://doi.org/10.1007/s11130-019-00771-5.
6. Cara Tomas, Julia Newton, and Stuart Watson, "A Review of Hypothalamic-Pituitary-Adrenal Axis Function in Chronic Fatigue Syndrome," *ISRN Neuroscience* (2013): 1–8, https://doi.org/10.1155/2013/784520.
7. "Foods That Fight Inflammation," Harvard Health, November 16, 2021, https://www.health.harvard.edu/staying-healthy/foods-that-fight-inflammation.

8. Razieh Jalal et al., "Hypoglycemic Effect of Aqueous Shallot and Garlic Extracts in Rats with Fructose-Induced Insulin Resistance," *Journal of Clinical Biochemistry and Nutrition* 41, no. 3 (2007): 218–23, https://doi.org/10.3164/jcbn.2007031; A. Gupta et al., "Effect of *Trigonella foenum-graecum* (Fenugreek) Seeds on Glycaemic Control and Insulin Resistance in Type 2 Diabetes Mellitus: A Double Blind Placebo Controlled Study," *Journal of the Association of Physicians of India* 49 (2001): 1057–61, https://pubmed.ncbi.nlm.nih.gov/11868855/; Jack N. Losso et al., "Fenugreek Bread: A Treatment for Diabetes Mellitus," *Journal of Medicinal Food* 12, no. 5 (2009): 1046–49, https://doi.org/10.1089/jmf.2008.0199.
9. Rajadurai Akilen et al., "Cinnamon in Glycaemic Control: Systematic Review and Meta Analysis," *Clinical Nutrition* 31, no. 5 (2012): 609–15, https://doi.org/10.1016/j.clnu.2012.04.003; Karalee J. Jarvill-Taylor, Richard A. Anderson, and Donald J. Graves, "A Hydroxychalcone Derived from Cinnamon Functions as a Mimetic for Insulin in 3T3-L1 Adipocytes," *Journal of the American College of Nutrition* 20, no. 4 (2001): 327–36, https://doi.org/10.1080/07315724.2001.10719053; Jennifer Imparl-Radosevich et al., "Regulation of PTP-1 and Insulin Receptor Kinase by Fractions from Cinnamon: Implications for Cinnamon Regulation of Insulin Signalling," *Hormone Research in Paediatrics* 50, no. 3 (1998): 177–82, https://doi.org/10.1159/000023270.
10. Kai Liu et al., "Effect of Green Tea on Glucose Control and Insulin Sensitivity: A Meta-Analysis of 17 Randomized Controlled Trials," *American Journal of Clinical Nutrition* 98, no. 2 (2013): 340–48, https://doi.org/10.3945/ajcn.112.052746.
11. Heather Basciano, Lisa Federico, and Khosrow Adeli, "Fructose, Insulin Resistance, and Metabolic Dyslipidemia," *Nutrition & Metabolism* 2, no. 1 (2005): 5, https://doi.org/10.1186/1743-7075-2-5; Kimber L. Stanhope et al., "Consuming Fructose-Sweetened, Not Glucose-Sweetened, Beverages Increases Visceral Adiposity and Lipids and Decreases Insulin Sensitivity in Overweight/Obese Humans," *Journal of Clinical Investigation* 119, no. 5 (2009): 1322–34, https://doi.org/10.1172/jci37385.
12. R. A. Anderson et al., "Elevated Intakes of Supplemental Chromium Improve Glucose and Insulin Variables in Individuals with Type 2 Di-

abetes," *Diabetes* 46, no. 11 (1997): 1786–91, https://doi.org/10.2337/diab.46.11.1786; J. Z. Martin et al., "Chromium Picolinate Supplementation Attenuates Body Weight Gain and Increases Insulin Sensitivity in Subjects with Type 2 Diabetes," *Diabetes Care* 29, no. 8 (August 2006): 1826–32, https://doi.org/10.2337/dc06-0254; Peter J. Havel, "A Scientific Review: The Role of Chromium in Insulin Resistance," *Diabetes Educator* 2004, Suppl.: 2–14, https://pubmed.ncbi.nlm.nih.gov/15208835/.

13. Benjamin B. Albert, "Higher Omega-3 Index Is Associated with Increased Insulin Sensitivity and More Favourable Metabolic Profile in Middle-Aged Overweight Men," *Scientific Reports* 4, no. 1 (2014): 6697, https://doi.org/10.1038/srep06697; Rohith N. Thota, Shamasunder H. Acharya, and Manohar L. Garg, "Curcumin and/or Omega-3 Polyunsaturated Fatty Acids Supplementation Reduces Insulin Resistance and Blood Lipids in Individuals with High Risk of Type 2 Diabetes: A Randomised Controlled Trial," *Lipids in Health and Disease* 18, no. 1 (2019), https://doi.org/10.1186/s12944-019-0967-x.
14. Bharti Kalra, Sanjay Kalra, and J. B. Sharma, "The Inositols and Polycystic Ovary Syndrome," *Indian Journal of Endocrinology and Metabolism* 20, no. 5 (September–October 2016): 720–24, https://doi.org/10.4103/2230-8210.189231.
15. F. Corrado et al., "The Effect of Myoinositol Supplementation on Insulin Resistance in Patients with Gestational Diabetes," *Diabetic Medicine* 28, no. 8 (2011): 972–75, https://doi.org/10.1111/j.1464-5491.2011.03284.x.
16. F. Guerrero-Romero et al., "Oral Magnesium Supplementation Improves Insulin Sensitivity in Non-Diabetic Subjects with Insulin Resistance. A Double-Blind Placebo-Controlled Randomized Trial," *Diabetes & Metabolism* 30, no. 3 (2004): 253–58, https://doi.org/10.1016/s1262-3636(07)70116-7; Mei Dou et al., "Combined Chromium and Magnesium Decreases Insulin Resistance More Effectively Than Either Alone," *Asia Pacific Journal of Clinical Nutrition* 25, no. 4 (2016): 747–53, https://doi.org/10.6133/apjcn.092015.48.
17. Jun Yin, Huili Xing, and Jianping Ye, "Efficacy of Berberine in Patients with Type 2 Diabetes Mellitus," *Metabolism* 57, no. 5 (2008): 712–17,

https://doi.org/10.1016/j.metabol.2008.01.013; Yan Li et al., "Effect of Berberine on Insulin Resistance in Women with Polycystic Ovary Syndrome: Study Protocol for a Randomized Multicenter Controlled Trial," *Trials* 14, no. 1 (2013): 226, https://doi.org/10.1186/1745-6215-14-226.

18. Mohammad Hassan Eftekhari et al., "The Relationship between Iron Status and Thyroid Hormone Concentration in Iron-Deficient Adolescent Iranian Girls," *Asia Pacific Journal of Clinical Nutrition* 15, no. 1 (2006): 50–55, https://pubmed.ncbi.nlm.nih.gov/16500878/.
19. Jan Calissendorff et al., "A Prospective Investigation of Graves' Disease and Selenium: Thyroid Hormones, Auto-Antibodies and Self-Rated Symptoms," *European Thyroid Journal* 4, no. 2 (2015): 93–98, https://doi.org/10.1159/000381768.
20. Salvatore Benvenga et al., "Usefulness Of L-Carnitine, a Naturally Occurring Peripheral Antagonist of Thyroid Hormone Action, in Iatrogenic Hyperthyroidism: A Randomized, Double-Blind, Placebo-Controlled Clinical Trial," *Journal of Clinical Endocrinology & Metabolism* 86, no. 8 (August 2001): 3579–94, https://doi.org/10.1210/jcem.86.8.7747.
21. Maurizio Nordio and Sabrina Basciani, "Treatment with Myo-Inositol and Selenium Ensures Euthyroidism in Patients with Autoimmune Thyroiditis," *International Journal of Endocrinology* 2017: 1–6, https://doi.org/10.1155/2017/2549491.
22. Ashok Kumar Sharma, Indraneel Basu, and Siddarth Singh, "Efficacy and Safety of Ashwagandha Root Extract in Subclinical Hypothyroid Patients: A Double-Blind, Randomized Placebo-Controlled Trial," *Journal of Alternative and Complementary Medicine* 24, no. 3 (2018): 243–48, https://doi.org/10.1089/acm.2017.0183.
23. Syed M. Meeran, Shweta N. Patel, and Trygve O. Tollefsbol, "Sulforaphane Causes Epigenetic Repression of *hTERT* Expression in Human Breast Cancer Cell Lines," *PLOS One* 5, no. 7 (2010): e11457, https://doi.org/10.1371/journal.pone.0011457; Maria Russo et al., "Nrf2 Targeting by Sulforaphane: A Potential Therapy for Cancer Treatment," *Critical Reviews in Food Science and Nutrition* 58, no. 8 (2017): 1391–405, https://doi.org/10.1080/10408398.2016.1259983; Yanyan Li et al., "Sulforaphane, a Dietary Component of Broccoli/Broccoli Sprouts, In-

hibits Breast Cancer Stem Cells," *Clinical Cancer Research* 16, no. 9 (May 2010): 2580–90, https://doi.org/10.1158/1078-0432.ccr-09-2937.

24. I. J. Rowe and R. J. Baber, "The Effects of Phytoestrogens on Postmenopausal Health," *Climacteric* 24, no. 1 (2021): 57–63, https://doi.org/10.1080/13697137.2020.1863356.

25. G. E. Abraham, "Nutritional Factors in the Etiology of the Premenstrual Tension Syndromes," *Journal of Reproductive Medicine* 28, no. 7 (1983): 446–64, https://www.unboundmedicine.com/medline/citation/6684167/Nutritional_factors_in_the_etiology_of_the_premenstrual_tension_syndromes.

26. Farzad Najafipour et al., "Review of Therapeutic Effects of Stinging Nettle (Urtica Dioica) in Women with Hyperandrogenism," *International Journal of Current Research and Academic Review* 2, no. 7 (July 2014): 153–60, http://www.ijcrar.com/vol-2-7/Farzad%20Najafipour,%20et%20al.pdf.

27. Masayuki Abe et al., "Pharmacologically Relevant Receptor Binding Characteristics and 5-alpha-Reductase Inhibitory Activity of Free Fatty Acids Contained in Saw Palmetto Extract," *Biological and Pharmaceutical Bulletin* 32, no. 4 (2009): 646–50, https://doi.org/10.1248/bpb.32.646; Jean-Pierre Raynaud, Henri Cousse, and Pierre-Marie Martin, "Inhibition of Type 1 and Type 2 5-alpha-Reductase Activity by Free Fatty Acids, Active Ingredients of Permixon," *Journal of Steroid Biochemistry and Molecular Biology* 82, nos. 2–3 (2002): 233–39, https://doi.org/10.1016/s0960-0760(02)00187-5.

28. Gokalp Oner and Iptisam Ipek Muderris, "Clinical, Endocrine and Metabolic Effects of Metformin vs N-Acetyl-Cysteine in Women with Polycystic Ovary Syndrome," *European Journal of Obstetrics, Gynecology, and Reproductive Biology* 159, no. 1 (2011): 127–31, https://doi.org/10.1016/j.ejogrb.2011.07.005.

29. Aitak Farzi, Esther E. Fröhlich, and Peter Holzer, "Gut Microbiota and the Neuroendocrine System," *Neurotherapeutics* 15, no.1 (2018): 5–22, https://doi.org/10.1007/s13311-017-0600-5.

30. Yasmine Belkaid and Timothy W. Hand, "Role of the Microbiota in Immunity and Inflammation," *Cell* 157, no. 1 (2014): 121–41, https://doi.org/10.1016/j.cell.2014.03.011.

31. Stephanie L. Brown, et al., "Social Closeness Increases Salivary Pro-

gesterone in Humans," *Hormones and Behavior* 56, no. 1 (2009): 108–11, https://doi.org/10.1016/j.yhbeh.2009.03.022.

Appendix 2: Cycle Symptom Relief

1. Fatemeh Shobeiri, Khodayar Oshvandi, and Mansour Nazari, "Clinical Effectiveness of Vitamin E and Vitamin B_6 for Improving Pain Severity in Cyclic Mastalgia," *Iranian Journal of Nursing and Midwifery Research* 20, no. 6 (2015): 723, https://doi.org/10.4103/1735-9066.170003.
2. Sandhya Pruthi et al., "Vitamin E and Evening Primrose Oil for Management of Cyclical Mastalgia: A Randomized Pilot Study," *Alternative Medicine Review* 15, no. 1 (2010): 59–67, https://pubmed.ncbi.nlm.nih.gov/20359269/.
3. Shobeiri, Oshvandi, and Nazari, "Clinical Effectiveness of Vitamin E."
4. Elsa H. Spencer, Hope R. Ferdowsian, and Neal D. Barnard, "Diet and Acne: A Review of the Evidence," *International Journal of Dermatology* 48, no. 4 (2009): 339–47, https://doi.org/10.1111/j.1365-4632.2009.04002.x; Christos C. Zouboulis, "Is Acne Vulgaris a Genuine Inflammatory Disease?," *Dermatology* 203, no. 4 (2001): 277–79, https://doi.org/10.1159/000051771.
5. "Feeling Close to a Friend Increases Progesterone, Boosts Well-Being and Reduces Anxiety and Stress," *ScienceDaily*, June 3, 2009, https://www.sciencedaily.com/releases/2009/06/090602171941.htm.
6. Seyedeh Zahra Masoumi, Maryam Ataollahi, and Khodayar Oshvandi, "Effect of Combined Use of Calcium and Vitamin B_6 on Premenstrual Syndrome Symptoms: A Randomized Clinical Trial," *Journal of Caring Sciences* 5, no. 1 (2016): 67–73, https://doi.org/10.15171/jcs.2016.007 (archived at https://web.archive.org/web/20160329040620/http://journals.tbzmed.ac.ir/JCS/Abstract/JCS_71_20160229112644); Nahid Fathizadeh et al., "Evaluating the Effect of Magnesium and Magnesium Plus Vitamin B_6 Supplement on the Severity of Premenstrual Syndrome," *Iranian Journal of Nursing and Midwifery Research* 15, Suppl. 1 (2010): 401–5, https://www.ncbi.nlm.nih.gov/pmc/articles/PMC3208934/.
7. Nahid Sohrabi et al., "Evaluation of the Effect of Omega-3 Fatty Acids

in the Treatment of Premenstrual Syndrome: 'A Pilot Trial,'" *Complementary Therapies in Medicine* 21, no. 3 (June 2013): 141–46, https://doi.org/10.1016/j.ctim.2012.12.008; Katri Peuhkuri, Nora Sihvola, and Riitta Korpela, "Dietary Factors and Fluctuating Levels of Melatonin," *Food & Nutrition Research* 56 (2012): PMC3402070, https://www.ncbi.nlm.nih.gov/pmc/articles/PMC3402070.

8. Vedat Cinar et al., "Effects of Magnesium Supplementation on Testosterone Levels of Athletes and Sedentary Subjects at Rest and after Exhaustion," *Biological Trace Element Research* 140, no. 1 (2010): 18–23, https://doi.org/10.1007/s12011-010-8676-3.

INDEX

ABOUT THE AUTHOR

Dr. Jolene Brighten is a women's hormone expert and prominent leader in women's medicine. She is a licensed naturopathic physician and clinical sexologist who is board-certified in naturopathic endocrinology and who takes an integrative approach in her clinical practice. A fierce patient advocate and completely dedicated to uncovering the root cause of hormone imbalances, Dr. Brighten empowers women worldwide to take control of their health and their hormones through her website and social media channels. She is the best-selling author of *Beyond the Pill* and *Healing Your Body Naturally After Childbirth.* Dr. Brighten is an international speaker, clinical educator, and medical adviser within the tech community and is considered a leading authority on women's health. She is a member of the mindbodygreen collective and the American Association of Sexuality Educators, Counselors and Therapists. Dr. Brighten serves as a faculty member for the American Academy of Anti-Aging Medicine. Her work has been featured in the *New York Post, Forbes, Cosmopolitan, HuffPost,* Bustle, the *Guardian, Sports Illustrated, Elle,* and ABC News.